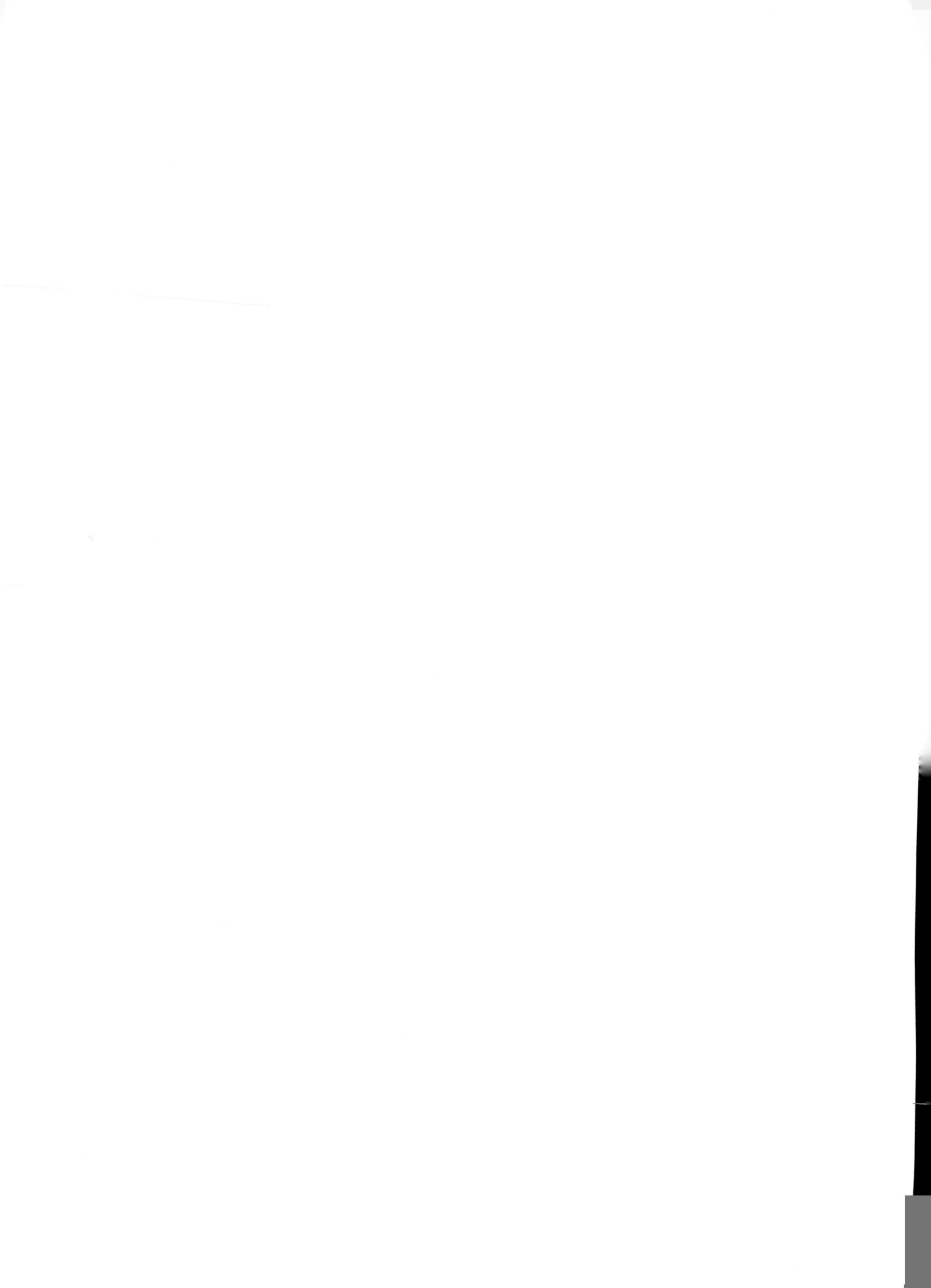

Orthodontics: Diagnosis and Treatment

Orthodontics: Diagnosis and Treatment

Editor: Kaley Ann

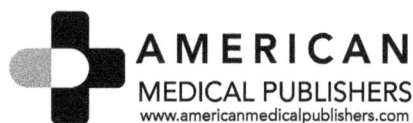

AMERICAN
MEDICAL PUBLISHERS
www.americanmedicalpublishers.com

AMERICAN
MEDICAL PUBLISHERS
www.americanmedicalpublishers.com

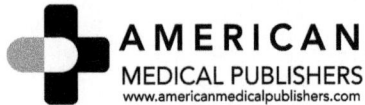

Cataloging-in-Publication Data

Orthodontics : diagnosis and treatment / edited by Kaley Ann.
    p. cm.
Includes bibliographical references and index.
ISBN 978-1-63927-060-6
1. Orthodontics. 2. Dentistry. I. Ann, Kaley.
RK521 .H36 2022
617.643--dc23

American Medical Publishers,
41 Flatbush Avenue,
1st Floor, New York,
NY 11217, USA

ISBN 978-1-63927-060-6 (Hardback)

Contents

Preface

In my initial years as a student, I used to run to the library at every possible instance to grab a book and learn something new. Books were my primary source of knowledge and I would not have come such a long way without all that I learnt from them. Thus, when I was approached to edit this book; I became understandably nostalgic. It was an absolute honor to be considered worthy of guiding the current generation as well as those to come. I put all my knowledge and hard work into making this book most beneficial for its readers.

The branch of dentistry that is concerned with the diagnosis, prevention and correction of malpositioned teeth and jaws is known as orthodontics. It is majorly used to treat malocclusions and deals with the control and modification of facial growth. Orthodontics primarily uses fixed appliances for the treatment as it consists of biomaterials that help in moving the teeth in dimensions and is considered significantly greater than the removable appliances. There are various types of fixed appliances that are used such as brackets, orthodontic bands and archwires. Orthodontics includes the use of fixed appliances, adjunctive therapy and post-treatment. In orthodontics aesthetics, oral health, stability and function are some aspects that should be kept in mind while planning treatment for the patient. The book studies, analyzes and upholds the pillars of orthodontics and its utmost significance in modern times. It presents researches and studies performed by experts across the globe. Students, researchers, experts and all associated with this domain will benefit alike from this book.

I wish to thank my publisher for supporting me at every step. I would also like to thank all the authors who have contributed their researches in this book. I hope this book will be a valuable contribution to the progress of the field.

Editor

The influence of protective varnish on the integrity of orthodontic cements

Érika Machado Caldeira[1], Antonio de Moraes Izquierdo[2], Felipe Giacomet[1], Eduardo Franzotti Sant'Anna[3], Antônio Carlos de Oliveira Ruellas[4]

Objective: The aim of the present study was to assess the influence of saliva contamination over the structural strength and integrity of conventional glass-ionomer cements used for cementing orthodontic bands in the absence and presence of a surface-protecting varnish. **Method:** 48 samples were prepared by inserting 3 types of glass-ionomer cements into standardized metallic matrixes of 10 mm of diameter and 2 mm of depth. The cements used were: Meron (VOCO), Ketac-Cem (3M ESPE) and Vidrion C (DFL), all of which comprised groups A, B and C, respectively. Subgroups A1, B1 and C1 comprised samples with no surface protection, whereas subgroups A2, B2 and C2 comprised samples of which surface was coated with Cavitine varnish (SS White), after cement manipulation and application, in order to protect the cement applied. All samples were stored in artificial saliva for 24 hours at 37°C. A Vickers diamond micro-durometer was used to produce indentations on the non-treated group (non-varnished) and the treated group (varnished). **Results:** Varnished materials had significantly higher microhardness values in comparison to non-varnished materials. Ketac-Cem had the highest microhardness value among the varnished materials. **Conclusion:** Varnish application is necessary to preserve the cement and avoid enamel decalcification. Glass-ionomer cements should be protected in order to fully keep their properties, thus, contributing to dental health during orthodontic treatment.

Keywords: Glass-ionomer cements. Artificial saliva. Microhardness.

[1] MSc in Orthodontics, Department of Pediatric Dentistry and Orthodontics, Federal University of Rio de Janeiro (UFRJ).

[2] Doctorate Student in Orthodontics, Department of Pediatric Dentistry and Orthodontics, Federal University of Rio de Janeiro (UFRJ).

[3] Adjunct professor, Department of Pediatric Dentistry and Orthodontics, Federal University of Rio de Janeiro (UFRJ).

[4] Adjunct professor, Department of Pediatric Dentistry and Orthodontics, Federal University of Rio de Janeiro (UFRJ).

» The authors report no commercial, proprietary or financial interest in the products or companies described in this article.

Programa de Pós-Graduação em Odontologia (Ortodontia) - Faculdade de Odontologia - Universidade Federal do Rio de Janeiro Rua Professor Rodolpho Paulo Rocco, 325 – Ilha do Fundão – Rio de Janeiro/ RJ — Brazil.

INTRODUCTION

Maintaining an adequate oral health is a constant challenge in Orthodontics, since the high number of retentive surfaces present in the orthodontic appliances hinders bacterial plaque removal. Some issues involving attachment material, such as poor sealing, inadequate structural and adhesive strength as well as cement solubility in oral fluids contribute to enamel decalcification.[1,2,3]

Failure in band cementation usually results in serious problems for orthodontic treatment. If any failure in cement seal occurring between the band and the tooth is not immediately detected, enamel demineralization may occur at the margins of the band.[4] In addition to attaching the bands, the cement protects the banded tooth against cavity. The resistance of these dental cements to oral fluids can be measured by their solubility and disintegration.[5]

Glass-ionomer cement is a generic denomination for a group of materials produced by the reaction between silicate glass powder and polyacrylic acid.[6] The main characteristics of this material are fluoride release, important for enamel remineralization of carious teeth, biocompatibility, and adhesion to the enamel, which occurs by chemical attraction between the apatite and the polyacrylic acid.[7]

Due to its capacity of adhering to the dental structure and its ability to release fluoride ions, the glass-ionomer cement is indicated not only for preventive restorations, but also as a filling and attaching material.[6] In addition, glass-ionomer cement can adhere to stainless steel, which favors its use as an attaching material.[8]

Bands attached with glass-ionomer cement require less recementations, present less decalcification in the surrounding enamel, and show higher amount of remnant cement after debonding.[9] On the other hand, the glass-ionomer cement has the disadvantage of being susceptible to humidity.[10]

During the initial curing phase of the glass-ionomer cement, any contamination can adversely affect its surface hardness, thus, altering its properties.[11,12] In clinical cases in which contamination control is difficult, its use is contra-indicated.[13] For this reason, it seems to be reasonable to isolate the glass-ionomer cement from the oral environment with impermeable materials during initial curing in order to avoid any undesired changes.

There are several studies in the literature relating materials and their adhesive capacity, particularly using composites and hybrid ionomers on shear bond tests,[14] in addition to those that emphasize bond strength and ts failures.[9,15,16] Other studies have correlated the fluoride-releasing ability of certain materials with their cariostatic effects.[3,9] However, no studies have been carried out on the need for isolating conventional glass-ionomer cements surfaces during cementation of orthodontic bands, even though this action is essential for the preservation and longevity of this type of cement in restorative Dentistry practice.[17]

In this study, Cavitine varnish was chosen for such protection. According to the manufacturer, it is a nitrocellulose-based (8%) varnish with some unique features, including excipients (ethyl acetate, ethanol) which cause it to be volatile and fast-drying. It is used as cavity liner and for protection of silicate restorations, since it prevents salivary action and avoids moisture during crucial reaction steps.

Microhardness is among the properties which may be affected by contamination during the initial curing phase. Surface microhardness is defined as being the microstructure and texture activities of a given material, which are used for predicting material strength as well as its ability of abrading opposite structures.[18] It is, in fact, one of the most important mechanical properties for comparative studies of dental materials.[11] Strength, curing time and erosion of the glass-ionomer cement have evolved as new hardness tests are performed.[19] Knowing the material surface microhardness behavior is crucial when choosing the best material, since this property changes when it is exposed to humidity — condition that is similar to that of the oral cavity.[18]

Therefore, the objective of the present study was to assess the effects of varnish isolation on microhardness of conventional glass-ionomer cements in the presence of salivary contamination during initial curing phase.

MATERIAL AND METHODS

In the present study, conventional glass-ionomer cements were assessed. They were manipulated according to the manufacturer's instructions and only one investigator tested the materials.

Three conventional glass-ionomer cements commonly available on the market were used, namely: Group A (Meron, VOCO, Cuxhaven, Germany, batch 109012051); Group B (Ketac-Cem, 3M ESPE, Seefeld, Germany, batch 221924); and Group C (Vidrion C, DFL, Rio de Janeiro, Brazil, batch 0060406 — powder, batch 0010106 — liquid). Each group was divided into two subgroups containing 8 samples each (Subgroups A1, A2, B1, B2, C1, and C2), in which number 1 refers to those samples without isolation after manipulation and application of the cement, and number 2 refers to those samples receiving protection against humidity. A total of 48 samples was obtained and humidity protection was achieved by means of applying Cavitine varnish (SS White, Rio de Janeiro, Brazil, batch 013) onto the cement surfaces.

The samples were obtained by inserting the materials into standardized metallic matrixes of 10 mm in diameter and 2 mm in depth. Insertion was performed by using Centrix syringe (DFL) in order to avoid air bubbles. A glass plate was put onto the matrixes so that a plane surface could be obtained, thus, preserving the surface layer as well as enabling the focus during microhardness test.

After the initial 10 minutes, all samples were immersed into artificial saliva, including those from subgroups A2, B2, and C2 which had been coated with Cavitine varnish by using microbrushes (Cavibrush – FGM). The material was kept in a stove at 37°C for 24 hours.[17]

All samples were kept under moist conditions in order to avoid dehydration and test the varnish efficiency. Artificial saliva was chosen because it increases surface hardness of glass–ionomer cements and simulates the conditions found within the oral environment, which would not happen if distilled water was used.[19]

The microhardness tests were performed by using a Vickers diamond microdurometer (E. LEITZ, Germany) with a 100 gf load being applied during 30 seconds in order to produce indentations, which were measured in Vickers hardness (HV). Five indentations were performed in each sample of each group, with a total of 80 indentations — 40 in varnish-coated samples and 40 in non-varnished ones. The microhardness values were obtained by measuring the diagonal of the imprints magnified

by 50 times with ZoomMagic 2.0 software (Peak-Star, USA). The results were calculated with the following formula: $HV = 1854.4 \, P/d^2$, where P = indentation load and d = diagonal obtained.[11]

Analysis of variance was employed to compare all the subgroups, whereas Tukey's test was used for multiple comparisons. The significance level was set at 1%.

RESULTS

Table 1 and Figure 1 show the microhardness values obtained for all subgroups. They demonstrate that varnish-coated samples had higher microhardness values in comparison to the non-varnished ones ($P < 0.01$). Ketac-Cem glass-ionomer cement (3M ESPE), either varnished or non-varnished, had the highest microhardness value after being stored in artificial saliva for 24 hours.

The varnish-coated samples were found to have smoother and more regular surfaces (Fig 2), as well as the highest microhardness values. On the other hand, cracks and rugosities were observed in the non-varnished samples which also presented inappropriate microhardness values (Fig 3).

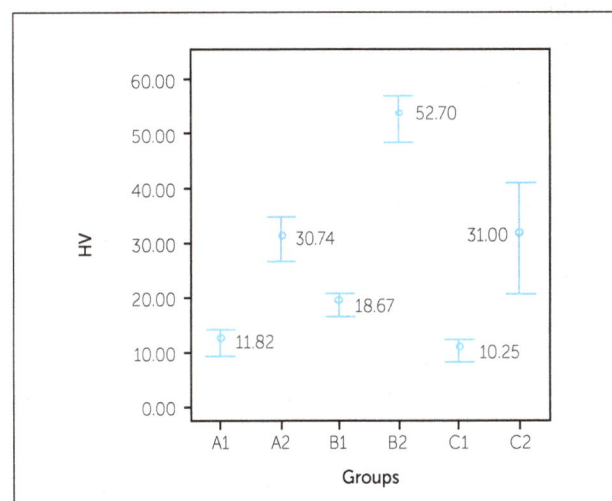

Figure 1 - Graphic representation of microhardness differences found for each subgroup.

Table 1 - Vickers microhardness values (kg/mm²) for different subgroups (mean ± standard deviation).

Group A (Meron, Voco)		Group B (Ketac-Cem, 3M ESPE)		Group C (Vidrion, DFL)	
A1[c]	A2[b]	B1[c]	B2[a]	C1[c]	C2[b]
HV = 11.82 ± 2.73	HV = 30.74 ± 4.88	HV = 18.67 ± 1.74	HV = 52.69 ± 4.27	HV = 10.24 ± 2.39	HV = 31.00 ± 12.21

Superscribed letters indicate statistically significant differences ($P < 0.01$) for a>b>c.

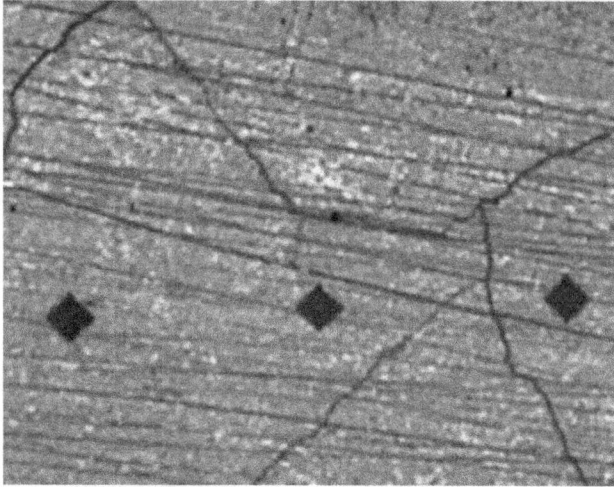

Figure 2 - Subgroup B1 sample surface (non-varnished). Presence of cracks, fissures, and large indentations . 50 times magnification.

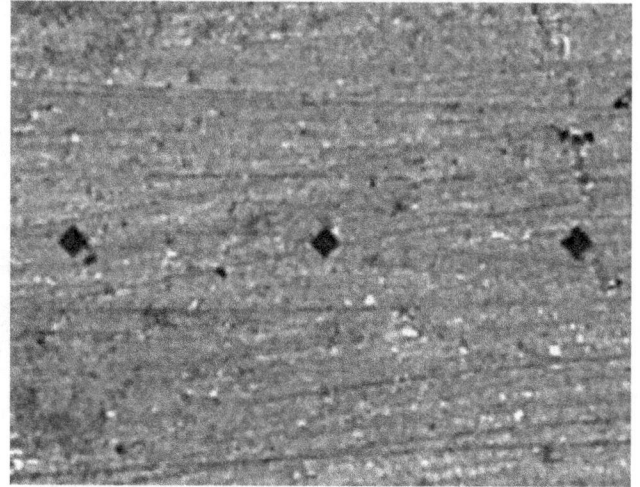

Figure 3 - Subgroup B2 sample surface (varnished). Smooth surface with small indentations. 50 times magnification.

DISCUSSION

Mechanical properties of materials are intimately related to their overall quality and integrity. Material's surface degradation is associated with an increase in rugosity and allows bacteria lodging and, as a consequence, causes undesirable tissue reactions. This explains the need for materials to preserve their mechanical properties, specially hardness.[20,21] Materials with better microhardness are more likely to withstand saliva biochemistry, constant pH variations, different temperatures and, specially, the resident oral microbiome.[22] This is the reason why the present study aimed at verifying surface behavior of 3 types of conventional glass-ionomer cements with regard to humidity and varnish-protection effects. Therefore, the methodology chosen has proved to be adequate.[17]

In the present study, a 10-minute curing time was adopted before saliva contamination, as stated in previous studies.[11,18] The curing time for conventional glass-ionomer cements ranges between 4.4 and 12.2 minutes.[23] The first 10 minutes of chemical reaction are the most important, since acid attack occurs during this period of time, thus, resulting in ion release (fluoride, sodium, calcium, aluminum, and phosphate).[24] Dehydration was also avoided in the first 10 minutes of chemical reaction by means of using glass plates on the samples, which prevented direct contact between the material and the air, in addition to making the surfaces smooth and uniform.

Total surface hardness of glass-ionomer cements is achieved nearly 24 hours after application and the testing procedures are usually carried out within this period of time to investigate the effects of storage on the cement properties.[23,25,26] As glass-ionomer cement is susceptible to humidity, it is recommended that its surface be coated during the initial curing phase, that is, soon after loosing its surface brightness.[10,18] However, glass-ionomer cements have a slow curing process and during this phase, they are susceptible to saliva and water attacks, which dissolve such materials.[27]

Water plays a crucial role during the curing phase of glass-ionomer cements. First, it serves as a reaction medium and then it slowly hydrates the cross-linked matrix, allowing formation of a stable gel structure which is more resistant and also less susceptible to humidity. If the newly-used cement is exposed to the environment with no protective layer, its surface will show cracks and fissures caused by dehydration. Both dehydration and excess humidity can damage the integrity of the material.[26,28]

If no protection is provided, the material surface will inevitably become porous and cracked, as observed in the non-varnished samples (subgroups A1, B1 and C1). This result can be explained by the nature of the material, because glass-ionomer cements, even when reinforced with composites, react in a more sensitive manner to moistness and abrasion.[29]

Since water balance is crucial to form a stable matrix, and, consequently, to cement maturation, surface protection is extremely important during the initial setting. Thus, due to the fact that glass-ionomer cements exhibit a high degree of solubility and disintegration in the oral environment, protecting the material surface, characterized by its rugosity, is essential to prevent degradation and avoid *S. mutans* colonization.[17,30]

Protecting the surface of glass-ionomer cement is a process that lasts for at least 1 hour, although the ideal time required to increase resistance to disintegration is 24 hours.[31] It is known, however, that in the oral environment, protective materials are lost within the first 24 hours because of friction.[17] That is the reason why in the methodology used for this study, Cavitine varnish was able to protect the surfaces of the materials within 24 hours.

Although varnishes are indicated as surface protection materials for cements,[13,32] there are reports in the literature in which the evaporation of the varnish solvent is associated with protective films with faulty lines, which does not ensure adequate protection.[17] On the other hand, according to the manufacturer's specifications and the results of this study, Cavitine varnish can be used in orthodontic practice. That is because it proved to be efficient with regard to protection, specially for cementation, since only a small amount of material is actually exposed to the oral environment when a correct adaptation of the band is achieved.

Subgroups A2, B2, and C2 (varnished with Cavitine) had the highest microhardness values. Among the commercially available materials assessed, Ketak-Cem proved to have the highest microhardness values, as previously observed.[33] Additionally, no statistically significant differences were observed in the microhardness values of the non-varnished samples. Therefore, surface protection of glass-ionomer cements during the initial curing phase was found to be useful.

Considering the complexity of the oral environment, preserving the integrity of the material is necessary,[30] since failures in cement bands may lead to tooth demineralization and delay treatment due to the need for recementation. Selecting appropriate materials and caring for their preservation is of professional responsibility, in view of the longevity of orthodontic treatments and commitment to patient health.

CONCLUSION

Protecting the surface of glass-ionomer cements with varnish during the initial curing phase promoted higher microhardness values 24 hours after its application, corroborating the fact that adequate cement preservation is necessary to avoid enamel decalcification. In addition, further clinical comparative studies are required to assess orthodontic bands cemented with either varnished or non-varnished glass-ionomer cements.

REFERENCES

1. Sadowsky PL, Retief DH. A comparative study of some dental cements used in orthodontics. Angle Orthod. 1976;46(2):171-81.
2. Gameiro GH, Nouer DF, Cenci MS, Cury JA. Enamel demineralization with two forms of archwire ligation investigated using an in situ caries model: a pilot study. Eur J Orthod. 2009;31(5):542-6.
3. Passalini P, Fidalgo TKS, Caldeira EM, Gleiser R, Nojima MCG, Maia LC. Preventive effect of fluoridated orthodontic resins subjected to high cariogenic challenges. Braz Dent J. 2010;21(3):211-5.
4. Noyes H. Dental caries and the orthodontic patient. J Am Dent Assoc. 1937;24:1243-54.
5. Cameron JC, Charbeneau GT, Craig RG. Some properties of dental cements of specific importance in the cementation of orthodontic bands. Angle Orthod. 1963;33(4):233-45.
6. Yli-Urpo H, Vallittu PK, Narhi TO, Forsback AP, Vakiparta M. Release of silica, calcium, phosphorus, and fluoride from glass ionomer cement containing bioactive glass. J Biomater Appl. 2004;19(1):5-20.
7. Vermeersch G, Leloup G, Vreven J. Fluoride release from glass-ionomer cements, compomers and resin composites. J Oral Rehabil. 2001;28(1):26-32.
8. Coury TL, Willer RD, Miranda FJ, Probst RT. Adhesiveness of glass-ionomer cement to enamel and dentin: a laboratory study. Oper Dent. 1982;7:2-6.
9. Caves GR, Millett DT, Creanor SL, Foye RH, Gilmour WH. Fluoride release from orthodontic band cements - a comparison of two in vitro models. J Dent. 2003;31(1):19-24.
10. Pellegrinetti MB, Imparato JCP, Bressan MC, Pinheiro SL, Echeverria S. Avaliação da retenção do cimento de ionômero de vidro. Pesq Bras Odontoped Clin Integr. 2005;5(3):209-13.
11. Ellakuria J, Triana R, Minguez N, Soler I, Ibaseta G, Maza J, et al. Effect of one-year water storage on the surface microhardness of resin-modified versus conventional glass-ionomer cements. Dent Mater. 2003;19(4):286-90.
12. McLean JW, Wilson AD, Prosser HJ. Development and use of water-hardening glass-ionomer luting cements. J Prosthet Dent. 1984;52(2):175-81.
13. Christensen GJ. Glass ionomer as a luting material. J Am Dent Assoc. 1990;120:59-62.
14. Reicheneder CA, Gedrange T, Lange A, Baumert U, Proff P. Shear and tensile bond strength comparison of various contemporary orthodontic adhesive systems: an in-vitro study. Am J Orthod Dentofacial Orthop. 2009;135(4):422.e1-6.
15. Passalini P, Fidalgo TKS, Caldeira EM, Gleiser R, Nojima MCG, Maia LC. Mechanical properties of one and two step fluoridated orthodontic resins submitted to different pH cycling regimes. Braz Oral Res. 2010;24(2):197-203.
16. Caldeira EM, Fidalgo TKS, Passalini P, Marquezan, M, Nojima MCG, Maia LC. Análise in vitro da influência da aplicação tópica de fluoreto nas propriedades mecânicas de uma resina ortodôntica sob ciclagem de pH. Pesq Bras Odontoped Clin Integr. 2011;11(1):47-52.
17. Zancopé BR, Novaes TF, Mendes FM, Imparato JCP, Benedetto MS, Raggio DP. Influência da proteção superficial na rugosidade de cimento de ionômero de vidro. ConScientiae Saúde. 2009;8(4):559-63.
18. Borges AFS, Puppin-Rontani RM, Sinhoreti MAC, Sobrinho LC. Influência do tempo de estocagem em meio úmido sobre a microdureza inicial de materiais restauradores estéticos. Ciênc Odontol Bras. 2004;7(4):79-86.
19. Okada K, Tosaki S, Hirota K, Hume WR. Surface hardness change of restorative filling materials stored in saliva. Dent Mater. 2001;17(1):34-9.

20. Silva KG, Pedrini D, Delbem ACB, Cannon M. Microhardness and fluoride release of restorative materials in different storage media. Braz Dent J. 2007;18(4):309-13.

21. Beyth N, Bahir R, Matalon S, Domb AJ, Weiss EI. Streptococcus mutans biofilm changes surface-topography of resin composites. Dent Mater. 2008;24(6):732-6.

22. Silva KG, Pedrini D, Delbem ACB, Cannon M. Effect of pH variations in a cycling model on the properties of restorative materials. Oper Dent. 2007;32(4):328-35.

23. Khouw-Liu VH, Anstice HM, Pearson GJ. An in vitro investigation of a poly (vinyl phosphonic acid) based cement with four conventional glass-ionomer cements. Part 2: Maturation in relation to surface hardness. J Dent. 1999;27(5):359-65.

24. Crisp S, Wilson AD. Reactions in glass ionomer cements: I. Decomposition of the powder. J Dent Res. 1974;53(6):1408-13.

25. Millett DT, Duff S, Morrison L, Cummings A, Gilmour WH. In vitro comparison of orthodontic band cements. Am J Orthod Dentofacial Orthop. 2003;123(1):15-20.

26. Aguiar DA, Silveira MR, Ritter DE, Locks A, Calvo MCM. Avaliação das propriedades mecânicas de quarto cimentos de ionômero de vidro convencionais utilizados na cimentação de bandas ortodônticas. Rev Dental Press Ortod Ortop Facial. 2008;13(3):104-11.

27. Algera TJ, Kleverlaan CJ, Prahl-Andersen B, Feilzer AJ. The influence of environmental conditions on the material properties of setting glass-ionomer cements. Dent Mater. 2006;22(9):852-6

28. Feilzer AJ, Kakaboura AI, De Gee AJ, Davidson CL. The influence of water sorption on the development of setting shrinkage stress in traditional and resin-modified glass ionomer cements. Dent Mater. 1995;11(3):186-90.

29. Cefaly DF, Wang L, Mello LLCP, Santos JL, Santos JR, Lauris, JRP. Water sorption of resin-modified glass-ionomer cements photoactivated with LED. Braz Oral Res. 2006;20(4):342-6.

30. Caldeira EM, Osório A, Oberosler ELC, Vaitsman DS, Alviano DS, Nojima MCG. Antimicrobial and fluoride release capacity of orthodontic bonding materials. J Appl Oral Sci. 2013;21(4):327-34.

31. Earl MSA, Ibbetson RJ. The clinical disintegration of a glass ionomer cement. Br Dent J. 1986;161(8):287-91.

32. Chain MC. Cimento de ionômero de vidro. RGO. 1993;38(5):351-7.

33. McComb D, Sirisko R, Brown J. Comparison of physical properties of commercial glass ionomer luting cements. J Can Dent Assoc. 1984;50(9):699-701.

Prevalence of mesiodens in orthodontic patients with deciduous and mixed dentition and its association with other dental anomalies

Tulio Silva Lara[1], Melissa Lancia[2], Omar Gabriel da Silva Filho[3], Daniela Gamba Garib[4], Terumi Okada Ozawa[5]

Objective: To determine the prevalence of mesiodens in deciduous and mixed dentitions and its association with other dental anomalies. **Material and Methods:** Panoramic radiographs of 1,995 orthodontic patients were analyzed retrospectively, obtaining a final sample of 30 patients with mesiodens. The following aspects were analyzed: gender ; number of mesiodens; proportion between erupted and non-erupted mesiodens; initial position of the supernumerary tooth; related complications; treatment plan accomplished; and associated dental anomalies. The frequency of dental anomalies in the sample was compared to reference values for the general population using the chi-square test (χ^2), with a significance level set at 5%. **Results:** The prevalence of mesiodens was 1.5% more common among males (1.5:1). Most of the mesiodens were non-erupted (75%) and in a vertical position, facing the oral cavity. Extraction of the mesiodens was the most common treatment. The main complications associated with mesiodens were: delayed eruption of permanent incisors (34.28%) and midline diastema (28.57%). From all the dental anomalies analyzed, only the prevalence of maxillary lateral incisor agenesis was higher in comparison to the general population. **Conclusion:** There was a low prevalence of mesiodens (1.5%) in deciduous and mixed dentition and the condition was not associated with other dental anomalies, except for the maxillary lateral incisor agenesis.

Keywords: Supernumerary tooth. Child. Prevalence.

[1] PhD in Orthodontics, UNESP.
[2] Masters student in Rehabilitation Sciences, Hospital for Rehabilitation of Craniofacial Anomalies/ University of São Paulo (USP).
[3] MSc in Orthodontics, UNESP.
[4] Full professor in Orthodontics, FOB-USP.
[5] PhD in Orthodontics, UNESP.

» The authors report no commercial, proprietary or financial interest in the products or companies described in this article.

Tulio Silva Lara
Hospital de Reabilitação de Anomalias Craniofaciais / Setor de Ortodontia
Rua Silvio Marchione, 3-20 – CEP: 17.012-900 – Bauru/SP — Brazil.
E-mail: tuliolara@hotmail.com

INTRODUCTION

The term mesiodens refers to supernumerary teeth located in the pre-maxilla region, precisely between the maxillary central incisors (Figs. 1 and 2). Mesiodens is the most frequent type of supernumerary tooth.[1,2] The prevalence of mesiodens reported in the literature varies from 0.15 to 7.8% (Table 1), with a higher prevalence in males, with a proportion of 2:1.[3-10] Although it has not been precisely established, its etiology seems to be related to genetic factors, given the records of family recurrence.[4,11-13] A dominant autosomal trait has been suggested, with incomplete penetrance in some generations[13] and x chromosome linked inheritance due to the higher prevalence among males.

The mesiodens is often unique[3,4,5,7,14] and anomalous in size and shape,[11] but may vary in morphology from a small rudimentary conical shape[4,7,8,9,14,18] to a complex form with several tubercles. It rarely erupts spontaneously,[8,10,14,17] which only occurs in situations in which the mesiodens faces the oral cavity. Most often, the mesiodens is inverted, with the crown positioned towards the nasal cavity and the root apex facing the oral cavity.[3,8,9] The presence of mesiodens can lead to local irregularities of which the most common are: delayed eruption or impaction of adjacent teeth, displacement or rotation of adjacent teeth, development of dentigerous cysts, resorption of adjacent roots, crowding, midline diastema or maxillary incisors root dilaceration.[1,3,4,5,7-11,14,17]

Studies have suggested a genetic and hereditary background in the etiology of dental anomalies of number, size and position. Such evidence comes from investigations carried out with families, monozygotic twins and the observation of associations in the occurrence of certain anomalies.[11,19,20] Tooth agenesis is often associated with other dental anomalies, such as microdontia, ectopia and delayed dental development.[19,20,21] Peck[20] has recently denominated the association of these occurrences as dental anomaly patterns (DAP), as a single mutant gene may be responsible for more than one morphological or functional trait.

Two previous studies verified the association between supernumerary teeth in general and other dental anomalies, including tooth agenesis, microdontia and ectopic eruption.[19,21] The findings revealed that the frequency of supernumerary teeth was not higher in patients with hypoplastic dental anomalies.[19,21] However, no previous study has investigated the exclusive association of mesiodens with other dental anomalies.

Thus, the aim of the present study was to verify the prevalence of mesiodens in children with deciduous and mixed dentitions and its association with other dental anomalies.

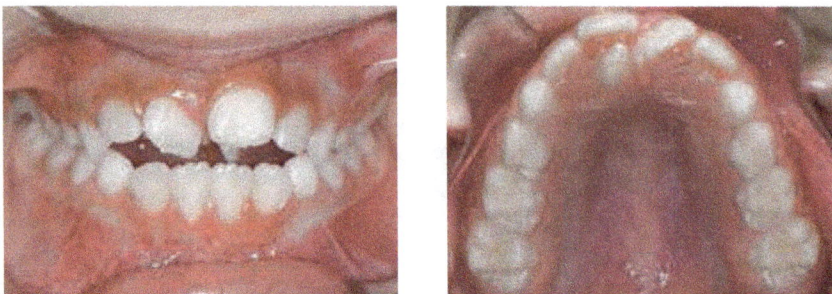

Figure 1 - Mesiodens erupted in the oral cavity.

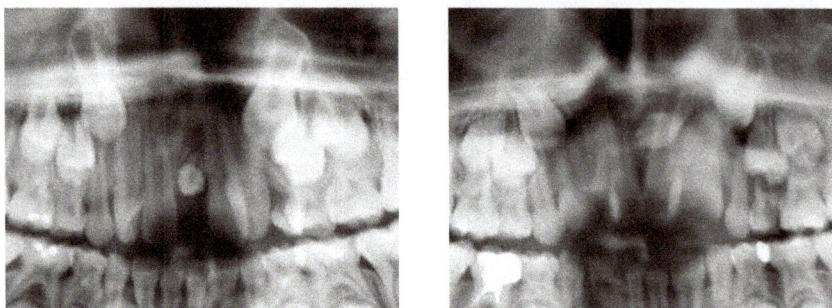

Figure 2 - Radiographic image showing mesiodens.

Prevalence of mesiodens in orthodontic patients with deciduous and mixed dentition and its association...

9

MATERIAL AND METHODS

The orthodontic records of 1,995 patients with deciduous and mixed dentition, taken from the archives of the Profis Preventive and Interceptive Orthodontics Course (Bauru, SP, Brazil) were retrospectively analyzed. Panoramic and periapical radiographs were analyzed by a single examiner. The inclusion criteria were: patients aged between 4 and 13 years old; with deciduous or mixed dentition; presence of at least one supernumerary tooth in the midsagittal region of the maxilla. The exclusion criteria were: presence of craniofacial anomalies; presence of syndromes; history of tooth extraction and incomplete documentation. After the initial analysis, a sample of 30 patients with mesiodens and a mean age of 8 years and 3 months was obtained.

The following aspects were analyzed in the orthodontic records of the sample: 1) sex; 2) number of mesiodens; 3) proportion between erupted and non-erupted mesiodens; 4) initial position of the supernumerary tooth; 5) related complications; 6) treatment planning accomplished; and 7) associated dental anomalies. The associated dental anomalies investigated included agenesis of permanent teeth, microdontia, ectopic eruption of permanent maxillary first molars, tooth transpositions, palatally displaced canines (PDC), distoangulation of mandibular second premolar, infraocclusion of deciduous molars, delayed tooth development and supernumerary teeth (in addition to mesiodens).

Diagnosis of palatally displaced maxillary canines followed the radiographic parameters suggested by Lindauer et al[22] confirmed by the interpretation of periapical radiographs by the tube shift method of object localization using two projections with significantly different x-ray tube angulations. Considering the findings of Ericson and Kurol[23] in which the attempt to determine the eruption path of maxillary canines radiographically is generally of little value in children under 10 years old, those subjects whose only diagnostic records were from an age under 10 years were excluded from the sample when evaluating palatally displaced canines. Diagnosis of distoangulation of mandibular second premolars followed the criteria described by Shalish et al[24] using the lower edge

Table 1 - Prevalence of mesiodens reported in previous studies and in our study sample.

Author	Number of subjects analyzed	Age range	Method	Origin of the sample	Prevalence of mesiodens
Montenegro et al[1]	36,057	5 to 56y	Analysis of patient's file	Unidad Ambulatoria de Cirurgía Bucal (Spain)	0.15%
Gündüz et al[14]	23,000	4 to 14y	Radiographic	Ondokuz Mayis University (Turkey)	0.3%
Buenviaje and Rapp[15]	2,439	2 to 20y	Radiographic	University of Pittsburgh (USA)	0.4%
Järvinen and Lehtinen[16]	1,141	3 to 4y	Clinical	University of Kuopio/ Public Health Centre (Finland)	0.4%
Tyrologou et al[9]	11,500	3 to 15y	Clinical and radiographic	Department of Paediatric Dentistry – Institute for Postgraduate Education (Sweden)	0.8%
Hurlen and Humerfelt[17]	63,029	9 m to 80y	Clinical and radiographic	University of Oslo (Norway)	1.4%
Salcido-García et al[18]	2,241	2 to 55y	Radiographic	Facultad de Odontología UNAM (Mexico)	1.6%
Kaller[6]	3,523	4 to 18y	Clinical and radiographic	Los Barrios Community Clinic – Hispanic area of Dallas (USA)	2.2%
Huang et al[5]	543	2.5 to 7y	Clinical and radiographic	Chang Gung Memorial Hospital (China)	7.8%
Present study	1,995	4 to 13y	Radiographic	Universidade de São Paulo (Brazil)	1.5%

of the mandible as a base line. The maxillary lateral incisor was considered as presenting microdontia when the maximal mesiodistal crown diameter was smaller than that of the opposing mandibular lateral incisor in the same patient.[19] This category also included conical maxillary lateral incisors.

The prevalence of dental anomalies in the sample was compared with reference values for the general population by means of the chi-square test (χ^2), with the significance level set at 5% (P < 0.05). The odds ratio (OR) was calculated with 95% of confidence intervals to measure the strength of associations between supernumerary mesiodens and the presence of other dental anomalies.

RESULTS

The prevalence rate of mesiodens in the sample corresponded to 1.5% with a male-female ratio of 1.5:1 (Tables 1 and 2). Among the affected patients, 80% had only one mesiodens and 20% had two mesiodens (Table 3). Three out of four mesiodens were unerupted and in an upright position (facing the oral cavity), and more than 80% had extraction indication (Table 5). The most common complications related to mesiodens included delayed eruption of maxillary central incisors and midline diastema (Table 5). No association was found between mesiodens and other dental anomalies, except for maxillary lateral incisor agenesis (Tables 6).

DISCUSSION

This study retrospectively assessed the complete orthodontic records of 1,995 patients who presented deciduous or mixed dentition at orthodontic treatment onset. A total of 36 mesiodens were diagnosed in 30 patients (average of 1.2 mesiodens per patient), corresponding to 1.5% of the overall sample. This prevalence was similar to that described in studies by Hurlen and Humerfelt[17] (1.4%) and Salcido-García et al[18] (1.6%), and is very close to the mean frequency observed for the prevalence values compiled in Table 1 (1.67%).

With regard to sex distribution, mesiodens was more common among males, with a male to female proportion of 1.5:1 (Table 2), which corroborates previous reports.[5-10,14] A retrospective study carried out in India,[8] on a sample of 30 patients with mesiodens, found the same male to female

proportion of 1.5:1, whereas a proportion of 2:1,[9] 2.5:1[5] and even 4:1[7] male-female proportions have been described in other studies. Sexual differences in the prevalence of mesiodens disagreed with what has been found for tooth agenesis. Tooth agenesis is more frequent among females, at an approximate proportion of 2:1.[19,25]

Table 2 - Gender distribution of the sample comprised of children with mesiodens.

Sex	Number of individuals	%
Male	18	60
Female	12	40
Total	30	100

Table 3 - Number of mesiodens per patient in the sample.

Number of mesiodens	Number of individuals	%
1	24	80
2	6	20
Total	30	100

Table 4 - Eruption condition, position and treatment planning for mesiodens in the sample.

Eruption condition	Number of mesiodens	%
Unerupted	27	75
Erupted	9	25
Total	36	100
Position	**Number of mesiodens**	**%**
Normal	27	75
Inverted	5	13.9
Horizontal	4	11.1
Total	36	100
Treatment	**Number of mesiodens**	**%**
Extraction	31	86.1
Follow-up	5	13.9
Total	36	100

Table 5 - Complications associated with mesiodens in the sample.

Complications	Number of cases (%)
Delayed eruption of maxillary permanent incisors	12 (34.28%)
Midline diastema	10 (28.57%)
Rotation or axial inclination of erupted permanent incisors	6 (17.14%)
Resorption of teeth adjacent to mesiodens	1 (2.85%)
Root anomaly	2 (5.57%)
None (asymptomatic)	4 (11.42%)
Total	35 (100%)

A single mesiodens was found in 80% of the sample, whereas the remaining 20% presented two mesiodens (Table 3). A very similar proportion was described in a clinical and radiographic study involving 90 patients and 113 mesiodens,[10] in which the majority of patients (78%) had a single mesiodens while the remaining patients had two. Kim and Lee[7] described a similar tendency with 75% of patients exhibiting only one mesiodens and 25% exhibiting two mesiodens. A patient with three mesiodens was described in a retrospective study involving Japanese children.[3]

Among the 36 mesiodens in the sample, 27 (75%) were unerupted while nine (25%) had erupted in the oral cavity (Table 4). Studies are unanimous in demonstrating that the majority of mesiodens remains impacted[6,8-10,14,18] and are often discovered only in routine radiographs requested for other reasons.[9] Mesiodens may also be identified in radiographs requested for follow-up of maxillary incisors trauma or due to delayed eruption of maxillary permanent incisors. These factors are the most common causes of mesiodens diagnosis.[9]

A mesiodens is most often in an upright position with the crown facing the oral cavity (normal position), but mesiodens can be found in inverted or even in a horizontal position.[4,5,9,14] In the present sample, the normal position (vertical, with the crown positioned towards the oral cavity) was found in 75% of the cases, followed by the inverted and horizontal positions (Table 4), which is in agreement with the literature.[4,9,14] These results, however, diverge from a study carried out with Korean children, in which the most common direction was the upright position with the crown facing the nasal cavity (inverted) observed in 52% of the sample, followed by normal (38%) and horizontal (10%) positions.[7] This same tendency was found in a sample of 200 Japanese children with 256 mesiodens, in which the inverted position (67%) predominated over normal (27%) and horizontal (6%).[3]

The most common treatment planning for mesiodens is extraction.[4,7] The removal of mesiodens in the deciduous dentition is not generally recommended due to the risk of injuring the developing maxillary incisors as well as due to lack of patient

Table 6 - Prevalence of dental anomalies in the sample compared with reference values.

Dental Anomaly	Prevalence rate in the sample	n	Reference values	n	χ^2	P	Odds Ratio	Confidence interval	
Tooth agenesis (excluding third molars)	10.00%	3/30	5.00% Grahnen[27]	53/1064	1.51	0.219	2.12	0.62	7.21
Mandibular second premolar agenesis	3.33%	1/30	3.00% Polder et al[25]	1479/48274	0.01	0.932	1.09	0.15	8.01
Maxillary second premolar agenesis	3.33%	1/30	1.50% Polder et al[25]	722/48274	0.69	0.407	2.27	0.31	16.70
Maxillary lateral incisor agenesis	10.00%	3/30	1.90% Le Bot and Salmon[28]	109/5738	10.28	0.001	5.74	1.71	19.20
Small maxillary lateral incisor	3.33%	1/30	4.70% Baccetti[21]	47/1000	0.12	0.726	0.70	0.09	5.24
Mandibular second premolar distoangulation	3.33%	1/30	0.19% Matteson et al[29]	52/26264	14.64	<0.001	17.38	2.32	129.99
Palatally displaced canines (PDC)	3.33%	1/30	1.70% Dachi and Howell[30]	25/1450	0.44	0.507	1.97	0.26	15.00
Supernumerary teeth	10.00%	3/30	3.90% Baccetti[21]	39/1000	2.77	0.096	2.74	0.80	9.41

cooperation during this stage.[4,9] Thus, the clinical and radiographic follow-up can also be indicated in cases in which the mesiodens is not causing a malocclusion or will not interfere in the orthodontic treatment.[9,14] In the present study, 86.1% of the mesiodens were surgically removed right after diagnosis, whereas the remaining 13.5% were followed-up radiographically due to the absence of any interference in the dental development (Table 4).

The main complications associated with mesiodens were: delayed eruption of permanent incisors (34.28%), midline diastema (28.57%) and rotation or axial inclination of permanent incisors (17.14%). Other local disorders were also associated with the presence of mesiodens as shown in Table 5. Similar findings have been previously reported.[7,9,14]

Regarding the presence of other dental anomalies associated with mesiodens, 22 patients (73.3% of the sample) did not exhibit any associated dental anomaly.

The other eight patients (26.7%) exhibited 12 associated dental anomalies including microdontia of maxillary lateral incisors, other supernumerary teeth, delayed development of second premolars, distoangulation of mandibular second premolars and tooth agenesis (Table 6).

The statistical analyses revealed that patients with mesiodens did not have an increased prevalence of permanent tooth agenesis in general or microdontia of the maxillary lateral incisors (Table 6). However, the prevalence of agenesis of maxillary permanent lateral incisors was approximately five times higher in the sample when compared with the general population. This uncommon association between a supernumerary mesiodens and the agenesis of max-

illary lateral incisor has been described in a case report previously published and the interpretation of the authors regarding this association was a possible transposition between a malformed lateral incisor and the central incisor.[26]

One patient (3.3%) in the sample exhibited distal angulation of the mandibular second premolars. Due to the small prevalence of this anomaly in the general population (0.19%), this result was considered statistically significant (Table 6). However, considering the small size of the sample, this result could have randomly occurred and should be interpreted with caution. Larger samples are needed to confirm such association.

Ectopic eruption of maxillary canines was diagnosed in one patient. However, since the patient was eight years old and the diagnosis of ectopia in panoramic radiographs is more reliable among patients over the age of 10,[23] this anomaly was not considered.

CONCLUSION

1. The prevalence of mesiodens in the deciduous and mixed dentition corresponded to 1.5%, with a male to female proportion of 1.5:1.
2. Mesiodens was associated with local disorders, such as maxillary incisor rotation, delayed eruption or impaction of maxillary incisors, midline diastema, permanent incisor root resorption and dilaceration.
3. Mesiodens was associated with other dental anomalies in 26.7% of the sample.
4. The prevalence of maxillary lateral incisor agenesis was higher in children with mesiodens in comparison to the general population.

REFERENCES

1. Montenegro PF, Castellón EV, Aytés LB, Escoda CG. Retrospective study of 145 supernumerary teeth. Med Oral Patol Oral Cir Bucal. 2006;11(4):339-44.
2. Stafne EC. Supernumerary teeth. Dental Cosmos. 1932;74:653-9.
3. Asaumi JI, Shibata Y, Yanagi Y, Hisatomi M, Matsuzaki H, Konouchi H, et al. Radiographic examination of mesiodens and their associated complications. Dentomaxillofac Radiol. 2004;33(2):125-7.
4. Ersin NK, Candan U, Alpoz AR, Akay C. Mesiodens in primary, mixed and permanent dentitions: a clinical and radiographic study. J Clin Pediatr Dent. 2004;28(4):295-8.
5. Huang WH, Tsai TP, Su HL. Mesiodens in the primary dentition stage: a radiographic study. ASDC J Dent Child. 1992;59(3):186-9.
6. Kaller LC. Prevalence of mesiodens in a pediatric Hispanic population. ASDC J Dent Child. 1998;55(2):137-8.
7. Kim SG, Lee SH. Mesiodens: a clinical and radiographic study. J Dent Child. 2003;70(1):58-60.
8. Roychoudhury A, Gupta Y, Parkash H. Mesiodens: a retrospective study of fifth teeth. J Indian Soc Pedod Prev Dent. 2000;18(4):144-6.
9. Tyrologou S, Koch G, Kurol J. Location, complications and treatment of mesiodentes – a retrospective study in children. Swed Dent J. 2005;29(1):1-9.
10. Von Arx T. Anterior maxillary supernumerary teeth: a clinical and radiographic study. Aust Dent J. 1992;37(3):189-95.
11. Gallas MM, Garcia A. Retention of permanent incisors by mesiodens: a family affair. Br Dent J. 2000;188(2):63-4.
12. Marya CM, Kumar BR. Familial occurrence of mesiodens with unusual findings: case reports. Quintessence Int. 1998;29(1):49-51.

Prevalence of mesiodens in orthodontic patients with deciduous and mixed dentition and its association...

13

13. Sedano HO, Gorlin RJ. Familial occurrence of mesiodens. Oral Surg Oral Med Oral Pathol. 1969;27(3):360-1.

14. Gündüz K, Celenk P, Zengin Z, Sümer P. Mesiodens: a radiographic study in children. J Oral Sci. 2008;50(3):287-91.

15. Buenviaje TM, Raap R. Dental anomalies in children: a clinical and radiographic survey. ASDC J Dent Child. 1984;51(1):42-6.

16. Järvinen S, Lehtinen L. Supernumerary and congenitally missing primary teeth in Finnish children. An epidemiologic study. Acta Odontol Scand. 1981;39(2):83-6.

17. Hurlen B, Humerfelt D. Characteristics of premaxillary hyperdontia. A radiographic study. Acta Odontol Scand. 1985;43(2):75-81.

18. Salcido-García JF, Ledesma-Montes C, Hernández-Flores F, Pérez D, Garcés-Ortíz M. Frequency of supernumerary teeth in Mexican population. Med Oral Patol Oral Cir Bucal. 2004;9(5):407-9, 403-6.

19. Garib DG, Peck S, Gomes SC. Increased occurrence of dental anomalies associated with second-premolar agenesis. Angle Orthod. 2009;79(3):436-41.

20. Peck S. Dental anomaly patterns (DAP): a new way to look at malocclusion. Angle Orthod. 2009;79(5):1015-6.

21. Baccetti T. A controlled study of associated dental anomalies. Angle Orthod. 1998;68(3):267-74.

22. Lindauer SJ, Rubenstein LK, Hang WM, Andersen WC, Isaacson RJ. Canine impaction identified early with panoramic radiographs. J Am Dent Assoc. 1992;123(3):91-2, 95-7.

23. Ericson S, Kurol J. Radiographic assessment of maxillary canine eruption in children with clinical signs of eruption disturbance. Eur J Orthod. 1986;8(3):133-40.

24. Shalish M, Peck S, Wasserstein A, Peck L. Malposition of unerupted mandibular second premolar associated with agenesis of its antimere. Am J Orthod Dentofacial Orthop. 2002;121(1):53-6.

25. Polder BJ, Van't Hof MA, Van der Linden FP, Kuijpers-Jagtman AM. A meta-analysis of the prevalence of dental agenesis of permanent teeth. Community Dent Oral Epidemiol. 2004;32(3):217-26.

26. Segura JJ, Jiménez-Rubio A. Concomitant hipohyperdontia: simultaneous occurrence of a mesiodens and agenesis of a maxillary lateral incisor. Oral Surg Oral Med Oral Pathol Oral Radiol Endod. 1998;86(4):473-5.

27. Grahnen H. Hypodontia in the permanent dentition. A clinical and genetical investigation. Odontol Revy. 1956;7:1-100.

28. Bot PL, Salmon D. Congenital defects of the upper lateral incisors (ULI): condition and measurements of the other teeth, measurements of the superior arch, head and face. Am J Phys Anthropol. 1977;46(2):231-43.

29. Matteson SR, Kantor ML, Proffit WR. Extreme distal migration of the mandibular second bicuspid. A variant of eruption. Angle Orthod. 1982;52(1):11-8.

30. Dachi S, Howell F. A survey of 3874 routine full-mouth radiographs. II. A study of impacted teeth. Oral Surg Oral Med Oral Pathol. 1961;14:1165-9.

3

Discoloration and force degradation of orthodontic elastomeric ligatures

Samaneh Nakhaei[1], Raha Habib Agahi[2], Amin Aminian[3], Masoud Rezaeizadeh[4]

Objective: The aim of the present study was to evaluate color changes and force degradation of orthodontic elastomeric ligatures in different stretching patterns during a 8-weeks period. **Methods:** Two elastomers with the minimum and two with the maximum color changing, and gray elastomers of two brands (American Orthodontics and Ortho Technology) were selected according to an opinion poll with clinicians and color changes after 4 weeks of intraoral use were evaluated. These elastomers were mounted on special jigs fabricated using a CAD-CAM technique, underwent different stretching patterns and the force was measured in 0, 24 hours, 2, 4 and 8 weeks. During *in vivo* part of the study, force levels of elastomers were measured after 4 weeks on a material testing machine. Data were analyzed with four-way ANOVA and Tukey *post hoc* tests. **Results:** All the elastomers showed color changing but the degree of color stability was significantly different. The mean force degradation was higher in 1-mm stretch groups. After 8 weeks, the average residual force of elastomers was $1.45 \pm 0.18\,N$ and the maximum force decay was seen in the elastomers that exhibited the maximum initial force. **Conclusion:** There is significant relationship between the stretching pattern and the amount of residual force of elastomers. Elastomers with higher initial forces exhibited higher percentages of force loss after 8 weeks. It seems that there is a relationship between initial color and color changing of elastomers.

Keywords: Color. Elastomers. Orthodontics. Force degradation.

[1] Assistant Professor, Department of Orthodontics, Birjand Dental School, Birjand University of Medical Science, Birjand, Iran.

[2] Oral and Dental Disease Research Center, Kerman Dental School, Kerman University of Medical Science, Kerman, Iran.

[3] Assistant Professor, Oral and Dental Diseases Research center, Department of Orthodontics, Kerman Dental School, Kerman University of Medical Science, Kerman, Iran.

[4] Assistant Professor, Graduate University of Advanced Technology, Mechanical Engineering Department , Kerman, Iran.

» The authors report no commercial, proprietary or financial interest in the products or companies described in this article.

Raha Habib Agahi
E-mail: raha2979@yahoo.com

INTRODUCTION

Clinicians may use pins, stainless steel ligature; self ligating clips and circular elastomers to ligate orthodontic archwires to the brackets.[1,2] Elastomeric ligatures are most commonly used by clinicians due to their several advantages including low cost, easy application, reduced chair time, patient comfort and satisfaction.[3]

These ligatures are manufactured by many companies in a variety of different colors that meet the growing global demand for esthetic orthodontic appliances. Also, the possibility of choosing the ligatures color facilitate young people adhesion to treatment.[4] Although adding pigments to ligatures seems to represent a great advantage, there is two concerns regarding colored elastomers. The first one is that clinicians and patients may choose ligatures of pleasing color at placement time, but this chosen color is susceptible to color degradation over time, which is a critical concern. Ardeshna et al[5] reported that food diet may affect elastomers color. The second question is whether force delivery is affected by adding pigments to elastomers. Oliveira et al[6] reported that elastomers of different colors have different initial force and residual force over time.

The important clinical issue about elastomers is force delivery and force degradation of these materials over time. The force exerted by elastomers depends on the initial force and force decay rate, many studies reported 50-70% force loss in the first 24 hours.[3,4,6]

Under clinical conditions, differently from usual laboratory conditions in force decay studies, the wire is not placed uniformly within the bracket slot and is not passive. Normally, during the early stages of treatment, high-stress areas that are under tension are produced in the ligature, depending on the extent of tooth misalignment and the differences in the buccolingual position of adjacent teeth. In studies carried out so far on elastomers, less attention has been paid to the exact simulation of the clinical situation and to the effect of stretching on the elastic properties of elastomers. In this study an attempt to evaluate the relationship between stretching pattern and the elastic properties of elastomeric modules as close to the clinical situation as possible was made by designing a specific instrument using CAD-CAM technology.

Knowledge about changes in the physical (like color changes) and mechanical properties (like force delivery) of elastomers is of great interest for their clinical application.[7] Since elastomers might remain in the oral cavity for an average of 30 days, it is very important to preserve their properties, including force consistency and color stability, and their relationship during this period.[5,8,9]

In this study, an attempt was made to evaluate color changes and force degradation of orthodontic elastomeric ligatures under different stretching conditions over a period of 8 weeks, and test the hypothesis that elastomeric ligatures of different color under different stretching pattern have different force decay rates.

MATERIAL AND METHODS

To determine the elastomers which exhibit the maximum and minimum color changes from one orthodontic treatment session to another, different colors of the most commonly used elastomeric ligatures (Unistick, American Orthodontics, USA; Power Sticks, Ortho Technology, USA) were selected and delivered to ten orthodontists, along with questionnaires. All the orthodontists had at least three years of experience working with those commercial brands. Based on the results of an opinion poll with these clinicians, two colored elastomers with maximum color changes and two colored elastomers with minimum color changes were selected from each brand, adding up to eight colored elastomers (Table 1). In the process of selecting the elastomers with the smallest and largest color changes, the next step was an intraoral stage: forty fixed orthodontic patients with good oral hygiene and no specific type of diet were assigned to two groups (n = 20), by simple randomization. Four selected colored elastomers of each brand were placed in the oral cavity of 20 patients from each group. Selected ligatures from each brand were placed in a crisscross pattern on teeth #4 and #5 in each quadrant to preserve esthetic appearance and to avoid the bias resulting from the patient's eating on only one side. After thirty days, the ligatures were removed from the oral environment, separated by quadrant and the brands were identified by numbers. A total of 168 photographs [8 at T_1 (not used elastomers), and 160 at T_2 (elastomers after 30 days use in oral cavity)], were obtained using a digital camera (Canon EF-S 18-55-IS II, Canon, Osaka, Japan), with a 10-megapixel resolution and color depth of 12 bits. All the photographs were taken manually by a single operator around noon under natural light, without the use of a flash, with 1/6 seconds speed, f/22 diaphragm aperture, ISO 200,

Table 1 - Percentage of color changing in elastomeric ligatures based on clinician's opinion* of digital photograph.

	American Orthodontics			Ortho Technology	
Color	Color changing score*	Percentage of color changing	Color	Color changing score*	Percentage of color changing
Red	1	63%	Red	1	58%
	2	27%		2	29%
	3	10%		3	13%
Blue	1	55%	Cobalt blue	1	51%
	2	28%		2	34%
	3	17%		3	15%
Pink	1	24%	Violet	1	21%
	2	30%		2	27%
	3	46%		3	52%
Bubble gum pink	1	15%	Fuchsia	1	10%
	2	28%		2	27%
	3	57%		3	63%

*Color changing score: 1 = unpigmented ligatures; 2 = pigmented ligatures; 3 = heavily pigmented ligatures.

self-timer mode set to trigger after 15 seconds. The images were stored in JPEG format (Fig 1). In order to carry out a visual analysis of the elastomeric ligatures, a Power Point presentation was created. The images were assessed independently by a panel of two orthodontists who rated the degree of discoloration of the elastomeric ligatures using a numerical scale ranging from 1 to 3, in which 1 was assigned to unpigmented ligatures, 2 to moderately pigmented ligatures, and 3 to heavily pigmented ligatures (Table 1). Finally, from each brand, one elastomer with the most color change and one elastomer with the least color change under clinical conditions were selected. The gray color elastomers from each brand served as control group.

Two types of storage jigs for '1-mm point stretch' and 'uniform stretch' groups were designed and fabricated by using a CAD-CAM technique (Fig 2) in which the designing process (CAD) was carried out with the software SolidWorks 2011 (3D design, SolidWorks Corp., USA) and the manufacturing phase (CAM) was carried out with a CNC machine (VMC Machine, model 850, Machine Sazi Tabriz corp., Iran) and Power MILL software (Delcam corp., UK). The 'uniform stretch' jig was prepared from a rectangular aluminum bar measuring 2.9×1.1 mm, equal to the width of a premolar bracket (Gemini Metal bracket, 0.022-in slot, 3M Unitek). The '1-mm point stretch' jigs were designed to

simulate the elastomers stretch condition during the first stage of fixed orthodontic treatment with malpositioned teeth. To create stretch and stress points in elastomers, 0.016-in SS wires were used (Fig 3). These holding jigs were used to store the elastomers during the study period in containers with artificial saliva in an incubator at $37 \pm 1°C$ under a traction force. All the elastomer groups were tested for force on a materials testing machine (model 10 KN, M350-10CT, Testometric Company, UK). The ligatures were stretched at a rate of 5 mm per minute until rupture according to Kovatch et al[10] study. As each elastomer was stretched, force (N) was constantly measured and recorded. Force–extension curve was plotted by WinTest Analysis Materials Testing software (Testometric Company, UK). The fixture of materials testing machine was designed by the CAD-CAM technique and was manufactured from two equal-sized aluminum cubes, with two semi-circular rods, measuring 1.1 mm in radius (Fig 4). At the beginning of the test the two halves of the fixture were placed next to each other with no space between them, hence producing a 2.2-mm diameter circle. To calculate distance between the two parts of fixture (Fig 4) at which the force levels of elastomeric modules were measured ('X' in Fig 4), the inner circumferences of the elastomer on the fixture of the testing machine were adjusted to match the inner cir-

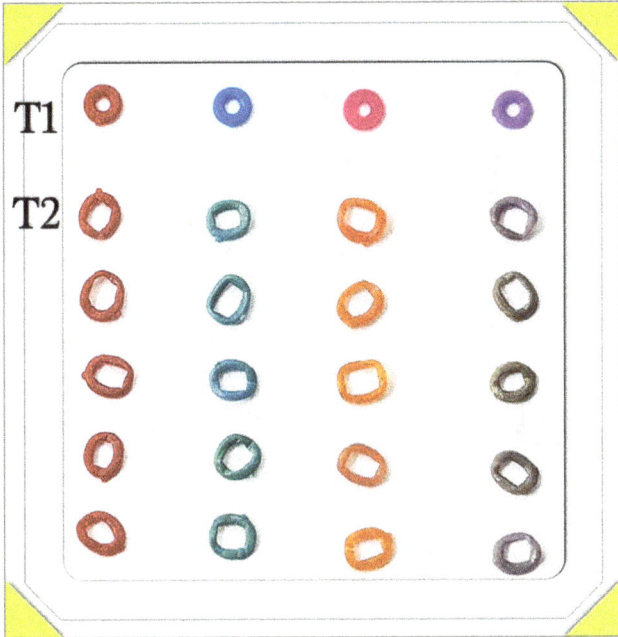

Figure 1 - Photographic evaluation of color changing of elastomers after intraoral use (T1: not used elastomers, T2: intraoral used elastomers).

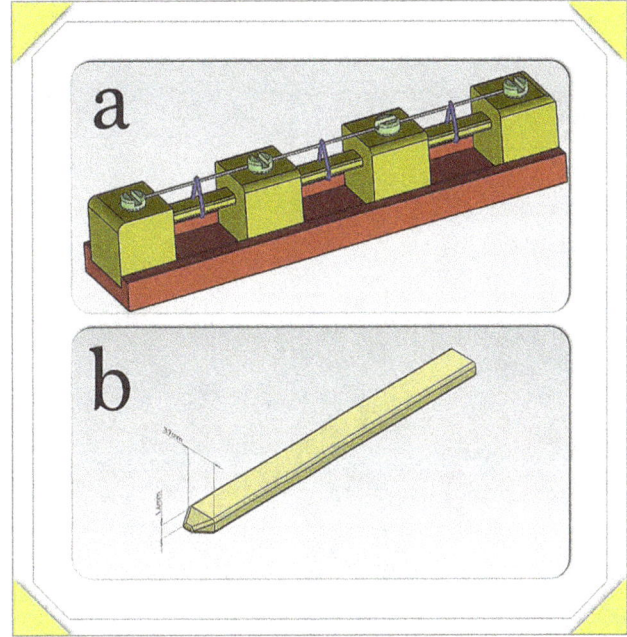

Figure 2 - CAD-CAM fabricated jigs (A = 1-mm point stretch jig, B = uniform-stretch jig).

cumferences of the specimens placed on the storage jigs of the relevant groups, and all the measurements were made at 0.1-mm accuracy, using SolidWorks software. The 'X' distance was calculated for all groups using the following formula:

$$X = \frac{y - 2z}{2}$$

Whereas:

y = the circumference of the elastomer on the storage jig;

z = the circumference of the half-circle of the fixture.

X was calculated at 1.5 mm in the 'uniform stretch' group and at 2 mm in the '1-mm point stretch' group. A total of 10 elastomers from each color were tested for the amount of initial force and residual force after 24 hours, 2, 4 and 8 weeks in the two groups with uniform and 1-mm point stretch patterns.

In order to confirm the accuracy of the results of the *in vitro* study with the results of the intraoral study, 10 elastomeric ligatures from each three selected colors (least color change, most color change, control) from both companies were placed on the premolar teeth of 10 patients using fixed appliances. They all used 3M-Unitek bracket system and were in the finishing stage with 0.016-in SS archwires. In order to make the *in vitro* and the oral cavity conditions as similar as possible, the elastomers were placed in both conditions with a ligature gun (Straight Shooter, TP Orthodontics, USA). The elastomers were retrieved from the oral cavity at a 4-week interval, rinsed with copious distilled water and placed in artificial saliva. The forces were measured in less than 30 minutes on a materials testing machine. Sixty samples were evaluated in the intraoral stage and a total of 600 samples were evaluated in the present study (Fig 5).

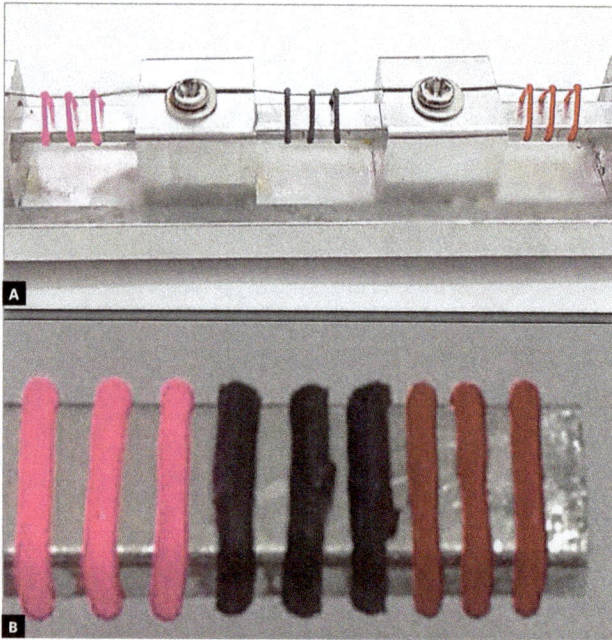

Figure 3 - The 1-mm point (**A**) and the uniform stretch (**B**) jigs.

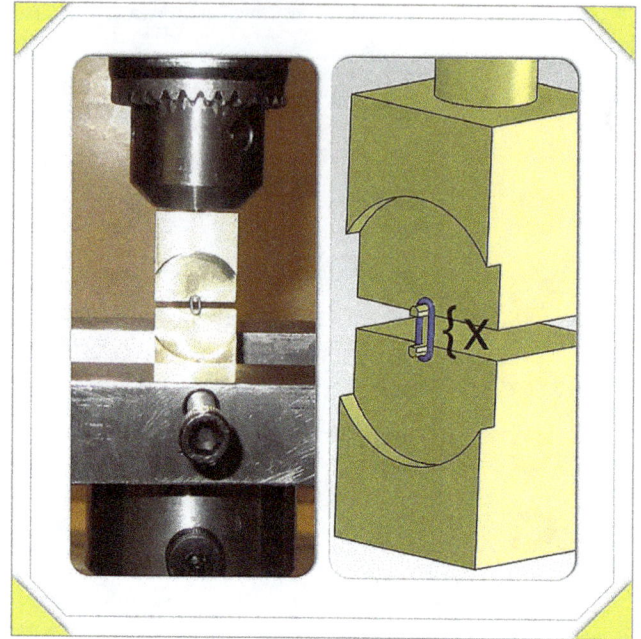

Figure 4 - Fixture fabricated for testometric machine.

A study of ethics in medical ethics committee reviewed and approved the research. The aim of the study was explained to the patients, which voluntarily participated in the study. Informed consent to participate in the study was obtained from patients before their involvement and they were given a choice to leave the study whenever they want. Patient's data were all kept confidential, and they did not had to pay any additional costs to take part in the study. Photographs were taken including only premolar of the patients, pictures of the face were not taken, to follow the ethical guidelines.

The SPSS software v. 18 (SPSS Inc. Chicago, IL, USA) was used for statistical analysis of data (at significance level of $p < 0.05$). Descriptive statistics were used to report the clinician's opinion regarding the most commonly used colored elastomers and photographic evaluation of elastomers with minimum and maximum color changes in the mouth. Results of force measurements were statistically analyzed with four-way ANOVA using brands, stretching pattern (uniform *versus* 1-mm), color and time as variables, followed by Tukey *post-hoc* tests.

RESULTS

According to results of the opinion poll, American Orthodontics (AO) red and blue elastomers, and Ortho Technology (OT) cobalt blue and red elastomers were selected as the ones with minimum color changes, and AO bubble-gum pink and pink elastomers, and OT violet and fuchsia elastomers were selected as the ones with maximum color changes. Based on photographic evaluation (Fig 1), red elastomers of both companies were rated as the ones with minimum color changes, and AO bubble-gum pink elastomer and OT fuchsia elastomer were rated as the ones with maximum color changes (Table 1).

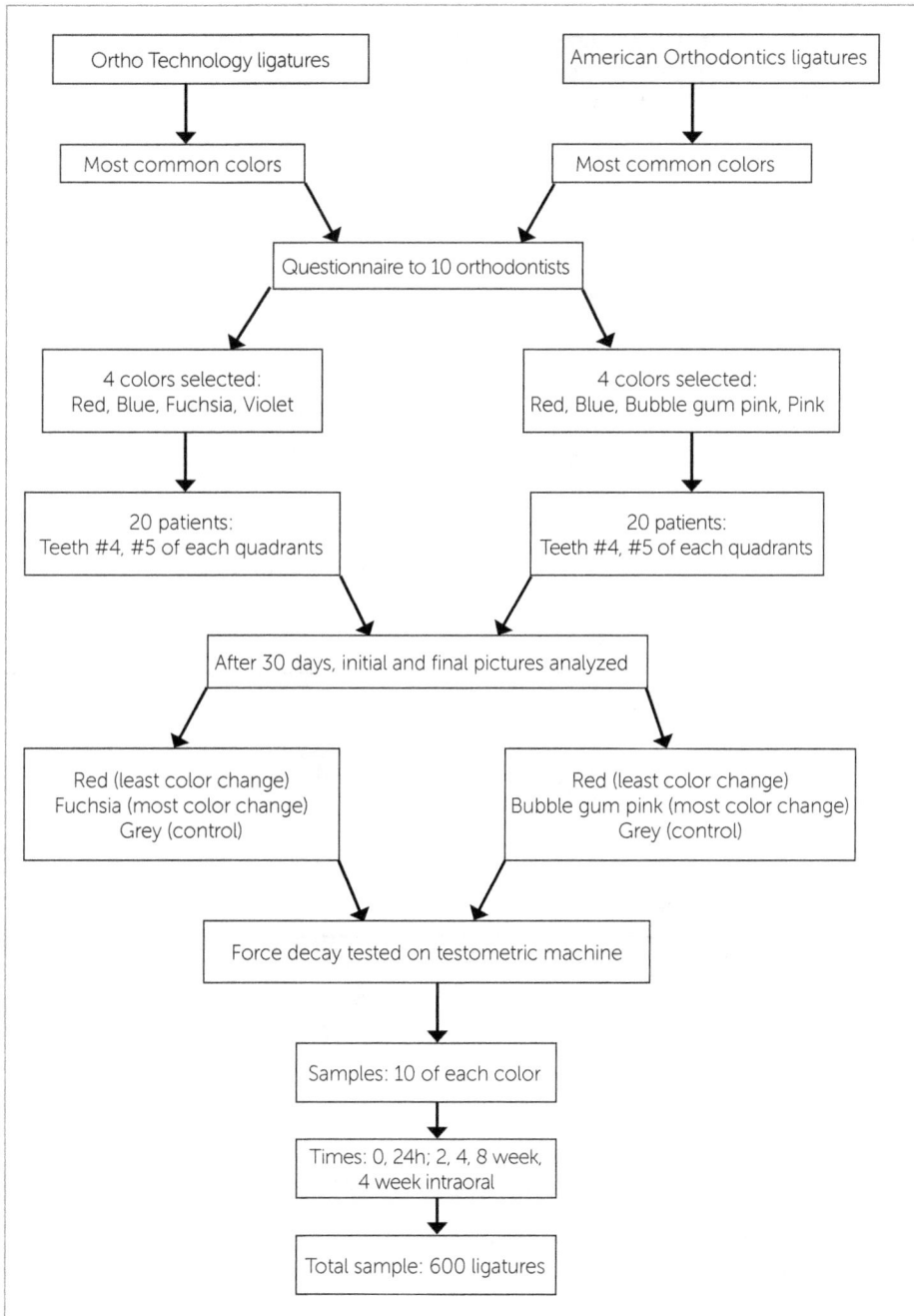

Figure 5 - Flow diagram of the study.

The results of four-way ANOVA showed that all four variables (commercial brand, color, time and stretching pattern) had significant effects on the force levels of the elastomers ($p < 0.001$) (Table 2).

The mean residual forces and mean percentages of force degradation for elastomeric ligatures of each brand are summarized in Table 3. Mean elastomers residual force in all experimental groups after 4 and 8 weeks were , respectively, in the following ranges: 1.07–2.28 N and 1.14–1.64 N. After 8 weeks, the minimum residual forces were recorded for the AO bubble-gum pink elastomers (1.29±0.56 N) and OT fuchsia elastomers (1.15±0.37 N) , with no significant differences. The maximum residual forces were also recorded for the gray elastomers of both companies (Table 3).

Table 2 - Test of between-subjects effects using 4-way ANOVA statistical analysis.

Subjects	Type III Sum of Square	fd	Mean Square	F-Value	P-Value
Color	.989	65	.494	7.215	.001
Brand	6.891	1	6.891	100.592	.000
Time	597.210	2	149.303	2.179	.000
Storage	4.275	1	2.137	31.199	.000
Color*Brand	.466	4	.233	3.404	.034
Color*Time	16.189	2	2.024	29.539	.000
Color*Tensile	1.658	2	.414	6.050	.000
Brand*Time	9.833	8	2.458	35.882	.000
Brand*Tensile	6.687	4	3.343	48.803	.000
Time*Tensile	10.452	4	2.613	38.142	.000
Color*Brand*Time	3.228	2	.403	5.890	.000
Color*Brand*Tensile	3.950	4	.988	14.415	.000
Color*Time*Tensile	3.671	8	.459	6.699	.000
Brand*Time*Tensile	2.298	4	.574	8.386	.000
Color*Brand*Time*Tensile	2.675	8	.334	4.880	.000
Total	3.919.722	621			

Table 3 - Mean residual force (N) and mean percentage of force decay for all test groups.

	Color	Type of traction	Residual force (mean ±SD)					Mean percentage of force decay (%)			
			0	24 hours	2 weeks	4 weeks	8 weeks	24 hours	4 weeks	8 weeks	4 weeks Intraoral
Ortho Technology	Red	0mm	3.598± .362	2.522± .362	2.054± .362	1.469± .128	1.272± .472	30	59	65	1.252± .125
		1mm	4.176± .338	2.363± .132	1.618± .135	1.423± .168	1.616± .175	43.5	66	61.5	65.21%
	Gray	0mm	3.162± .391	2.134± .362	1.658± .202	1.782± .327	1.089± .107	32.6	43.7	65.6	1.780± .289
		1mm	3.577± .416	1.958± .180	1.641± .132	1.480± .154	1.641± .158	45.3	58.7	54.2	43.71%
	Fuchsia	0mm	3.803± .232	2.127± .358	1.685± .135	1.702± .100	1.148± .129	44	55.3	69.9	1.055± .783
		1mm	4.247± .240	1.722± .106	1.608± .152	1.071± .615	1.150± .375	59.5	74.8	72.8	72.26%
American Orthodontics	Red	0mm	4.684± .217	2.385± .230	2.036± .141	1.545± .247	1.493± .371	49	67	68	1.348± .115
		1mm	5.269± .228	2.309± .096	2.224± .147	1.713± .086	1.598± .278	56	67.5	69.7	71.2%
	Gray	0mm	3.883± .469	2.635± .315	2.080± .170	2.285± .511	1.613± .126	32.2	41.2	58.5	1.143± .713
		1mm	4.418± .464	2.315± .133	2.016± .165	1.952± .212	1.588± .132	47.7	55.9	64.1	63.15%
	Bubble-gum pink	0mm	4.541± .513	2.518± .319	1.812± .075	1.580± .107	1.295± .567	44.6	65.3	71.5	1.442± .116
		1mm	5.191± .554	2.530± .133	2.313± .143	1.701± .133	1.411± .131	51.3	67.3	72.82	68.25%

In all ligatures of both companies and two different stretch pattern groups, the greatest rate of force decay occurred during the first 24 hours. At 0–4-week interval, the percentages of force degradation in all the elastomers were higher in the '1-mm stretch' groups than the 'uniform stretch' groups. Comparison of the residual forces in the intraoral elastomers with those of the *in vitro* evaluation at 4-week interval showed that the residual forces in the intraoral elastomers in all the groups were smaller than those studied *in vitro*; however, the differences were clinically significant only in the OT fuchsia elastomers (0.7 N) and AO gray elastomers (1.14 N).

DISCUSSION

The results of the present study confirmed that elastomeric ligatures with different color under different stretching patterns have different force decay rates.

OT fuchsia elastomers and AO red elastomers, which had the maximum initial forces, exhibited maximum force degradation during the first 24 hours followed by less force decay or relative force stability at subsequent intervals, compared to other elastomers, corroborating previous studies, which showed that elastomers producing higher initial forces displayed more force decay.[9,11,12,13]

The advantages of differentiating the elastomers with the minimum and the maximum color changes after exposure to oral environment not only provides results closer to the reality but also can help patient and clinician to choose the color and brand of elastomers that show greater esthetic stability during the period between two orthodontic follow-up appointments. In order to do so, in the process of selecting elastomers with maximum and minimum color changes —after a opinion poll with the clinicians that had used these products for a considerable time—, and for higher data accuracy, the elastomers were placed in the oral cavity and all the factors affecting color change process (through simple staining and chemical degradation, including foodstuffs, temperature changes and oral bacterial flora) were taken into account and the results were very close to real clinical situations.[3]

The aim of this study was to determine clinically noticeable discoloration of elastomers. Digital camera was used because it is a more cost-effective and simpler process than the use of traditional methods such as spectrophotometry.[14,15] Also, there is a very high and statistically significant correlation between the traditional method and digital camera.[16] Another reason to use digital photography to evaluate color change, compared with other complex procedures, is that it is a practical method, reproducible by professional in clinical conditions. For these reasons, digital photographs were used to compare discolorations of elastomeric ligatures before and after exposure to the oral environment.

Lam et al[17] results were similar to the findings of the present study: they reported that addition of pigments to elastomers can change their mechanical properties. Since the fuchsia and bubble-gum pink elastomers exhibited maximum color changes in the oral cavity and also maximum force loss under the circumstances of the present study, it might be hypothesized that there is correlation between elastomer color changes and the amount of force loss, but this theory also needs to be evaluated in different brands of elastomers and different study condition.

The force degradation pattern of elastomers in the intra- and extraoral stages of the study was the same. However, the amount of intraoral residual forces in AO gray and OT fuchsia elastomers exhibited a significant decrease, compared to *in vitro* conditions. Eliades et al[18] evaluated the tensile properties of elastomeric chains and showed no significant differences between the intraoral and laboratory conditions, consistent with the results of the present study. However, Ash et al[19] showed significantly lower residual forces in the elastomeric chains placed in the oral cavity compared to samples placed under atmospheric conditions; although there were minor differences in forces in elastomers placed in water and in the oral cavity. Such differences might be attributed to the lack of similarity between the conditions of *in vitro* and *in vivo* studies.

The dimensional accuracy of the storage jigs, and also the use of artificial saliva and conserving the elastomers at 37 °C resulted in the similarity of the results of intra- and extraoral stages of study. It should be pointed out that the elastomers were placed in the oral cavity on the premolar teeth in the finishing stage of treatment, during which the teeth exhibit sufficient leveling and alignment, which is similar to the *in vitro* conditions in the uniform stretch pattern. It was not possible to simulate the 1-mm point stretch condition in the oral cavity due to differences in teeth positions in the early stages of treatment and it was not possible to match the tension and stress conditions in the elastomers.

During the first stage of fixed orthodontic treatment, some stress concentration points are created in elastomers due to the misalignment of the dentition and differences in the buccolingual positions of adjacent teeth. In the present study, 1-mm point stretch storage jigs were designed and fabricated using a CAD-CAM technique, with the dimensional accuracy of up to 0.1 mm, to simulate the first stage of treatment.

Another advantage of the present study in comparison to some previous studies[13,18,20] was selection of the 0–8-week interval. Sims et al[21] stated that a single elastic module produces a ligation force of 50–150 g. Therefore, the results of the present study showed that the residual forces in all the tested groups after 8 weeks (142 ± 23 g and 149 ± 11 g in OT and AO elastomers, respectively) were adequate to hold the wire within the bracket slot and make it possible to arrange inter-appointment intervals longer than four weeks during the early stages of orthodontic treatment (in cases where there is no concern regarding plaque accumulation), which makes the treatment process more cost-effective for both the patient and the clinician. Peterson et al[22] reported that if ligation or normal forces decrease, there will be a corresponding decrease in frictional resistance, so in other words higher forces in elastomers result in higher frictional forces in the system, decreasing tooth movement rate in early stage of treatment.[23] Contrarily, this high amount of force decays after 8 weeks. The elastomeric modules are not good candidates for remaining in oral cavity more than 4 weeks in the final stages of fixed orthodontic treatment, in which the wire should be completely and actively seated in the bracket slot.

Under the terms of our study on two brands of elastomers, it seems that incorporation of different pigments into elastomers affects force degradation rates by affecting the amount of the initial forces. Therefore, further studies on other brands of elastomers are required to evaluate the correlation between the characteristics of elastomers, which can be observed in the clinic and the mechanical properties of these elastic materials. It is possible to match the results of *in vitro* and *in vivo* studies by exact simulation of *in vitro* conditions of studies. However, to determine the amount of ligation force produced by elastomers and force decay rate and their correlation with elastomer size, elastomer brand, color, time, stage of treatment, etc, further intraoral studies are required.

CONCLUSION

1. All the ligatures showed an unwanted color changes after exposure to intraoral environment, although American Orthodontics (AO) red and blue elastomers and Ortho Technology (OT) cobalt blue and red elastomers showed minimum color changes.

2. The results of the present study showed a significant relationship between the stretching pattern and the amount of residual force of elastomeric ligatures.

3. Elastomers with higher initial forces exhibited higher percentages of force decay after 8 weeks.

4. In the elastomers evaluated in this study, the maximum force decay occurred during the first 24 hours continuing at lower rates during the 8 weeks period.

REFERENCES

1. Carneiro GKM, Roque JA, Garcez Segundo AS, Suzuki H. Evaluation of stiffness and plastic deformation of active ceramic self-ligating bracket clips after repetitive opening and closure movements. Dental Press J Orthod. 2015 July-Aug;20(4):45–5.

2. Walton DK, Fields HW, Johnston WM, Rosenstiel SF, Firestone AR, Christensen JC. Orthodontic appliance preferences of children and adolescents. Am J Orthod Dentofacial Orthop. 2010 Dec;138(6):698.e1-12; discussion 698-9.

3. Buchmann N, Senn C, Ball J, Brauchli L. Influence of initial strain on the force decay of currently available elastic chains over time. Angle Orthod. 2012 May;82(3):529-35.

4. Eliades T, Bourauel C. Intraoral aging of orthodontic materials: the picture we miss and its clinical relevance. Am J Orthod Dentofacial Orthop. 2005 Apr;127(4):403-12.

5. Ardeshna AP, Vaidyanathan TK. Colour changes of orthodontic elastomeric module materials exposed to in vitro dietary media. J Orthod. 2009 Sept;36(3):177-85.

6. Oliveira AS, Kaizer MR, Salgado VE, Soldati DC, Silva RC, Moraes RR. Influence of whitening and regular dentifrices on orthodontic clear ligature color stability. J Esthet Restor Dent. 2015 Mar-Apr;27 Suppl 1:S58-64.

7. Kim SH, Lee YK. Measurement of discolouration of orthodontic elastomeric modules with a digital camera. Eur J Orthod. 2009 Oct;31(5):556-62.

8. Silva DL, Mattos CT, Araújo MV, Ruellas ACO. Color stability and fluorescence of different orthodontic esthetic archwires. Angle Orthod. 2013 Jan;83(1):127-32.

9. Masoud AI, Bulic M, Viana G, Bedran-Russo AK. Force decay and dimensional changes of thermoplastic and novel thermoset elastomeric ligatures. Angle Orthod. 2016 Sept;86(5):818-25.

10. Kovatch JS, Lautenschlager EP, Apfel DA, Keller JC. Load-extension-time behavior of orthodontic alastiks. J Dent Res. 1976 Sept-Oct;55(5):783-6.

11. Stevenson JS, Kusy RP. Force application and decay characteristics of untreated and treated polyurethane elastomeric chains. Angle Orthod. 1994;64(6):455-64; discussion 465-7.

12. Tonks M, Millett P, Cai W, Wolf D. Analysis of the elastic strain energy driving force for grain boundary migration using phase field simulation. Scr Mater. 2010;63(11):1049-52.

13. Dowling PA, Jones WB, Lagerstrom L, Sandham JA. An investigation into the behavioural characteristics of orthodontic elastomeric modules. Br J Orthod. 1998 Aug;25(3):197-202.

14. Cal E, Sonugelen M, Guneri P, Kesercioglu A, Kose T. Application of a digital technique in evaluating the reliability of shade guides. J Oral Rehabil. 2004 May;31(5):483-91.

15. Dozić A, Kleverlaan CJ, El-Zohairy A, Feilzer AJ, Khashayar G. Performance of five commercially available tooth color-measuring devices. J Prosthodont. 2007 Mar-Apr;16(2):93-100.

16. Jarad FD, Russell MD, Moss BW. The use of digital imaging for colour matching and communication in restorative dentistry. Br Dent J. 2005 July 9;199(1):43-9; discussion 33.

17. Lam TV, Freer TJ, Brockhurst PJ, Podlich HM. Strength decay of orthodontic elastomeric ligatures. J Orthod. 2002 Mar;29(1):37-43.

18. Eliades T, Eliades G, Silikas N, Watts DC. Tensile properties of orthodontic elastomeric chains. Eur J Orthod. 2004 Apr;26(2):157-62.

19. Ash JL, Nikolai RJ. Relaxation of orthodontic elastomeric chains and modules in vitro and in vivo. J Dent Res. 1978 May-June;57(5-6):685-90.

20. Dechkunakorn S, Viriyakosol N, Anuwongnukroh N, Suddhasthira T, Laokijcharoen P, Churnjitapirom P, et al. Residual force of orthodontic elastomeric ligature. Adv Mat Res. 2011;378-379:674-680.

21. Sims AP, Waters NE, Birnie DJ, Pethybridge RJ. A comparison of the forces required to produce tooth movement in vitro using two self-ligating brackets and a pre-adjusted bracket employing two types of ligation. Eur J Orthod. 1993 Oct;15(5):377-85.

22. Petersen A, Rosenstein S, Kim KB, Israel H. Force decay of elastomeric ligatures: influence on unloading force compared to self-ligation. Angle Orthod. 2009 Sept;79(5):934-8.

23. Bortoly TG, Guerrero AP, Rached RN, Tanaka O, Guariza-Filho O, Rosa EA. Sliding resistance with esthetic ligatures: an in-vitro study. Am J Orthod Dentofacial Orthop. 2008 Mar;133(3):340.e1-7.

4

Macroscopic and microscopic evaluation of flapless alveolar perforations on experimental tooth movement

Jose Luis Munoz Pedraza[1], Mariana Marquezan[2], Lincoln Issamu Nojima[3,4], Matilde da Cunha Gonçalves Nojima[3,4]

Objective: The aim of this study was to evaluate a flapless surgical technique as an alternative to traditional alveolar corticotomy used to accelerate orthodontic tooth movement (OTM). **Methods:** To induce OTM in Wistar rats, 40 cN of orthodontic force were applied to the maxillary left first molars. Forty rats were distributed into control groups (CG1, CG3, CG7 and CG14) and experimental groups ($n=5$), in which alveolar perforations were made using a spear-shaped guide bur (EG1, EG3, EG7, EG14). Euthanasia dates were set at 1, 3, 7 and 14 days, respectively, after tooth movement began. The amount of OTM was measured with a caliper, and osteoclasts present in the periodontal ligament of the mesial root of the moved tooth were counted by means of histological evaluation (tartrate-resistant acid phosphatase staining, TRAP). **Results:** Although there was no difference in the amount of OTM within subgroups of corresponding experimental periods ($p>0.05$), when EG14 and CG14 were compared, a larger number of osteoclasts was counted in the experimental group ($p<0.00$). **Conclusion:** The authors concluded that flapless cortical alveolar perforations led to more intense osteoclastic activity on the fourteenth day; nevertheless, no evidence of accelerated OTM could be noted.

Keywords: Tooth movement techniques. Orthodontics. Bone remodeling.

[1] Private practice (Rio de Janeiro/RJ, Brazil).

[2] Universidade Federal de Santa Maria, Departamento de Estomatologia, Disciplina de Ortodontia (Santa Maria/RS, Brazil).

[3] Universidade Federal do Rio de Janeiro, Faculdade de Odontologia, Departamento de Ortodontia e Odontopediatria (Rio de Janeiro/RJ, Brazil).

[4] Case Western Reserve University, Department of Orthodontics (Cleveland, USA).

Matilde da Cunha Gonçalves Nojima
Universidade Federal do Rio de Janeiro, Av. Professor Rodolpho Rocco, 325
Ilha do Fundão, Rio de Janeiro/RJ – CEP: 21.941-617
E-mail: matildenojima@uol.com.br

INTRODUCTION

In some clinical situations, orthodontic tooth movement (OTM) can be a complex task due to the severity of malocclusions, or to diminish the biologic responses commonly seen in periodontally compromised adults and patients with general health problems.[1,2] Therefore there is demand for therapeutic approaches that facilitate OTM whenever a factor involving difficulty is associated, thus reducing the time of active orthodontic treatment. Selective alveolar bone corticotomy before beginning with orthodontic treatment is outstanding among the available alternatives,[3-9] because increased local tissue metabolism in response to surgical trauma can accelerate OTM.[5,10]

According to Köle,[11] alveolar corticotomy is a surgical procedure in which incisions limited to the bone cortex are made. For treating severe dentoskeletal discrepancies, the author suggested a clinical combination of interdental cuts and subapical osteotomies, followed by use of a removable orthodontic appliance. Later, the surgical approach was restricted to alveolar corticotomy in association with orthodontic therapy, shortening treatment duration.[12] Ever since it was first reported, the success of alveolar corticotomy was related to outlining the bone blocks connected by cancellous bone only, thereby offering less resistance to orthodontic forces.[11]

The combination of orthodontic movement with selective alveolar corticotomy was addressed again in 2001.[13] According to the authors, the increased efficiency of orthodontic treatment did not result from facilitated bone block movement, outlined by the corticotomy, but from an increment in bone metabolism. This concept was described as the Regional Acceleratory Phenomenon (RAP).[13] Change in bone physiology would result in a local reduction of trabecular bone density, offering less resistance to moving the desired teeth. It has been demonstrated, in a systematic review, a reduction of the time varying between 28 and 66% for accomplishment of the orthodontic movement.[14]

In spite of the success of accelerated OTM, the aggressive nature of traditional corticotomy resulted in reluctance by both patients and the dental community to proceed with this technique.[15] To overcome the disadvantages of corticotomy, less invasive and flapless techniques were developed, such as corticision[10,16] and micro-osteoperforations.[17] In corticision, a reinforced scalpel is used as a thin chisel to separate the interproximal cortices transmucosally without reflecting a flap.[10,16] In micro-osteoperforations, a disposable device with cutting edge designed for this purpose (Propel Orthodontics, Ossining, NY) can be used.[17] Kits for miniscrew placement often have tips for cortical perforation that could be used as an alternative to this device. The aim of this study was to evaluate the macroscopic and microscopic effects of a flapless cortical alveolar perforation technique, using a spear-shaped guide bur from a miniscrew placement kit, during OTM.

MATERIAL AND METHODS
Experimental model

This *in vivo* study used 40 male Wistar rats (*Rattus norvegicus*), weighing 250-280 g and approximately 90 days old. Animals were kept in a vivarium of the *Universidade Federal do Rio de Janeiro* (UFRJ), under ideal conditions throughout the experiment. The research project had been previously approved by the Ethics Committee for Animal Research at the Health Sciences Center of UFRJ.

Animals were randomly distributed into control (CG) and experimental groups (EG), split into 4 subgroups of 5 animals each, namely CG1, CG3, CG7 and CG14; EG1, EG3, EG7 and EG14, according to the date of euthanasia set at 1, 3, 7 and 14 days, respectively, after tooth movement began. In the experimental subgroup animals, the maxillary left first molar was moved in a mesial direction and flapless perforations were made on the buccal and palatal cortical plates, limited by the adjacent alveolar process. Control group animals were submitted exclusively to orthodontic movement, following the same protocol described for the experimental groups.

Animals were sedated via intraperitoneal injection of 1ml/Kg anesthetic solution, made up of equal parts of 100 mg/ml ketamine hydrochloride and 20 mg/ml xylazine hydrochloride, for placement of the orthodontic device.

A 7-mm NiTi closed coil spring (Dental Morelli Ltda; Sorocaba, São Paulo, Brazil) stretched up to the maxillary incisors (Fig 1) applied a force of 40 cN to the first molar, measured with a tension gauge (Dentaurum, Ispringen, Baden-Württemberg, Germany). The mandibular incisors were trimmed for the purpose of preserving the integrity of orthodontic devices.

Once the devices were placed, two cortical alveolar perforations were made on the buccal plate and another two on the palatal plate of all animals in EG1, EG3, EG7 and EG14. Perforations were made in the attached gingiva of mesial and distal portions of the maxillary left first molar (Fig 1), using a spear-shaped guide bur (FML 70, S.I.N., Sistema de Implante Nacional Ltd., São Paulo, Brazil), attached to a miniscrew manual driver (CDM 02, S.I.N., Sistema de Implante Nacional Ltd., São Paulo, Brasil) (Fig 2). No flaps were raised during this procedure. Perforations of all groups were performed only at baseline.

Quantification of OTM

The amount of OTM was measured with an orthodontic caliper (Odin, Orthopli, Philadelphia, Pennsylvania, USA), positioned from a point marked on the composite covering the maxillary incisors to the cervical portion of the mesial surface of the maxillary left first molar. Distances were measured immediately after placement of the devices and before euthanasia of each animal with an overdose of anesthetic solution composed of ketamine hydrochloride and xylazine hy-drochloride. The amount of OTM was calculated by subtracting the final from initial distances. All measurements were repeated twice by the same examiner, and a mean value was obtained and registered.

Histological analysis

The maxillary bones were dissected and the anatomical blocks were fixed in 4% formaldehyde buffered solution. Bone structures were demineralized using Allkimia® (Campinas, São Paulo, Brazil) and were subsequently embedded in paraffin blocks (Paraplast, Sigma-Aldrich Co, St. Louis, MO, USA). Cross-sections 5-μm thick were obtained from the cervical third of the root, placed on glass slides, deparaffinized, hydrated in water, and then stained. Tartrate-resistant acid phosphatase (TRAP) histochemistry stain (TRAP kit n. 387, Sigma Chemicals, Saint Louis, Missouri, USA) was used to count the number of osteoclasts on the adjacent alveolar bone surface throughout the entire extension of the periodontal ligament of the mesial root of the maxillary left first molar, and to estimate the degree of bone resorption. Cells were considered osteoclasts if they were multinucleated, TRAP positive (red-brownish color), and located on or close to bone surfaces (Fig 3). Counting was done manually under light microscopy (microscope Nikon Eclipse E600, 400x magnification).

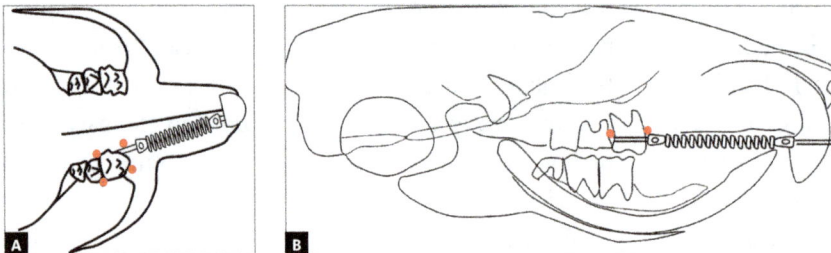

Figure 1 - Schematic drawing of the orthodontic coil spring and perforation points (circles) in occlusal (A) and lateral (B) views.

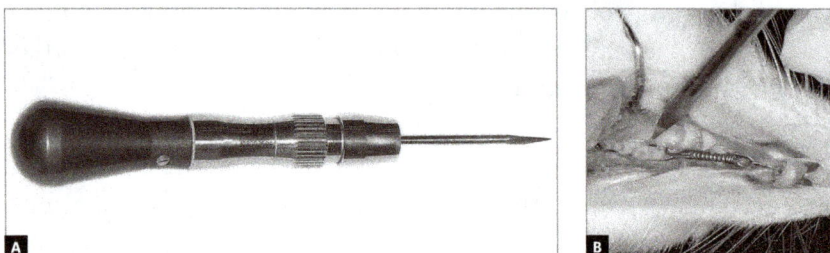

Figure 2 - Spear-shaped guide bur (FML 70) (A) used to perform perforations in attached gingiva (B).

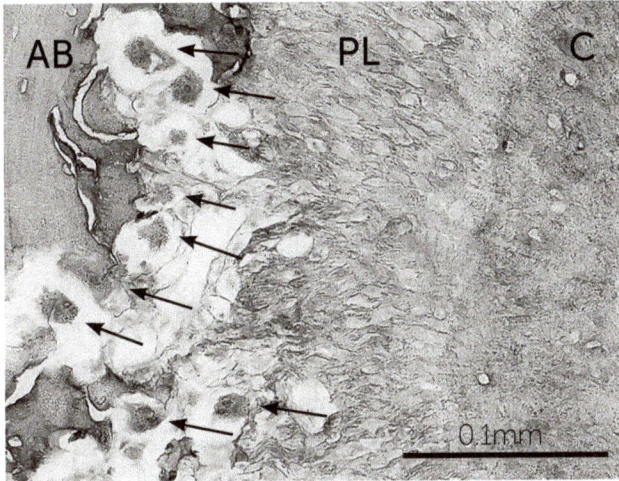

Figure 3 - Micrograph of the mesial root of a first molar and its supporting tissue processed for TRAP histochemistry to identify osteoclast cells (arrows) (400x magnification). AB = alveolar bone; PL = periodontal ligament; C = cementum; bar: 0.1 mm.

Table 1 - Mean and standard deviation (SD) of amount of OTM and number of osteoclasts and results of ANOVA/Tukey tests.

	OTM (mm)	Number of osteoclasts
CG1	0.41 ± 0.10^a	$27.60 \pm 8.20^{a,b}$
CG3	$0.76 \pm 0.05^{a,b,c}$	$37.60 \pm 10.03^{a,b}$
CG7	$0.76 \pm 0.10^{a,b,c}$	$47.80 \pm 17.56^{a,b}$
CG14	1.1 ± 0.30^c	50.60 ± 15.46^b
EG1	$0.67 \pm 0.25^{a,b}$	12.60 ± 3.91^a
EG3	$0.73 \pm 0.28^{a,b}$	62.00 ± 28.15^b
EG7	$0.68 \pm 0.07^{a,b}$	48.40 ± 16.68^b
EG14	$0.78 \pm 0.07^{b,c}$	107.20 ± 24.38^c
	P=0.001	P=0.000

Different letters indicate statistical difference at α=0.05% (ANOVA/Tukey). Each column refers to an independent statistical test.

Statistical analysis

Statistical Package for the Social Science software (version 17, SPSS Inc., Chicago, Illinois, USA) was used for analyzing the results. Reproducibility of the osteoclast count measurements was tested by the Intraclass Correlation Coefficient (ICC = 0.981), and 30% of total sample measurements were repeated after a 15-day interval. Data were submitted to descriptive statistical analysis. Normality and homogeneity of variables were assessed by Shapiro-Wilk and Levene tests, respectively, to a level of significance of 0.05. Since normal and homogenous distribution were verified, the Analysis of Variance (ANOVA) and Tukey multiple comparisons tests were used to evaluate intergroup differences. The level of significance adopted was of 0.05.

RESULTS

The amount of OTM showed no significant differences between control and experimental subgroups after the same periods of activation. In the control group, a difference was detected between the first and fourteenth day of orthodontic movement ($p = 0.001$) (Table 1).

Histological analysis demonstrated a significant difference in the number of osteoclasts between control and experimental subgroups on the fourteenth day after tooth movement began, with increased quantities of osteoclasts in EG14 ($p < 0.000$) (Table 1).

DISCUSSION

OTM is a process of bone remodeling in response to mechanical loading. The velocity of OTM is influenced by bone turnover, bone density, and the degree of hyalinization of the periodontal ligament in response to the forces applied.[10] The elimination of cortical resistance or increased local tissue metabolism might prevent excessive pressure buildup in the periodontal ligament and subsequent hyalinization.[8] In this context, surgical techniques performed in alveolar bone can accelerate OTM by increasing bone turnover and reducing hyalinization in the periodontal ligament.[10]

Ever since Local Alveolar Corticotomy (LAC) was first used by Heinrich Köle[11] (in 1959) to facilitate orthodontic movement, new surgical interventions have been proposed to decrease the considerable risks to the periodontium and maintaining vitality of the associated teeth.[18] The aim was to attain better treatment results in a reduced period of time; therefore, with this focus, less invasive and extensive variations of the original surgical technique have proved effective in achieving more complex tooth movements.[4,19] The association between local alveolar corticotomy and lyophilized bone grafts has been described as a method to shorten conventional orthodontic treatment time,[13,15,20] together with other minimally invasive methods, such as smaller cortical incisions, either associated or not with piezosurgery.

However, these approaches have been described in the literature mainly as case reports.[4,12,16,19,21,22] Thus, the biological responses derived from rapid OTM have not been fully understood. Thus, the aim of this experimental study was to evaluate the amount of OTM and periodontal reactions that resulted from a flapless surgical technique involving cortical alveolar perforation, considered less invasive from a biological standpoint. The experimental periods were chosen with the purpose of contemplating the three phases of orthodontic movement: dental movement within the periodontal ligament (1 to 3 days), lag phase (7 days), and frontal bone resorption (14 days).[23]

The results showed no statistically significant difference in the amount of OTM between the experimental and control subgroups. This result was in agreement with a previous experimental study that evaluated the effect of two distinct magnitudes of force applied with and without corticision on the rate of OTM in rats. Corticision was unable to induce clinical changes after two weeks of OTM, irrespective of the force magnitude.[10] On the other hand, this result disagreed with a previous clinical study using flapless cortical microperforations.[17] The site of perforations must have influenced the result. While we performed four perforations — two on buccal and two on lingual side — all in cervical third of the roots, Alikhani et al[17] performed three perforations along the root length on the buccal surface. The purpose of the choice to perform the perforations on the buccal and lingual surfaces of the bone tissue was to increase bone turnover, based on conventional corticotomy techniques, in which cuts were performed buccally and lingually.[24,25] However, it seemed to be important to perform perforations along the root length to obtain better results.

Specifically on the fourteenth day of OTM (although there was no statistical difference) there was an important numerical difference in the rate of OTM between the control and experimental groups. The control group obtained 0.32 mm more OTM. Studies with larger samples could better clarify this issue.

The TRAP enzyme is an osteoclast marker that can be used to quantify them in different tissues. Changes in bone resorption are usually associated with changes in the osteoclast count, suggesting that TRAP could be a useful marker for bone resorption.[26] Multinucleated TRAP-positive cells adhered or close to bone were considered osteoclasts and therefore counted, throughout the periodontal ligament. The present results showed a gradual progression in the number of osteoclasts in the control subgroups during the experiment. However when analyzing the effect of alveolar perforations, an expressive response with a statistically significant increase in osteoclast counts was verified over two specific time intervals during the experiment, from the first (EG1) and seventh (EG7) days, to the third (EG3) and fourteenth (EG14) days of orthodontic movement. Intergroup analysis also showed evidence of a significant difference in osteoclast counts on the fourteenth day of tooth movement, with higher numbers in the experimental subgroup (EG14) than in control subgroup (CG14), suggesting that the tissue responded favorably to the surgical procedure performed in this study. Previous studies using surgical techniques to accelerate OTM in rats showed little differences in their results. While Wang et al[27] found an increase in osteoclast number on the third day after corticotomy, Murphy et al[10] found no difference in osteoclast number and activity after 14 days of tooth movement in rats, despite of corticision being performed or not. These results must be explained by methodological differences, including differences in surgical techniques.

The strength of the present study lies in accomplishing the evaluation of an innovative technique in research, previously cited only in clinical cases. Research in animals has greatly contributed to knowledge in the field of etiology, prevention and treatment of oral diseases. There are advantages to using animals, such as the possibility of better local control, less genetic diversity when using litters, ease of sample collection, higher number of replications and ease of microscopic analysis.[28] However, some biological differences should be considered between humans and animals, such as the faster metabolism of rats. Therefore, clinical results in our patients could be expected in a longer period of time, compared to those found in experimental studies. Moreover, animal studies are at the bottom of the pyramid of scientific evidence and their findings should be extrapolated into clinical practice with caution.

As science is a cumulative process, this paper significantly improves the knowledge base beyond what is already published on the topic through histological findings. However, further researches with similar methodology as presented in this study and longer observation periods are necessary in order to verify whether the significant difference in osteoclast count found between groups on the fourteenth day of the experiment will continue to evolve and result in a clinically significant difference in amount of OTM. Moreover, the authors suggest that further studies performing perforations along the entire root length should be conducted to verify the histological reactions; in addition, a positive control group should be used, in which traditional corticotomy (the gold standard technique) should be performed.

CONCLUSIONS

It could be concluded that flapless cortical alveolar perforations led to more intense osteoclastic activity on the fourteenth day of tooth movement (verified microscopically); nevertheless, no evidence of accelerated OTM could be noted macroscopically.

Author's contribution (ORCID®)

Jose Luis M. Pedraza (JLMP): 0000-0002-9232-1949®
Mariana Marquezan (MM): 0000-0001-6078-5194®
Lincoln Issamu Nojima (LIN): 0000-0001-8486-9704®
Matilde C. G. N. (MCGN): 0000-0002-8830-939X®

Conception or design of the study: JLMP, MCGN. Data acquisition, analysis or interpretation: JLMP, MM, LIN, MCGN. Writing the article: MM. Critical revision of the article: JLMP, MM, LIN, MCGN. Final approval of the article: JLMP, MM, LIN, MCGN. Obtained funding: JLMP. Overall responsibility: MCGN.

REFERENCES

1. Yamaguchi K, Nanda RS. Blood flow changes in gingival tissues due to the displacement of teeth. Angle Orthod 1992;62(4):257-64.

2. Machado CC, Nojima Mda C, Rodrigues e Silva PM, Mandarim-de-Lacerda CA. Histomorphometric study of the periodontal ligament in the initial period of orthodontic movement in Wistar rats with induced allergic asthma. Am J Orthod Dentofacial Orthop. 2012;142(3):333-8.

3. Anholm JM, Crites DA, Hoff R, Rathbun WE. Corticotomy-facilitated orthodontics. CDA J. 1986;14(12):7-11.

4. Hwang HS, Lee KH. Intrusion of overerupted molars by corticotomy and magnets. Am J Orthod Dentofacial Orthop 2001;120(2):209-16.

5. Bhattacharya P, Bhattacharya H, Anjum A, et al. Assessment of corticotomy facilitated tooth movement and changes in alveolar bone thickness - A CT Scan Study. J Clin Diagn Res. 2014;8(10):ZC26-30.

6. Gkantidis N, Mistakidis I, Kouskoura T, Pandis N. Effectiveness of non-conventional methods for accelerated orthodontic tooth movement: a systematic review and meta-analysis. J Dent. 2014;42(10):1300-19.

7. Hassan AH, Al-Saeed SH, Al-Maghlouth BA, Bahammam MA, Linjawi AI, El-Bialy TH. Corticotomy-assisted orthodontic treatment. A systematic review of the biological basis and clinical effectiveness. Saudi Med J. 2015;36(7):794-801.

8. Hoogeveen EJ, Jansma J, Ren Y. Surgically facilitated orthodontic treatment: a systematic review. Am J Orthod Dentofacial Orthop. 2014 Apr;145(4 Suppl):S51-64.

9. Liem AM, Hoogeveen EJ, Jansma J, Ren Y. Surgically facilitated experimental movement of teeth: systematic review. Br J Oral Maxillofac Surg. 2015 July;53(6):491-506.

10. Murphy CA, Chandhoke T, Kalajzic Z, Flynn R, Utreja A, Wadhwa S, et al. Effect of corticision and different force magnitudes on orthodontic tooth movement in a rat model. Am J Orthod Dentofacial Orthop. 2014 July;146(1):55-66.

11. Kole H. Surgical operations on the alveolar ridge to correct occlusal abnormalities. Oral Surg Oral Med Oral Pathol. 1959;12(5):515-29 concl.

12. Generson RM, Porter JM, Zell A, Stratigos GT. Combined surgical and orthodontic management of anterior open bite using corticotomy. J Oral Surg. 1978;36(3):216-9.

13. Wilcko WM, Wilcko T, Bouquot JE, Ferguson DJ. Rapid orthodontics with alveolar reshaping: two case reports of decrowding. Int J Periodontics Restorative Dent. 2001;21(1):9-19.

14. Hoogeveen EJ, Jansma J, Ren Y. Surgically facilitated orthodontic treatment: a systematic review. Am J Orthod Dentofacial Orthop. 2014;145(4 Suppl):S51-64.

15. Cassetta M, Pandolfi S, Giansanti M. Minimally invasive corticotomy in orthodontics: a new technique using a CAD/CAM surgical template. Int J Oral Maxillofac Surg. 2015;44(7):830-3.

16. Kim SJ, Park YG, Kang SG. Effects of Corticision on paradental remodeling in orthodontic tooth movement. Angle Orthod. 2009;79(2):284-91.

17. Alikhani M, Raptis M, Zoldan B, Sangsuwon C, Lee YB, Alyami B, et al. Effect of micro-osteoperforations on the rate of tooth movement. Am J Orthod Dentofacial Orthop 2013;144(5):639-48.

18. Bell WH, Levy BM. Revascularization and bone healing after maxillary corticotomies. J Oral Surg. 1972;30(9):640-8.

19. Chung KR, Oh MY, Ko SJ. Corticotomy-assisted orthodontics. J Clin Orthod. 2001;35(5):331-9.

20. Wilcko WM, Ferguson DJ, Bouquot JE, Wilcko MT. Rapid orthodontic decrowding with alveolar augmentation: case report. World J Orthod. 2003;4(3):197-205.

21. Germec D, Giray B, Kocadereli I, Enacar A. Lower incisor retraction with a modified corticotomy. Angle Orthod. 2006;76(5):882-90.

22. Sebaoun JD, Surmenian J, Dibart S. [Accelerated orthodontic treatment with piezocision: a mini-invasive alternative to conventional corticotomies]. Orthod Fr. 2011;82(4):311-9.

23. Reitan K. Tissue behavior during orthodontic tooth movement. Am J Orthod Dentofacial Orthop. 1960;46(12):881-900.

24. Shoreibah EA, Salama AE, Attia MS, Abu-Seida SM. Corticotomy-facilitated orthodontics in adults using a further modified technique. J Int Acad Periodontol. 2012;14(4):97-104.

25. Wilcko MT, Wilcko WM, Pulver JJ, Bissada NF, Bouquot JE. Accelerated osteogenic orthodontics technique: a 1-stage surgically facilitated rapid orthodontic technique with alveolar augmentation. J Oral Maxillofac Surg. 2009;67(10):2149-59.

26. Halleen JM, Tiitinen SL, Ylipahkala H, Fagerlund KM, Vaananen HK. Tartrate-resistant acid phosphatase 5b (TRACP 5b) as a marker of bone resorption. Clin Lab. 2006;52(9-10):499-509.

27. Wang L, Lee W, Lei DL, Liu YP, Yamashita DD, Yen SL. Tisssue responses in corticotomy- and osteotomy-assisted tooth movements in rats: histology and immunostaining. Am J Orthod Dentofacial Orthop. 2009 Dec;136(6):770.e1-11; discussion 770-1.

28. Valladares Neto JV, Souza JB. Ética em Pesquisa. In: Estrela C, editor. Metodologia Científica. São Paulo: Artes Médicas; 2001. Cap. 16, p. 257.

5

Occlusal assessment in surgically assisted unilateral cleft lip and palate patients

Leanne Matias Portela Leal[1], Marcus Vinicius Neiva Nunes do Rego[2], Cosme José Albergaria da Silva Filho[3], Leopoldino Capelozza Filho[4], Mauricio de Almeida Cardoso[5]

Objective: The aim of this study was to assess the magnitude of occlusal changes in individuals with unilateral cleft lip and palate (CLP). The study was conducted on study casts of 25 subjects, 14 men and 11 women aged from 7 to 20 years, without previous orthodontic treatment and with surgical repair carried out at São Marcos Hospital, Teresina, Piauí State, Brazil. **Methods:** The casts were assessed by three orthodontists based on the occlusal scores established by Atack et al., whose scores range from 1 to 5, according to the magnitude of transverse and sagittal changes. **Results:** Intra and inter-observer reproducibility of occlusal scores was satisfactory and statistically significant according to the Spearman Correlation test with significance level set at 5%. With regard to the distribution of occlusal scores, 30.67% of the subjects achieved scores 1 and 2, 22% score 3 and 47.53% achieved scores 4 and 5. **Conclusions:** Four was the score most frequently assigned by the observers, disclosing a high degree of transverse and sagittal disorders in the occlusion of patients.

Keywords: Growth. Malocclusion. Cleft lip.

[1] Masters student in Orthodontics, Sacred Heart University (USC).

[2] Professor of Orthodontics at the Graduate and Postgraduate programs, UNINOVAFAPI. Professor of Orthodontics at the Postgraduate program, Federal University of Piauí (UFPI).

[3] Graduated in Dentistry, UNINOVAFAPI.

[4] PhD in Orthodontics, College of Dentistry — Bauru/USP. Professor of Orthodontics at the Graduate and Postgraduate (specialization and Masters courses) programs, USC.

[5] PhD in Orthodontics, State University of São Paulo (UNESP). Professor of Orthodontics at the Graduate and Postgraduate (specialization and Masters courses) programs, USC.

» The authors report no commercial, proprietary or financial interest in the products or companies described in this article.

Mauricio de Almeida Cardoso
Rua Arnaldo de Jesus Carvalho Munhoz, 6-100 – Bauru/SP, Brazil
CEP: 17018-520 – E-mail: maucardoso@uol.com.br

INTRODUCTION

Individuals with cleft lip and palate exhibit functional and morphological changes and may, in some cases, manifest psychosocial changes given that the affected region is highly visible, causing a negative esthetic impact. As for their morphological diversity, lip and palate clefts yield different levels of severity and consequences, requiring not only changes in treatment protocol, but also an interdisciplinary team composed of an orthodontist, pediatrician, plastic surgeon, speech pathologist, psychologist, geneticist and social worker, to promote adequate esthetic and functional rehabilitation as well as seamless social and psychological integration to patients.[6]

In Brazil, clefts are currently classified on the basis of a system proposed by Spina,[18] which uses the incisive foramen, the only single structure connecting the primary and secondary palates during intrauterine life, as anatomical reference. These palates ultimately formed the midface. Thus, this classification defines clefts based on length, in line with their embryonic origin.[17] According to this classification, clefts are divided into four different groups: Group I = Pre-foramen clefts; Group II = Trans-foramen incisor clefts; Group III = Post-foramen incisor clefts; and Group IV = Rare facial clefts.[14]

Some treatments should be provided as soon as patients with this anomaly are born in order to improve the quality of life of these individuals. Soon after the third month of life, the lip should be reconstructed (cheiloplasty) and in the twelfth month, the palate should be reconstructed (palatoplasty). These surgeries are called primary surgeries as they are aimed at restoring the anatomic integrity left unfinished in intrauterine life. If necessary, secondary surgeries are performed to close the fistulas, as well as pharyngoplasty while finishing touches are applied to the primary surgeries.

The craniofacial growth of individuals with unilateral cleft lip and palate (CLP) should be constantly monitored due to the adverse effects of primary surgeries on the anteroposterior and transverse growth of the maxilla. Some changes in the occlusion are frequently found, especially anterior crossbite and posterior crossbite.[12]

The impact of primary plastic surgery on the midface growth makes it important to study the magnitude of occlusal changes undergone by patients with unilateral cleft lip and palate (CLP) subjected to surgery at São Marcos Hospital in Teresina, Piauí State (PI), Brazil, an institution recognized by the Ministry of Health as a reference center in the Northeastern region of Brazil.

MATERIAL AND METHODS
Sample characterization

The NOVAFAPI Institutional Review Board (CEP/NOVAFAPI) reviewed this research project and found that it met the provisions of resolution No. 196/96, issued by the National Council of Health (CNS/MS). Therefore, the project was authorized and filed under number 0430-08.

The sample comprised 25 individuals aged from 7 to 20 years old, with unilateral CLP, subjected to primary plastic surgery at the São Marcos Hospital in the city of Teresina, Piauí State, Brazil. Out of 25 patients who participated in this study, 14 (56%) were men while 11 (44%) women. Patients' age range was 14 years and 3 months (Table 1). According to the number of primary plastic surgeries and the time when they were performed, the first lip repair was carried out by means of the Millard's technique, on average, when the patient was 7 months old; whereas

Table 1 - Mean, median and standard deviation of ages (in years) of patients with unilateral CLP who underwent surgery at São Marcos Hospital. Data displayed according to sex.

Sex	Mean ± standard deviation	Median
Feminine	14.24 ± 5.97	14.00
Masculine	14.23 ± 3.55	15.00
TOTAL	14.25 ± 5.30	15.00

Table 2 - Distribution of the 25 patients with unilateral CLP who underwent surgery at São Marcos Hospital. Data displayed according to the number of surgeries and the time when the first plastic surgeries were performed (in months).

Surgery	Mean ± standard deviation	Median
Number of procedures		
cheiloplasty	1.29 ± 0.62	1.00
palatoplasty	1.29 ± 0.62	1.00
Age (months)		
1st cheiloplasty	7.63 ± 8.24	3.00
1st palatoplasty	30.17 ± 31.29	20.00

palatoplasty was performed at 30 months of age, using a modified version of Von Langenback's technique (Table 2).

The following inclusion criteria were applied: Plastic surgeries performed at São Marcos Hospital; cheiloplasty (lip surgery) before 2 years of age; palatoplasty (surgery of the palate) before 3 years of age; no prior orthopedic treatment performed to achieve expansion and/or reverse traction of the maxilla; no syndrome in the craniofacial region; no alveolar bone graft in the cleft area.

Assessment of occlusal characteristics in the study casts

The occlusal characteristics of the 25 patients with unilateral CLP were evaluated on study casts (Fig 1) by 3 examiners (orthodontists and professors at the NOVA-FARI Specialization Course in Orthodontics) using the occlusal index proposed by Atack et al.[2] (Table 3).

The casts were carefully arranged in ascending order on a bench concealing the patients' personal identification data. This evaluation was performed individually with no communication between examiners, who were previously calibrated for application of the occlusal index, while changing the numbering on the casts in both assessments to prevent memorization.

In order to verify method reliability, all casts were reassessed 15 days after the first evaluation.[8]

Statistical analysis
Method reliability

Evaluation results were exported to a database created with SPSS software, version 13.0. Inter-examiner correlation was determined in both assessments

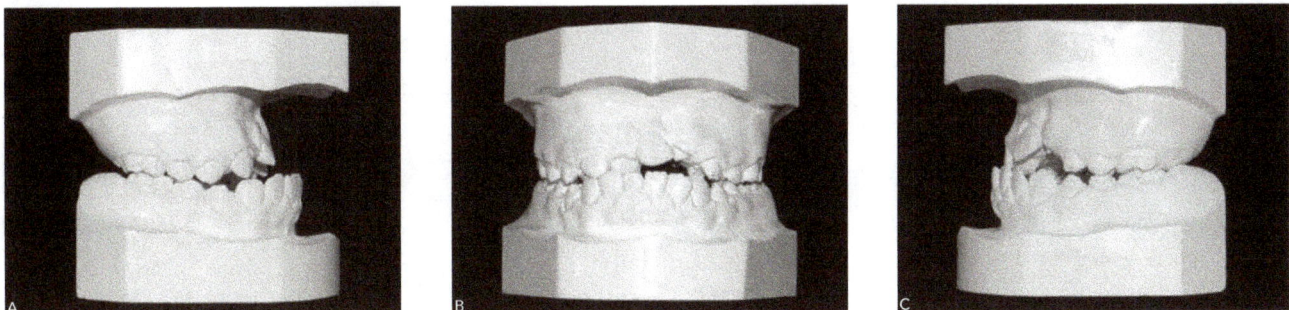

Figure 1 - Study casts of an individual from the sample used in this study, showing unilateral CLP. A) Right lateral view. B) Frontal view. C) Left lateral view.

Table 3 - Evaluation index of the occlusal characteristics using casts (inter-arch relationship) in individuals with unilateral CLP.[3]

Group	Occlusal characteristics	Long-term outcome prognosis
1	– Positive overjet with normal inclination or lingual inclination of the incisors; – Absence of crossbite and open bite; – Satisfactory morphology of the upper dental arch	Excellent
2	– Positive overjet with normal inclination or labial inclination of the incisors; – Unilateral crossbite / tending towards crossbite; – Tendency towards open bite adjacent to the cleft	Good
3	– End-on relationship with normal inclination or labial inclination of the incisors, or negative overjet with incisors inclined lingually; – Tendency towards open bite adjacent to the cleft	Regular
4	– Negative overjet with normal inclination or labial inclination of the incisors; – Tendency towards unilateral/bilateral crossbite; – Tendency towards open bite adjacent to the cleft	Bad
5	– Negative overjet with labial incisor inclination – Bilateral crossbite; – Substantially changed upper jaw morphology	Very bad

(initial and after 15 days), as well as intraexaminer correlation with the purpose of verifying method reliability using Spearman's correlation test with a significance level set at 5% (p < 0.05).

To define the degree of agreement, the scale proposed by Altman[2] was applied to the values shown in Table 4. Only "good" and "very good" scores were considered satisfactory.

RESULTS

Intra and inter-observer agreement in determining the occlusal index

Table 5 depicts a correlation between the first and second scores assigned to each observer (p), and shows whether the degree of agreement is acceptable. A statistically significant correlation (R) was found for all examiners.

As regards inter-observer correlation, the degree of agreement ranged between "good" and "very good" (Table 6). The good repeatability accomplished in the test was expected because all examiners were orthodontists and the index designed by Atack et al.[3] proved to be easy to apply.

Magnitude of occlusal changes exhibited by the patients with CLP

The results showed that 30.67% of patients were included in indices 1 and 2, 22% in index 3, and 47.33% were included in indices 4 and 5 (Fig 2).

Table 4 - Relevance of the level of agreement as described by Altman.[2]

Value	Level of agreement (LA)
≤ 0.2	Poor
0.21 to 0.40	Regular
0.41 to 0.60	Mild
0.61 to 0.80	Good
0.81 to 1.00	Very good

Table 5 - Intraobserver agreement in determining the occlusal index in the 25 patients with unilateral CLP who underwent surgery at São Marcos Hospital. Teresina, Piauí State, Brazil.

Examiner	Correlation		
	P	R	LA
Orthodontist 1	0.000*	0.896	VG
Orthodontist 2	0.000*	0.627	G
Orthodontist 3	0.000*	0.917	VG

Spearman correlation. N = 25, *significant at p < 0.05.
Captions for Level of Agreement: P - Poor, M - Mild, R - Regular, G - Good, VG - Very good.

P column= correlation between the first and second score assigned to each observer. R column = correlation for all examiners.

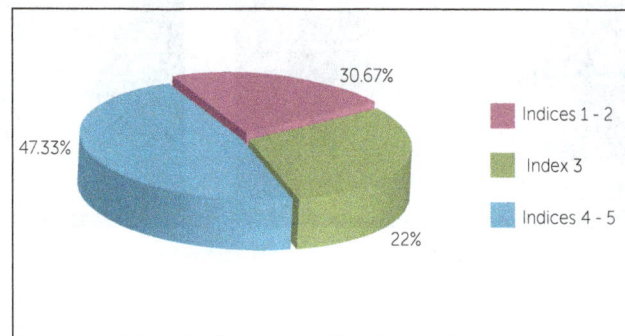

Figure 2 - Distribution of occlusal indices in the 25 patients with unilateral CLP who underwent surgery at São Marcos Hospital.

Table 6 - Inter-observer agreement in the first and second evaluations in determining the occlusal index in the 25 patients with unilateral CLP who underwent surgery at São Marcos Hospital.

Examiner 1st Evaluation	Orthodontist 1			Orthodontist 2			Orthodontist 3		
	p	R	LA	p	R	LA	p	R	LA
Orthodontist 1	-	-	-	0.000*	0.667	G	0.000*	0.785	G
Orthodontist 2	0.000*	0.667	G	-	-	-	0.000*	0.809	VG
Ortodontist 3	0.000*	0.785	G	0.000*	0.809	VG	-	-	-
Examiner 2nd Evaluation	**Orthodontist 1**			**Orthodontist 2**			**Orthodontist 3**		
	p	R	LA	p	R	LA	p	R	LA
Orthodontist 1	-	-	-	0.000*	0.700	G	0.000*	0.892	VG
Orthodontist 2	0.000*	0.700	G	-	-	-	0.000*	0.651	G
Orthodontist 3	0.000*	0.892	VG	0.000*	0.651	G	-	-	-

Spearman correlation. N = 25, *significant at p < 0.05. LA (Level of Agreement): P - Poor, M - Mild, R - Regular, BG- Good, VG - Very good.
P column= correlation between the first and second score assigned to each observer. R column = correlation for all examiners.

DISCUSSION

Lip and palate clefts are a congenital defect with diverse clinical manifestations. Its involvement can range from a small notch in the lip vermilion or mucosa of the uvula to a complete breakdown of the maxilla. In summary, from an embryonic point of view, clefts can affect the primary and secondary palate with different levels of severity. Given their higher prevalence, this study aimed at assessing the behavior of post-surgical complete unilateral clefts involving the primary and secondary palate, also known as unilateral cleft lip and palate (CLPs). Corroborating the literature,[3] this study also showed a higher prevalence of unilateral CLP in males.

According to surveys conducted at the Hospital for Rehabilitation of Craniofacial Anomalies (HRAC-USP), these clefts account for approximately 33% of occurrences.[16] Among unilateral CLPs, there are numerous variables that influence their anatomical configuration and differentiate one patient from another, such as cleft width, the presence of Simonart's band and degree of nose asymmetry. Simonart's band is formed by a bridge of soft tissue that joins the mesial and distal edges of a complete lip and palate cleft, which can positively affect the morphology of postoperative upper dental arches when the band is bulky.[11]

Primary plastic surgery reconstructs lesions in the lip and palate and in so doing influences the behavior of the nasomaxillary complex, of which expression of genetic growth potential is restricted. The more numerous the morphological variables inherent in clefts are, the greater will be the number of therapeutic variables that may influence the patient's face and occlusion in the long-term. Among these variables, one could mention the amount of time required to complete surgery, surgical techniques, number of repetitive surgeries as well as the extra-surgical care provided pre- and postoperatively. Undoubtedly, the surgeon's skill in manipulating young tissue plays a key role in ultimately shaping the face.[11,13,14]

The current surgical protocol adopted at São Marcos Hospital recommends the performance of lip repair at 6 months of postnatal life and palatoplasty at 18 months. However, the protocol used at the Hospital for Rehabilitation of Craniofacial Anomalies (HRAC-USP) recommends that such procedures be carried out at 3 and 12 months of postnatal life, respectively.[11]

Choosing a straightforward occlusal index is of paramount importance since it interferes in method reliability and in determining the number of examiners. The results of this study agree with those of Okada,[11] who also found the occlusal index of Atack et al.[3] to be straightforward and easy to apply, since there was no statistically significant intraobserver differences, even when different groups of examiners were used, such as oral maxillofacial surgeons, plastic surgeons and orthodontists. Therefore, the ease with which the occlusal assessment method was applied precluded the need for a greater number of examiners.

The quality of a given rehabilitation protocol used by a reference center in treating patients with cleft lip and palate can be measured by the magnitude of occlusal changes that occur, especially in patients with CLP, since sequelae inherent to the morphology of the clefts as a result of the surgical repair procedure, involve significant changes in the transverse and anteroposterior growth of the maxilla. Results showed that cases considered "very bad" (indices 4 and 5) accounted for almost half of the sample, confirming the negative effect of primary plastic surgery in the growth of midface structures, for which there seems to be consensus in the literature.[1,5,7,9-12]

On assessing the magnitude of occlusal alterations observed in patients rehabilitated at São Marcos Hospital (Teresina, Piauí State), this magnitude was found to be close to results achieved by reference centers both in Brazil and abroad - such as the Hospital for Rehabilitation of Craniofacial Anomalies, Bauru, São Paulo State, and the Rehabilitation Center of Oslo, Norway. The indices found in this study were compared to those obtained by Okada,[11] which were assessed by the Bauru and Oslo centers. For indices 1 and 2, the data showed a percentage of 30.67% in Teresina, 34% in Bauru and 60% in Oslo. As for index 3, the percentage was 22% in Teresina, 27.72% in Bauru and 22% in Oslo. For indices 4 and 5 (which represent the major occlusal sequelae and comprise the cases requiring orthognathic surgery) the percentages were 47.33% in Teresina, 38.20% in Bauru and 18% in Oslo. Thus, it can be asserted that the Oslo Center results were higher than those of the Brazilian centers, especially when comparing the percentage of cases with greater occlusal sequelae.

With regard to the average occlusal index based on all scores assigned by examiners in both assessments, there was an index of 3.28 in Teresina, 3.07 in Bauru and 2.52 in the Oslo Center. In examining the median scores assigned by examiners in the present study, index 4 proved to be the most frequent, indicating a high degree of transverse and anteroposterior changes in the occlusion of the patients.

How can one explain Oslo's higher results in terms of occlusion conditions? Many variables certainly play a role in the diversity of the outcomes, but according to Shaw et al.[13] one major factor is the standardization of the protocol and the surgical techniques adopted, along with a small number of surgeons, with surgeries being performed by virtually one single surgeon.

When the results obtained in Teresina were compared to those of Bauru, a higher percentage of cases with greater occlusal sequelae were found in Teresina. However, age is yet another key factor to be taken into account when interpreting these results. The vast majority of patients in this study were at the permanent dentition stage, whereas those assessed by Okada[11] in Bauru were at the early mixed dentition stage. Given that plastic surgery cumulatively affects the growth of the midface, patients at the stage of occlusal maturity tend to produce more sequelae in transverse and anteroposterior maxillary growth

compared to younger patients. It is worth noting that variables such as the anatomical extent of the cleft, the presence of Simonart's band, surgical procedure variables such as the surgical technique, surgeon skills and pre and postoperative care were not assessed.

The findings of this study confirmed the assumption that the maxillomandibular relationship of a patient with cleft lip and palate undergoes — starting from the stage of embryo formation — the strains imposed by the cleft and the resulting functional deviations. Furthermore, maxillomandibular relationship is potentially undermined by reconstructive surgeries (lip repair and palatoplasty), which hinder maxillary growth to varying degrees, resulting in changes in craniofacial growth and deficiencies in the intra and inter-arch relationships.

CONCLUSIONS

» With regard to the magnitude of occlusal changes, it was found that 30.67% of the subjects exhibited indices 1 and 2, 22% index 3 and 47.53% exhibited indices 4 and 5.

» On examining the scores assigned by examiners, occlusal index 4 proved to be the most frequent, indicating a high degree of transverse and anteroposterior changes in the occlusion of the patients.

REFERENCES

1. Aiello CA, Silva Filho OG, Freitas JAS. Fissuras labiopalatais: uma visão contemporânea do processo reabilitador. In: Mugayar LRF, colaboradores. Pacientes portadores de necessidades especiais. Manual de odontologia e saúde bucal. São Paulo: Pancast, 2000. p. 111-39.

2. Altman DG. Practical statistics for medical research. p. 403-409. London: Chapman & Hall; 1991.

3. Atack N, Hathorn IS, Semb G, Dowell T, Sandy JR. A new index for assessing surgical outcome in unilateral cleft lip and palate subjects aged five: reproducibility and validity. Cleft Palate Craniofac J. 1997;34(3):242-6.

4. Capelozza Filho L, Cavassan AO, Silva Filho OG. Avaliação do crescimento craniofacial em portadores de fissuras transforame incisivo unilateral. Estudo transversal. Rev Bras Cirur. 1987;77(2):97-106.

5. Cavassan AO, Silva Filho OG. Abordagem ortodôntica. In: Trindade IEK, Silva Filho OG. Fissuras labiopalatinas: uma abordagem interdisciplinar. São Paulo: Ed. Santos; 2007. cap. 4, p. 213-38.

6. Correia JP, Carvalho LRR, Rego MVNN. Fissuras labiais. In: Carreirão S. Cirurgia plástica. São Paulo: Atheneu; 2005. p. 220-30.

7. Faraj JORA, André M. Alterações dimensionais transversas do arco dentário com fissuras labiopalatinas, no estágio de dentadura decídua. Rev Dental Press Ortod Ortop Facial. 2007;12(5):100-8.

8. Gravely JF, Benzies PM. The clinical significance of tracing error in cephalometry. Br J Orthod. 1974;1(3):95-101.

9. Houston WJ. The analysis of errors in orthodontic measurements. Am J Orthod. 1983;83(5):382-90.

10. Mazzottini R. Variações nas dimensões do arco dentário superior em fissurados unilaterais, em função da época do tratamento cirúrgico [tese]. Bauru (SP): Universidade de São Paulo; 1985.

11. Okada TO. Avaliação dos efeitos da queiloplastia e palatoplastia primária sobre o crescimento dos arcos dentários de crianças com fissura transforame incisivo unilateral dos 5-6 anos de idade [tese]. Araraquara (SP): Universidade Estadual Paulista; 2001; 205 p.

12. Ribeiro AA, Leal L, Thuin R. Análise morfológica dos fissurados de lábio e palato do centro de tratamento de anomalias craniofaciais do Estado do Rio de Janeiro. Rev Dental Press Ortod Ortop Facial. 2007;12(5):109-18.

13. Mars M, Asher-McDade C, Battström V, Dahl E, McWilliam J, Molsted K, et al. A six-centre international study of treatment outcome in patients with clefts of the lip and palate: Part 3. Dental arch relationships. Cleft Palate Craniofac J. 1992;29:405-408.

14. Silva Filho OG. Crescimento facial. In: Trindade IEK, Silva Filho OG. Fissuras labiopalatinas: uma abordagem interdisciplinar. São Paulo: Ed. Santos; 2007. p. 173-98.

15. Silva Filho OG, Freitas JAS. Caracterização morfológica e origem embrionária. In: Trindade IEK, Silva Filho OG. Fissuras labopalatinas: uma abordagem interdisciplinar. São Paulo: Ed. Santos; 2007. p. 17-49.

16. Silva Filho OG, Freitas JAS, Okada T. Fissuras labiopalatais: diagnóstico e uma filosofia interdisciplinar de tratamento. In: Pinto VG. Saúde bucal coletiva. 4ª ed. São Paulo: Ed. Santos; 2000. p. 481-527.

17. Silva Filho OG, Ferrari Júnior FM, Rocha DL, Freitas JAS. Classificação das fissuras labiopalatais: breve histórico, considerações clínicas e sugestão de modificação. Rev Bras Cir. 1992;82(2):59-65.

18. Spina V, Psillakis JM, Lapa FS, Ferreira MC. Classificação das fissuras lábio-palatinas: sugestão de modificação. Rev Hosp Clin Fac Méd. 1972;27(1):5-6.

6

Protein biomarkers of external root resorption: A new protein extraction protocol - Are we going in the right direction?

Giovanni Modesto Vieira[1]

Objective: The aim of this study is to determine a protocol of gingival crevicular fluid protein extraction used for the first dimension of 2-DE gels. It also aims at conducting a review on the current candidates for protein markers of this pathology, all of which may be used to prevent the disease. **Methods:** Gingival crevicular fluid was collected from two groups of 60 patients each, with and without external root resorption. Samples were extracted by means of various methods of protein extraction. SDS-PAGE gels were used to assess the quality of the method which was subsequently tested during isoelectric focusing of 2-DE gels taken from samples of patients with and without the disease. **Results:** Milli-Q ultrapure ice cold water, without precipitation for gingival crevicular fluid protein extraction, proved the method with greatest sharpness to detect protein bands. Additionally, it allowed two-dimensional electrophoresis to be performed. **Conclusion:** The new protein extraction protocol does not interfere in isoeletric focusing of 2-DE gels. Furthermore, it provides the greatest sharpness in detecting protein bands of SDS-PAGE gels. This will allow mapping and searching of new external root resorption markers, particularly due to the difficulty in carrying out molecular tests with the current candidates for protein markers.

Keywords: Root resorption. Molecular diagnosis technique. Gingival crevicular fluid. Electrophoresis. Isoelectric focusing.

[1] PhD resident in Medical Sciences, University of Brasília (UnB).

Giovanni Modesto Vieira
STN Conj. O – Centro Clínico Life Center – Sala 21 – Plano Piloto – Asa Norte
Brasília/DF – Brazil — E-mail: giovanni.modesto.vieira@gmail.com

» The author reports no commercial, proprietary or financial interest in the products or companies described in this article.

INTRODUCTION

The high prevalence of inflammatory external root resorption (IERR) associated with orthodontic treatment (95 to 100%)[1] poses the need to integrate basic research, supported by scientific evidence, with daily clinical practice in order to minimize the biological costs (IERR) of orthodontic treatment itself.

The expression of gingival crevicular fluid markers (GCF) is mainly used in Dentistry to estimate the immune response of the host to periodontal disease.[2] The potential use of GCF markers proves a non-invasive technique employed to clinically track the activity of osteoclasts, bone remodeling and external root resorption occurring during orthodontic treatment.[2]

Evans et al[3] demonstrated the presence of gingival crevicular fluid proteins, particularly the dentin matrix protein (DMP-1), in patients undergoing orthodontic treatment. Since then, the study of these proteins has significantly deepened, and research correlating their presence with root resorption has markedly increased.[3]

Because they are part of the dental tissue, more specifically the dentin, these proteins are not routinely released into periodontal ligament spaces, unless active external root resorption is present.[4]

The search for IERR markers was intensified by the discovery of dentin-specific proteins (dentin phosphoprotein-DPP and dentin sialoprotein-DSP) which appeared as by-products of root resorption in the gingival crevicular fluid. They were analyzed by enzyme-linked immunosorbent assays (ELISA) by James Mah[5] (DPP), and subsequently confirmed (DPP and DSP) by Laura Balducci et al[4] by means of one-dimensional electrophoresis (SDS-PAGE), Western blot and ELISA; and Shalene et al[6] (DSP) also by Western blot and ELISA.[4,5,6]

In all these researches, protein extraction was performed through sodium phosphate buffer, which hinders visualization of protein bands in SDS-PAGE gel and its later use in proteomic techniques of higher resolution (two-dimensional electrophoresis-2DE) to precisely identify the proteins contained in the samples.

The present article aims at reporting the use of a new method of GCF protein extraction, which provides better visualization of samples and does not interfere in the isoelectric focusing of 2DE gels, as in the classical extraction technique. This new protocol will enable accurate mapping of proteins related to IERR. The present study also discusses whether the current candidates for dentin protein markers reported in the literature can actually be used as molecular diagnostic kits for the prevention of IERR sequelae in patients undergoing orthodontic treatment.

MATERIAL AND METHODS:

Sampling

The sample comprised 60 patients (22 men and 38 women) aged between 15 and 30 years old who did not have systemic disease, periodontal disease, gingivitis or tooth decay. In addition, they did not take any systemic medication. Patients were divided into two groups: Group 1 (control) comprising 30 patients who had been undergoing orthodontic treatment for at least six months without IERR being revealed by periapical radiographs; and Group 2 comprising 30 patients who had been undergoing orthodontic treatment for at least six months with mild to moderate IERR, according to the classification by Levander and Malmgren, as shown in radiographic examination[7] (Fig 1).

Gingival fluid collection

Sterile absorbent paper cones were used according to the method proposed by Burke et al[8] and Bang et al.[9]

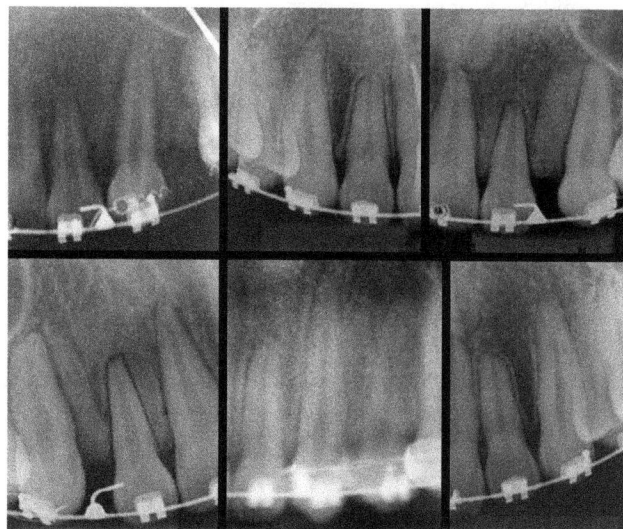

Figure 1 - Periapical radiograph of patients comprising the mild to moderate IERR group.

Protein extraction

Protein extraction was performed without protein precipitation. The cones containing gingival fluid samples from both groups (Fig 2) were collected to form a pool of proteins from each group. A total of 100 µl of ultrapure ice cold water (Milli-Q RG, Millipore) and protease inhibitor (PMSF-phenyl methyl sulfonyl fluoride) were added to every pair of absorbent paper cones which were then centrifuged twice at 13.400 rpm for 5 minutes. The process was repeated and the supernatant with eluted proteins was lyophilized and stored for subsequent electrophoretic analysis.

Protein quantification was carried out by the 2-DE Quant kit (Amersham biosciences-GE Healthcare), following the manufacturer's instructions (Fig 3). The major advantage of this technique lies in the application of copper ions which bind to the main protein chain. It differs from conventional protein quantification techniques that do not use this ion and bind to arginine and hydrophobic radicals that may be in accessory chains of protein amino acids. Therefore, the new technique is more reliable and of greater accuracy.

One-dimensional gel electrophoresis: SDS-PAGE

Analysis of the composition of gingival crevicular fluid proteins in patients with IERR was performed by denaturant electrophoresis in 12% polyacrylamide SDS-PAGE gel at room temperature (Fig 4) and as described by Kojima et al.[10] Invitrogen (Bench Marcker, Protein Ladder) protein markers were used. Subsequently, the gel was stained with Coomassie G-250 brilliant blue.

Isoelectric focusing

The first dimension was performed at 15°C, in Ettan IPGphor 3 (GE Healthcare) appliance, following the manufacturer's instructions (GE Healthcare) and under the following conditions: 500 V for one hour, 1000 V for two hours, 1000 V gradient at 8000 V up to one hour and forty minutes, 8000 V for five hours, totaling 50,000 V/H with upper limit of electric current of 50 mA and potential of 5 W totaling nine hours and 40 minutes. After isoelectric focusing, the strips were stored at -80 °C until the second dimension was carried out.

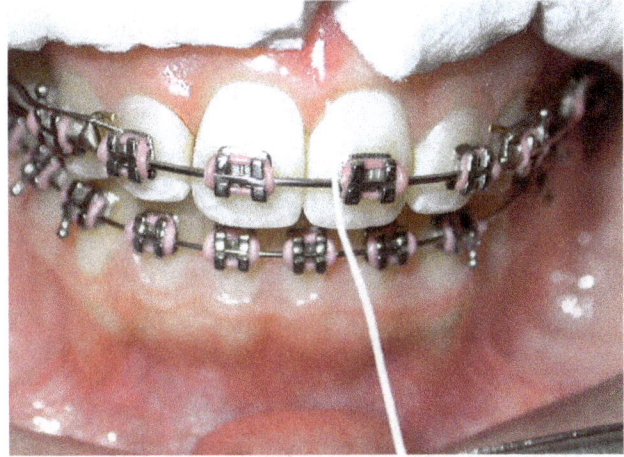

Figure 2 - Patient subjected to prophylaxis followed by relative isolation with cotton rolls and the use of ejector. GCF sample collection with absorbent paper cones.

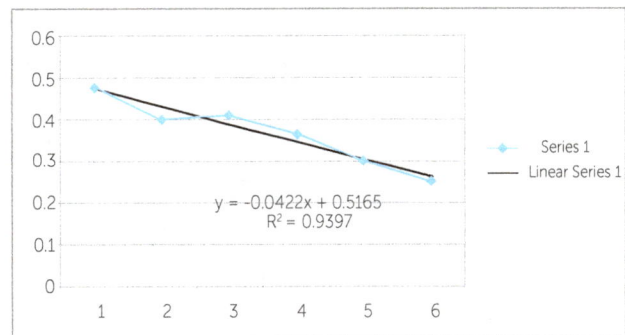

$$y = -0.0422x + 0.5165$$
$$R^2 = 0.9397$$

Figure 3 - 2-DE Quant kit curve depicting 12µg/µl and 8 µg/µl of proteins for samples with and without IERR.

RESULTS

The gel performing protein extraction by means of sodium phosphate buffer solution (Fig 5) showed traces of salt and did not achieve the first dimension of isoelectric focusing (Fig 6) in the two-dimensional electrophoresis.

Several classic methods of protein extraction were used, namely: ammonium acetate precipitation with and without dialysis, as well as precipitation by trichloroacetic acid and acetone (TCA acetone). However, in either one of the methods (Fig 7), the resolution of protein bands was satisfactory in terms of sharpness and amount of bands. Additionally, they interfered in isoelectric focusing (during the first dimension) (Fig 6).

Protein extraction without precipitation, but by means of Milli-Q ultrapure ice cold water, was the only protein extraction method that did not interfere

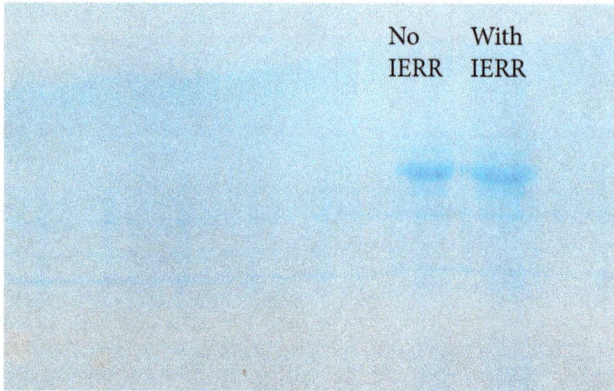

Figure 4 - 12% SDS-PAGE gel for the GCF of patients with and without IERR obtained by means of the new extraction method.

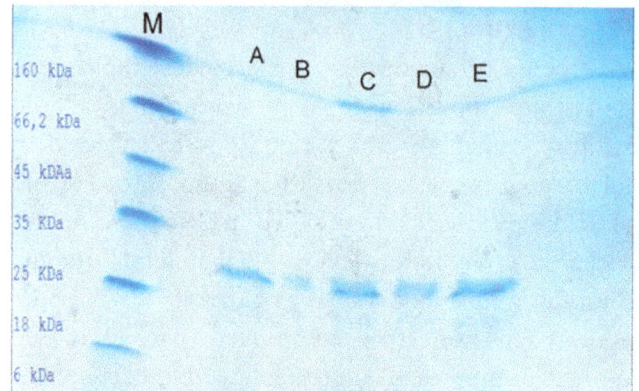

Figure 5 - One-dimensional 12% SDS-PAGE gel. Protein extraction by means of sodium phosphate buffer solution stained with Coomassie G-250 blue. M: Molecular marker; A,C,E: mild to moderate external root resorption groups; B,D: groups without external root resorption. Note the traces of salt. 16 µg of samples were applied to each pool of gel.

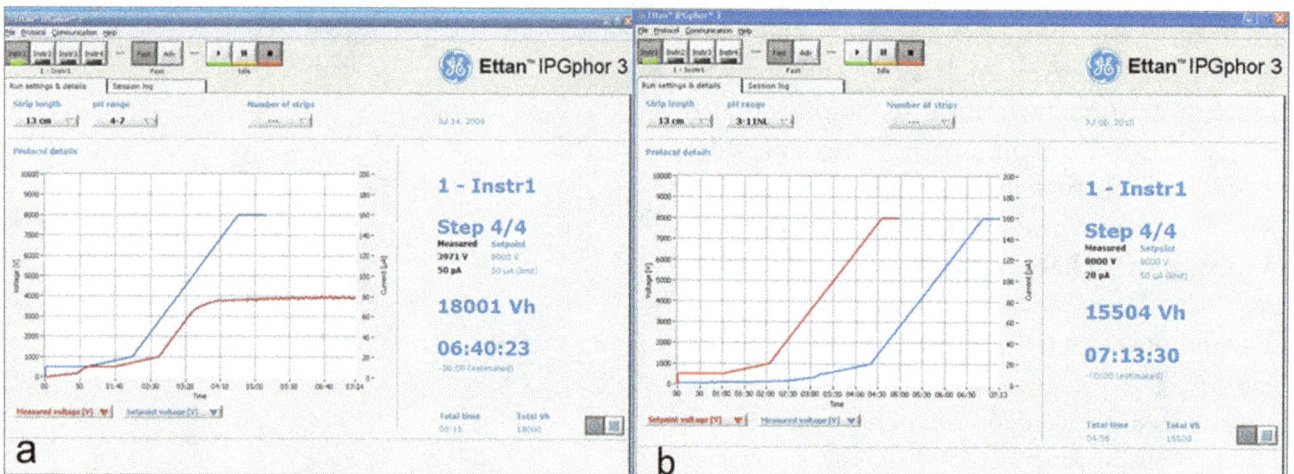

Figure 6 - A) Electrophoretic patterns of gel with phosphate buffer; difficulty in carrying out the first dimension due to traces of salt which affected isoelectric focusing. B) Electrophoretic profile with three strips: one control and two strips embedded into two different samples wherein isoelectric focusing carried out by means of the new protein extraction method proved successful.

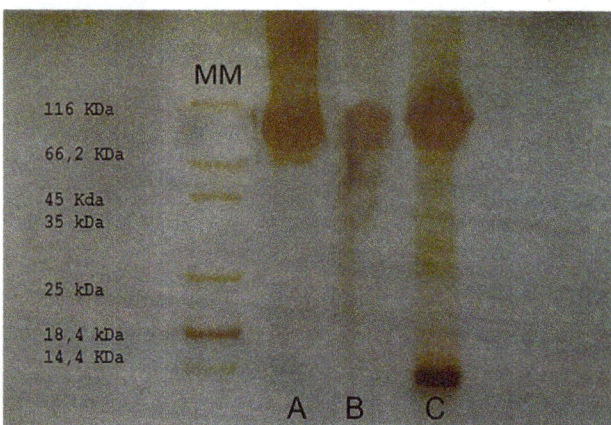

Figure 7 - 12% SDS-PAGE one-dimensional gel stained with silver nitrate. GCF proteins of different protein precipitation methods. MM, molecular marker; A, IERR sample precipitated with ammonium acetate/dialysis/lyophilization; B, sample without IERR precipitated with ammonium acetate/dialysis/lyophilization; C, sample without IERR precipitated with TCA/acetone, 50 µl of the lyophilized sample was applied to each pool.

in isoelectric focusing during the first dimension of 2-DE gels (Fig 6). Moreover, this method presented better resolution in terms of size and quantity of protein bands, which differs from other techniques.

DISCUSSION

According to Wellington Rody,[2] the dental procedure used to collect samples of GCF consists in removing subgingival plaque (prophylaxis) with a plastic scraper without touching the gingiva, followed by careful drying of the gingiva for 10 seconds with compressed air (syringe) and relative isolation of saliva with cotton rolls. Subsequently, the strips are inserted into the gingival sulcus of teeth for 30 to 60 seconds. The strips are labelled and taken to Eppendorf tubes with phosphate saline buffer, and immediately sent to a laboratory where they are agitated for 15 seconds at room temperature, and centrifuged for 5 minutes at 3.000 g so as to eliminate bacterial biofilm and cellular elements. The supernatant is then stored at -80 °C for further analysis as a biomarker.[11]

This protein extraction method was used by all authors who have studied external root resorption through SDS-PAGE gel; however, the presence of salt in the sample solution (even if dialyzed) hinders isoelectric focusing in the first dimension, when two-dimensional electrophoresis is used. This hampers analysis of electrophoretic and protein profile of the sample (Fig 6).

The presence of contaminants, even after constant washing and dialysis of several methods of protein extraction, probably prevented proper focusing of samples during the first dimension phase. Even with the use of the new method for protein extraction (Milli-Q ultrapure ice cold water), focusing was only possible with increased IPG-Buffer (ampholyte) which is usually used at 0.5%. The use of 2% IPG-Buffer is required to increase conductivity of electrical current during the focusing process, thereby increasing voltage and allowing it to take place normally (Fig 6).

During orthodontic movement, the cementum is reabsorbed and subsequently repaired. Moreover, the products of cementum degradation in the GCF were detected by most researches in both control and treatment groups. Thus, cementum proteins may not be indicative of permanent loss of root structure, which somehow disqualifies them as IERR markers.[5,12,13]

Although small areas of dentin resorption have been proved to undergo repair, larger apical areas do not undergo repair, thereby rendering dentin loss significant in root structure loss.[5]

Laura Balducci et al[4] identified and quantified dentin extracellular matrix proteins: dentin matrix protein 1 (DMP1), dentin phosphoprotein (DPP) and dentin sialoprotein (DSP) in gingival crevicular fluid of individuals undergoing orthodontic treatment.

DMP-1, a non-collagen protein found in dentin and bone mineral matrix, was found in large amounts in the gingival crevicular fluid during the process of resorption. This can be attributed to the presence of this protein which is removed from bone and dentin during IERR. By means of SDS-PAGE gel,

Balducci et al[4] proved that the total concentration of protein in the IERR group was greater than that of the control group, particularly due to degradation of protein matrix during IERR.

In Western Blot analysis, the size of bands was equal in both groups, but more intense for the IERR group.[4] In the enzyme-linked immunosorbent assay (ELISA), the distribution of values occurred with normal concentrations (DMP-1, DPP, DSP) within all groups; however, the DMP-1 antibody showed high concentrations in the IERR group in comparison to the control group, which did not occur among groups with mild to moderate and severe IERR.[4]

Although there is statistically significant difference between the control and the study group (IERR), DMP-1 is not specific to the dentin and its presence is not only due to the IERR process, but also due to increased bone remodeling during orthodontic movement.[12] DMP-1 is not a good root resorption marker, since it does not allow us to distinguish between normal and pathological activity.[4]

Balducci et al[4] also studied DPP and DSP proteins, and found larger concentrations of DPP and DSP in the severe IERR group, followed by the mild IERR group and the control group. However, the authors used polyclonal antibodies that react to proteins with similar epitopes (antigenic recognition sites), and may indicate the presence of small amounts of DPP and DSP in the control group.[14] Even so, the authors suggest that since concentrations found in severe and mild to moderate IERR were statistically different, including in comparison with the control group, DPP and DSP might be considered as molecular markers for early detection and dynamic monitoring of IERR.[4]

Mah and Neelanjani[5] related IERR-treated groups and control groups by means of enzyme-linked immunosorbent assay (ELISA), and also found small amounts of DPP in the control group. The authors suggested that this may be due to the high sensitivity of the ELISA method, even if the antibody used for this purpose was developed with DPP of rats — counterparts of human beings. Finding human antibodies for DPP is a challenge due to protein folding and extensive post-translational changes that affect the molecule which, in turn, is shielded by many phosphate and carbohydrate groups.[5] These phosphate groups are commonly found in other proteins and are not particularly antigenic, thereby hindering the production of human antibodies against DPP.

In addition, the experimental group used by the authors comprised individuals aged between 12 and 16 years old. That is the period when the apex of maxillary incisors is formed (rizogenesis), with odontoblasts and odontoclasts working similarly to osteoblasts and osteoclasts, thereby forming, reabsorbing, remodeling and maintaining dentin.[5] Dentin remodeling has not yet been proved; however, some researches have demonstrated that dentin tissue is not homogeneous and protein components change with age and root maturation.[15]

Shalene et al[6] also found DSP in the control group, but by means of Western Blot. They believed DSP was related to complex structural and cell changes happening within the periodontium, which involved the front of mineralization when root maturation takes shape. They also cited that the basal turnover of dentin matrix proteins occurs during the process of root structuring from deciduous to adult dentition, and that DSP may have been released from the pulp cells when the apex of teeth were still open.[6,16]

Nevertheless, a research conducted by Quin et al[17] may explain the presence of these proteins (DSP, DPP) in the control group of all aforementioned researches. DSP and DPP were transcribed in a single RNA messenger, a transcript derived from a large precursor protein known as DSPP, traditionally considered to be specific to the dentin. The authors found that the DSPP gene was also expressed in osteoblastic cells. DSP was detected in the extracts of long bones of rats in the ratio of 1: 400 in relation to the dentin.[17] By means of polymerase chain reaction of reverse transcriptase and primers specific to the 5' DSP portion and the 3' DPP sequence, DSPP mRNA was detected in osteoblastic-like cells and osteoblasts of rat calvarium, even if this gene was expressed in a much lower level in dentin osteoblasts than odontoblasts.[6,16]

This may indicate that different regulatory mechanisms control the expression of DSPP and are involved in bone tissue and dentin.[6]

The literature does not reach a consensus regarding DPP and DSP proteins as molecular markers due to the presence of these proteins in control groups (even if in small quantities). Evidence shows that these proteins are not unique to the dentin, but are also expressed in bone tissue. Moreover, they might be present in gingival crevicular fluid due to the physiological process of bone remodeling, which is typically increased in patients undergoing orthodontic treatment, and not due to root resorption.[4,5,6,14,17]

In addition, some studies suggest that dentin remodeling does occur. Furthermore, they also suggest that the dentin is not a homogeneous tissue and its protein components change with age and root maturation even if significant dentin repair does not occur, thereby leading to significant dentin loss.[5,15] Thus, it is possible that these alleged proteins be present in gingival crevicular fluid in the absence of disease or not be present in GCF due to tissue aging process.

Some authors believe in the use of these proteins as molecular markers. According to them, logical argumentation is based on the characteristics of the immune system which does not recognize the global structure of proteins, but discrete sites known as epitopes. Large molecules with more than 10 kDa feature a greater number of epitopes capable of potentially increasing the existence of receptors for some of these determinants in lymphocyte cells.[18] Antigen molecular complexity also increases antigenicity (for instance, with an aromatic ring possessing above three amino acids) which enables DSP (55 kDa) and DPP (140 kDa) dentin proteins of high mass and molecular complexity to be considered as good candidates for antigenic determinants.[18]

The higher the phylogenetic distance between the receiver and the antigen, the greater the antigenicity. Although it does not occur in recognition of dentin (DSP and DPP) by lymphocytes, because both are human, they have sizes and molecular complexity conducive to good immune recognition, including DPP with its extensive post-translational changes that interfere in antigenicity.[19] The largest post-translational change in DPP is in the phosphate groups which are essential for dental biomineralization.[20,21]

It is known that inorganic substances never activate lymphocytes, and dentin is covered with hydroxyapatite, totaling 50% of its total weight. Suppa et al[22] compared the antigenicity of secondary dentin (affected by caries) and normal dentin by means of highly specific monoclonal antibodies. They floated the possibility of protein epitopes being masked by mineral apatite in the region of hyper-mineralized peritubular secondary dentin.[22] In fact, they found decreased antigenicity, and later found this to be due to denaturation of protein components, thereby disabling identification by the antibody used in the research, with high specificity to intact molecule.[22]

Perhaps, differential mineralization among different individuals and in certain dentin areas is responsible for the extensive variations in IERR presented in the literature, which hinders the presentation of these antigens to the immune system, as it does not recognize the global structure of proteins, but discrete sites known as epitopes.[18] In this case, the spatial conformation of DPP protein, a post-translational feature, could not only manifest as a sub-clinical deficiency, since differences in detectable situations occur at clinical level, but also cause antigenicity to vary among individuals.

Thus, we could establish risk groups for IERR based on post-translational variations of DPP if the latter was correlated with haplotypes for DPP, since these haplotypes exist in large quantities for this protein[23] and are seen in the normal population as single silent nucleotide polymorphisms (SNPs). In other words, extensive variations in SNPs for DDP and its alleged post-translational modifications could be correlated. There could also exist some correlation with the degree of IERR, whether affecting or not dentin biomineralization at the molecular level, but not to the clinical one.

In 2007, Kimchi-Sarfaty et al[24] found SNPs which do not alter the genetic code, but change the function of the protein in which they occur This was reported in the gene of multidrug resistance — and the change of its product: P-glycoprotein (P-gp), which results in changes in the inhibition to drugs.

This was explained by conformational changes, with the hypothesis that SNPs alter the time of cotranslational protein folding and P-gp insertion within the membrane, thereby altering the structure of the substrate and the sites of inhibition.

In an insight about the subject, Komar[25] reported that despite the fact that the codon was degenerated, meaning that many amino acids are represented by more than a triple nucleotide (and these codons are synonymous with respect to translational process), these SNPs are considered silent. This changes the composition of the constituent amino acids of the protein they refer to, and there is no discernible effect on the function of the gene or on the phenotype, there is a change in mRNA translation kinetics in ribosomes, which leads to changes in the final protein structure ("folding") and, therefore, in its function.[25] The author concludes that SNPs mufflers can contribute to the development and progress of certain diseases.[25]

CONCLUSION

To date, molecular diagnostic kits for detection of IERR at the clinical level have not yet been developed. No consensus has been reached on the use of these dentin proteins as IERR markers. Further high-resolution protein research methods searching for new molecular markers are still necessary. Two-dimensional electrophoresis followed by mass spectrometry (MALDI-TOF) is the technique of choice for this task.

This new protein extraction technique opens up the possibility to use two-dimensional electrophoresis, since the traditional extraction method used by several authors does not allow isoelectric focusing, necessary for 2-DE gels, to be carried out.

REFERENCES

1. Massler M, Malone AJ. Root resorption in human permanent teeth. Am J Orthod. 1954;40(8):619-33.

2. Wellington Rody J Jr. Gingival crevicular fluid (GCF): Is it the link between clinical Orthodontics and biological research? American association of Orthodontists: info. 2009.

3. Evans CA, Srinivasan R, George A. Detection of dentin proteins in human gingival crevicular fluid. In: Davidovitch Z, Mah J, editors. Biological mechanisms of tooth movement and craniofacial adaptation. Concord: Harvard Society for the Advancement of Orthodontics; 2000. p. 201-5.

4. Balducci L, Ramachandran A, Hao J, Narayanan K, Evans C, George A. Biological markers for evaluation of root resorption. Arch Oral Biol. 2007;52(3):203-8.

5. Mah J, Prasad N. Dentine phosphoprotein in gingival crevicular fluid during root resorption. Eur J Orthod. 2004;26(1):25-30.

6. Kereshanan S, Stephenson P, Waddington R. Identification of dentine sialoprotein in gingival crevicular fluid during physiological root resorption and orthodontic tooth movement. Eur J Orthod. 2008;30(3):307-14.

7. Levander E, Bajka R, Malmgren O. Early radiographic diagnosis of apical root resorption during orthodontic treatment: a study of maxillary incisors. Eur J Orthod. 1998;16:223-8.

8. Burke JC, Evans CA, Crosby TR, Mednieks MI. Expression of secretory proteins in oral fluid after orthodontic tooth movement. Am J Orthod Dentofacial Orthop. 2002;121(3):310-5.

9. Bang SJ, Cimasoni G. Total protein in human crevicular fluid. J Dent Res. 1971;50(6):1683.

10. Kojima T, Andersenl E, Sanchez JC, Wilkins MR, Hochstrasser DF, Pralong WF, et al. Human gingival crevicular fluid contains MRP8 (S1 0A8) and MRP14 (S100A9), Two Calcium-binding Proteins of the S100 Family. J Dent Res. 2000;79(2):740-7.

11. Schierano G, Pejrone G, Brusco P, Trombetta A, Martinasso G, Preti G, et al. TNF-alpha TGF-beta-2 and IL-1beta levels in gingival and perimplant crevicular fluid before and after de novo plaque accumulation. J Clin Periodontol. 2008;35(6):532-8.

12. Liu YC, Evans CA, Narayanan AS, George A. Immunodetection of dentin and cementum proteins in crevicular fluid. J Dent Res. 2000;79:613. Abstract.

13. Owmann-Moll P. Orthodontic tooth movement and root resorption with special reference to force magnitude and duration: a clinical and histological investigation in adolescents. Swed Dent J Suppl. 1995;105:1-45.

14. Wehrbein H, Fuhrmann R, Diedrich PR. Human histological tissue response after long-term orthodontic tooth movement. Am J Orthod Dentofacial Orthop. 1995;107(4):360-71.

15. Clarkson BH, Chang SRH. Phosphoprotein analysis of sequential extracts of human dentin and determination of the subsequent remineralization potential of these dentin matrices. Caries Res. 1998;32(5)357-64.

16. Chang SR, Chiego JRD, Claerkson BH. Characterization and identification of a human dentin phosphophoryn. Calcif Tissue Inst. 1996;59(3):149-53.

17. Qin C, Brunn JC, Jones J, George A, Ramachandran A, Gorski JP. The expression of dentin sialophosphoprotein gene in bone. J Dent Res. 2002;81:392-4.

18. Hidalgo MM. Estudo sobre o potencial imunogênico da dentina [tese]. Bauru (SP): Universidade de São Paulo; 2001.

19. Yasuo Yamakoshi, Jan C.C.Hu, Takanori Iwata, Kazuyuki Kobayashi, Makoto Fukae, P.Simmer James. Dentin Sialophosphoprotein is processed by MMP-2 and MMP-20 in vitro and in vivo. J Biol Chem. 2006;281(50):38235-43.

20. He G, Ramachandran A, Dahl T, George S, Schultz D, Cookson D, Phosphorylation of phosphophoryn is crucial for its function as a mediator of biomineralization. J Biol Chem. 2005;280(39):33109-14.

21. Qin C, Baba O, Butler WT. Post-translational modifications of sibling proteins and their roles in osteogenesis and dentinogenesis. Crit Rev Oral Biol Med. 2004;15(3):126-36.

22. Suppa P, Ruggeri A Jr, Tay FR, Prati C, Biasotto M, Falconi M, et al. Reduced antigenicity of type I collagen and proteoglycans in sclerotic dentin. J Dent Res. 2006;85(2):133-7.

23. Song YL, Wang CN, Fan MW, Su B, Bian Z. Dentin phosphoprotein frameshift mutations in hereditary dentin disorders and their variation patterns in normal human population. J Med Genet. 2008;45(7):457-64.

24. Kimchi-Sarfaty C, Oh JM, Kim IW. A "Silent" Polymorphism in the MDR1 Gene changes substrate specificity. Science. 2007;315(5811):525-8. Epub 2006 Dec 21.

25. Komar AA. SNPs, silent but not invisible. Science. 2007;315(5811):466-7.

7

Peri-implant evaluation of osseointegrated implants subjected to orthodontic forces: Results after three years of functional loading

Bruna de Rezende Marins[1], Suy Ellen Pramiu[2], Mauro Carlos Agner Busato[3], Luiz Carlos Marchi[3], Adriane Yaeko Togashi[4]

Objective: The objective of this study was to clinically and radiographically assess the peri-implant conditions of implants used as orthodontic anchorage. **Methods:** Two groups were studied: 1) a test group in which osseointegrated implants were used as orthodontic anchorage, with the application of 200-cN force; and 2) a control group in which implants were not subjected to orthodontic force, but supported a screw-retained prosthesis. Clinical evaluations were performed three, six and nine months after prosthesis installation and 1- and 3-year follow-up examinations. Intraoral periapical radiographs were obtained 30 days after surgical implant placement, at the time of prosthesis installation, and one, two and three years thereafter. The results were compared by Kruskal-Wallis test. **Results:** There was no statistically significant difference in clinical probing depth ($p = 0.1078$) or mesial and distal crestal bone resorption ($p = 0.1832$) during the study period. After three years of follow-up, the mean probing depth was 2.21 mm for the control group and 2.39 mm for the test group. The implants of the control group showed a mean distance between the bone crest and implant shoulder of 2.39 mm, whereas the implants used as orthodontic anchorage showed a mean distance of 2.58 mm at the distal site. **Conclusion:** Results suggest that the use of stable intraoral orthodontic anchorage did not compromise the health of peri-implant tissues or the longevity of the implant.

Keywords: Bones. Dental implants. Orthodontic appliances. Osseointegration.

[1] Graduate student in Oral and Maxillofacial Surgery, Universidade Estadual do Oeste do Paraná (UNIOESTE), School of Dentistry, Cascavel, Paraná, Brazil.

[2] Undergraduate student, Universidade Estadual do Oeste do Paraná (UNIOESTE), School of Dentistry, Cascavel, Paraná, Brazil.

[3] Professor, Universidade Estadual do Oeste do Paraná (UNIOESTE), Department of Orthodontics, School of Dentistry, Cascavel, Paraná, Brazil.

[4] Professor of Periodontology and Oral Implantology, Universidade Estadual do Oeste do Paraná (UNIOESTE), Department of Implantology, School of Dentistry, Cascavel, Paraná, Brazil.

» The authors report no commercial, proprietary or financial interest in the products or companies described in this article.

Adriane Yaeko Togashi
Rua Universitária, 2069 – Jd. Universitário, Cascavel/PR – Brasil
CEP: 85.814-110 – E-mail: adriane.togashi@unioeste.br

INTRODUCTION

Osseointegrated titanium implants were initially used as abutment for prosthetic reconstruction in fully edentulous patients in order to increase masticatory function.[1,2,3] The implants were later used extensively to replace missing teeth in partially edentulous patients, allowing for preservation of the remaining dental structures.[1,4,5,6] Other indications have been proposed for osseointegrated implants, such as orthodontic or maxillofacial anchorage,[7-11] since decayed or missing teeth can impair orthodontic treatment due to absence of appropriate dental anchorage for orthodontic movement.

The advantage of osseointegrated implants for orthodontic anchorage is the absolute immobility of the implant, as the periodontal ligament is inexistent, allowing for the application of controlled orthodontic forces without bone resorption. This phenomenon is known as "absolute anchorage."[12] Thus, the implant will first function as intraoral orthodontic anchorage and later as prosthetic anchorage, providing stability, biocompatibility and comfort.[13]

Since several studies have demonstrated that anchorage of orthodontic forces on implants seems to be a good alternative in partially edentulous patients who require orthodontic treatment,[7,14-18] the present study proposed to assess the long-term peri-implant behavior of implants subjected to orthodontic anchorage. Thus, the objective of this study was to clinically and radiographically assess implants used as orthodontic anchorage, as well as the success rate of such implants over a period of three years after the installation of prostheses over them.

MATERIAL AND METHODS
Patient selection and study design

A prospective clinical study using titanium implants as orthodontic anchorage was conducted. The patients were recruited from the Undergraduate and Postgraduate clinics of the Department of Dental Implantology, School of Dentistry, Universidade Estadual do Oeste do Paraná (UNIOESTE), Brazil. The study was approved by the Ethics Committee of the same university (Process 301/2008-CEP) and were asked to sign a free informed consent form after receiving detailed information about the study.

After patient selection according to inclusion and exclusion criteria, the sample was randomly divided into two groups: 1) test group in which osseointegrated implants were used as orthodontic anchorage (n = 26 implants);

and 2) control group in which the implants were only used as support for prostheses (n = 24 implants).

Criteria for inclusion in the study were: 18 years of age or older (mean patient age was 41 years, with a range of 35 to 56 years old); willingness to cooperate with the requirements of the study; no systemic health condition; good oral hygiene; good periodontal health; sufficient alveolar bone volume at the implant recipient site (width: ≥ 6 mm and height: ≥ 8 mm) exclusively for the study group; and type I-III bone quality. Exclusion criteria were: pregnancy or breast-feeding; smoking and use of alcohol or drugs; previous reconstruction at the implant recipient site; insufficient alveolar bone volume at the implant recipient site (width: < 6 and height: < 8 mm); presence of residual roots at the recipient site; type IV bone quality; keratinized mucosa < 2 mm at the implant recipient site; stomatological and periodontal diseases; and clinical signs of temporomandibular dysfunction and bruxism.

The implants were installed according to the number of missing teeth and bone availability in the posterior region of the mandible, which required prosthetic rehabilitation and dental movements.

Surgical procedures

Titanium implants were placed under local anesthesia by a dental surgeon and within a single intervention. The surgical procedure consisted of an incision in the alveolar ridge crest for preservation of the keratinized mucosa. Subsequently, lingual and buccal mucoperiosteal flaps were carefully elevated from the top of the alveolar crest. The implants were placed supracrestally, according to the protocol of the system, and primary stability was always achieved. The mucoperiosteal flaps were repositioned for healing by first intention. After one week, the sutures were removed and postoperative control was performed. The patient was advised to properly clean the treated area.

The surgical phase of implant installation consisted of the use of self-tapping external hexagon titanium implants (Dentoflex Comércio e Indústria de Materiais Odontológicos, São Paulo, Brazil), installed according to Branemark's surgical protocol.[19] Implants with a diameter of 3.75 or 4.0 mm and 8, 10 and 11.5 mm in length were used according to bone availability.

Patients were advised to avoid any trauma to the implant sites and to rinse the mouth with 0.12% chlorhexidine digluconate for at least one minute, twice a day, for one week.

Clinical sequence

Four months after implant placement, the period corresponding to osseointegration, reopening and placement of healing abutments were performed. Subsequently, the implant was transferred and the crowns were screwed in place with a torque of 45 Nm. Molds of each patient were taken and each case was planned by an implantodontist and two orthodontists participating in the study.

Occlusion of the provisional acrylic resin screw-retained restorations was established with contact in maximum intercuspation and no contact in excursive movements. In the test group, provisional screw-retained restorations received the following orthodontic accessories: TMA wire cantilever (0.018x0.025-in, Morelli, Sorocaba, Brazil) and NiTi spring (0.25 mm diameter – Morelli, Sorocaba, Brazil). The maximum force applied to the implants was 200 cN. Orthodontic force was used in order to correct minor dental movements, such as molar uprighting and incisor relationship, and to improve the occlusal relationship with the objective of obtaining prosthetic space for implant placement. Orthodontic treatment period varied between 9 and 12 months. At the end of orthodontic treatment, provisional restorations were replaced with definitive prostheses.

Clinical evaluation

Clinical evaluations were performed three, six and nine months after prosthesis installation. The 1- and 3-year follow-up examinations included the following parameters: 1) modified plaque index (mPlI)[20] for all implants; 2) modified bleeding index (mBlI)[20] for all implants; 3) pocket probing depth (PPD): distance between the gingival margin and pocket depth in millimeters;[21,22] and 4) keratinized mucosa width (KMW): distance between the keratinized gingival-mucosa junction and the free gingival margin in millimeters for implants. All measurements were performed at six aspects of each implant site by means of a Hu-Friedy PCP-UNC probe (Hu-Friedy, Chicago, IL, USA) .

Radiographic evaluation

Intraoral periapical radiographs were obtained before implant placement and 30 days after surgery for implant placement at the time of prosthesis installation and one, two and three years thereafter (Fig 1). The paralleling technique was used. Radiographs were taken with the aid of a digital radiographic sensor (Kavo-Kerr), an individual acrylic positioning device, and an exposure time of 0.4 seconds. For the evaluation of changes in peri-implant crestal

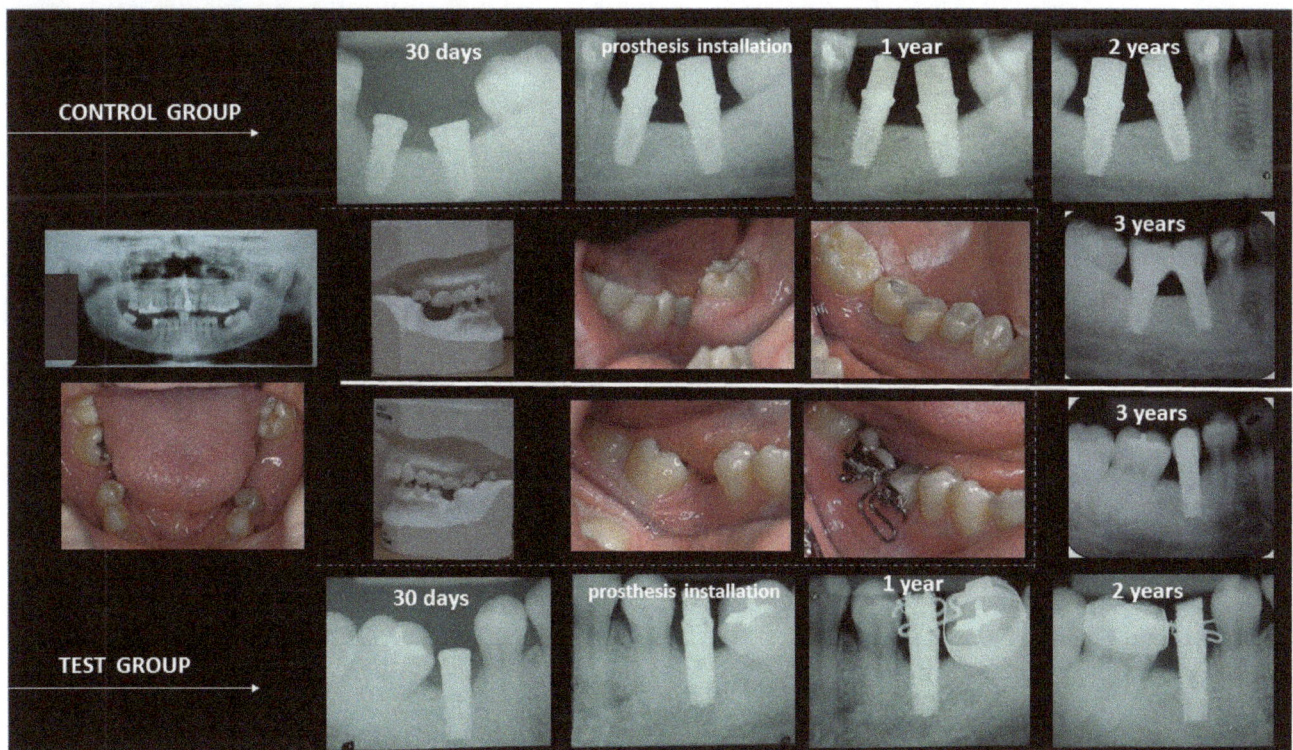

Figure 1 - Intraoral periapical radiographs of the control and test groups before implant placement, 30 days after implant installation, at the time of prosthesis installation, and one, two and three years thereafter.

bone height, a single examiner measured the linear distance (in mm) from the implant shoulder to the most coronary part of the mesial and distal bone crest,[23] using the Image Tool analysis program (UTHSCSA, Texas, USA).

Crestal bone measurements were made on the periapical radiographs obtained for the 8-mm, 10-mm and 11.5-mm implants. The length of the implant represents the reference to compensate for radiographic distortion. Subsequently, crestal bone measurements were obtained on the mesial and distal side for all implants at the pre-established intervals.[24]

Follow-up and maintenance

Periodic visits were held for maintenance and reinforcement of oral hygiene instructions at 3-month intervals during the first year after prosthesis installation, and at 6-month intervals during the subsequent two years.

Clinical parameters were evaluated at three, six and nine months and one and three years after prosthesis installation. Radiographic analysis was performed 30 days after surgery for implant placement at the time of prosthesis installation and one, two and three years thereafter.

Success criteria established for the present study followed those of Karoussis et al;[21] i.e., absence of mobility, absence of subjective complaints (pain, foreign body sensation, and/or paresthesia), no probing depth of 5 mm or more and positive modified sulcus bleeding index (mSBl), absence of continuous radiolucency around the implant, and an annual vertical bone loss not exceeding 0.2 mm after the first year since installation.

The results of the clinical parameters as well as bone crestal distance mesially and distally were compared by

Kruskal-Wallis test. A p-value < 0.05 was considered to indicate statistical significance, and all calculations were performed by means of GraphPad InStat and GraphPad Prisma 5 software (GraphPad Software Inc, USA).

RESULTS

Clinical, radiographic and peri-implant parameters showed that the biological response of gingival tissue and bone structure surrounding the implant subjected to orthodontic anchorage was similar to control. Peri-implant health was maintained for approximately one year of anchorage on the implant and over a period of three years of follow-up.

The mean bone crest/shoulder distance of the implant during a period of 30 days after implant installation, at the time of prosthesis installation, and one, two and three years thereafter revealed similar bone

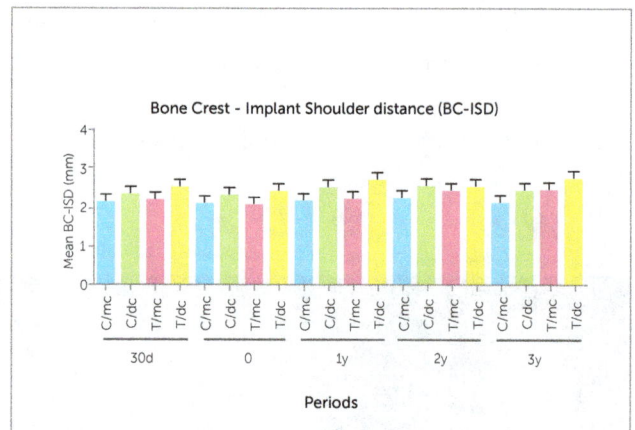

Figure 2 - Comparison of the bone crest-implant shoulder distance of the implant during a period of 30 days after implant installation, at the time of prosthesis installation and after one, two and three years. Crestal bone measurements were obtained on the mesial (mc) and distal (dc) side for all implants, on groups Control (C) and Test (T), at the pre-established time points.

Table 1 - Mean values of the bone crest/shoulder distance of the implant during a period of 30 days after implant installation, at the time of prosthesis installation and one, two and three years thereafter. Crestal bone measurements were obtained on the mesial (mc) and distal (dc) side for all implants at the pre-established time points.

	Bone crest/shoulder distance of the implant (mm) mean ±SD										
	Periods										
Group	30 days		0		1 year		2 years		3 years		p
	mc	dc	mc	dc	mc	dc	mc	dc	mc	dc	
Control	2,13 (0.72)	2.33 (0.79)	2.09 (0.74)	2.27 (0.84)	2.15 (0.52)	2.47 (0.78)	2.22 (0.64)	2.53 (0.71)	2.14 (0.63)	2.39 (0.79)	0.1832 (NS)
Test	2.17 (0.74)	2.45 (1.02)	2.08 (0.59)	2.28 (1.03)	2.22 (0.68)	2.06 (0.96)	2.32 (1.02)	2.41 (1.11)	2.36 (0,92)	2.58 (1.19)	

Data are expressed as mean (SD). Kruskal-Wallis test, * $p < 0.05$; NS = non significant ($p > 0.05$). Crestal bone measurements: mesial (mc) and distal (dc) sides.

remodeling of the implant crests for the test and control groups, with no statistically significant difference between groups, since the time of implant placement, during the application of orthodontic force and throughout the study period (Fig 2 and Table 1). However, the mean bone crest/implant shoulder distance was 2.58 ± 1.19 mm on the distal surface for the test group and 2.39 ± 0.79 mm for the control group after three years of follow-up.

There was no significant difference in pocket probing depth between groups throughout the study period (Fig 3 and Table 2). The mean probing depth was 2.57 ± 0,40 mm and 2.39 ± 0.45 mm three months and three years after prosthesis installation, respectively, for implants of the test group, and 2.30 ± 0.54 mm and 2.21 ± 0.47 mm for the control group, showing that mean probing depth was unchanged throughout the study period.

Keratinized mucosa width (KMW) did not differ significantly between groups during the study, with mean values of 1.43 ± 0.21 mm for the control group and 1.54 ± 0.40 mm for the test group, three months after prosthesis installation, and of 1.51 ± 0.47 mm and 1.56 ± 0.51 mm, respectively, after three years of follow-up (Fig 4 and Table 3). Thus, keratinized mucosa width remained stable and in sufficient quantity to protect the implant and the health of peri-implant tissue, providing better safety regarding the maintenance of peri-implant health.

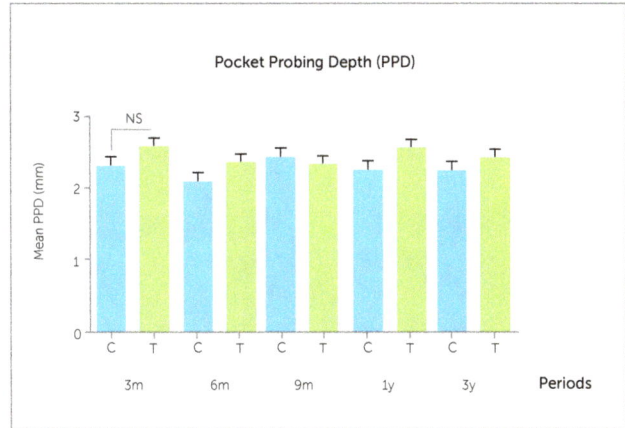

Figure 3 - Comparison of pocket probing depth (PPD) measurements of implant at 3, 6 and 9 months and at 1 and 3 years after prosthesis installation, on Control (C) and Test (T) groups.

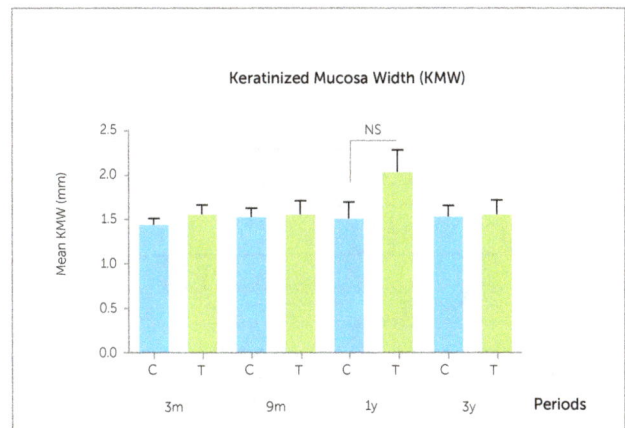

Figure 4 - Comparison of keratinized mucosa width (KMW) measurements of the implant at 3 and 9 months and at 1 and 3 years after prosthesis installation, on Control (C) and Test (T) groups.

Table 2 - Comparison of pocket probing depth (PPD) measurements of the implant at three, six and nine months and at one and three years after prosthesis installation.

Group	Pocket probing depth (mm)					p
	Periods					
	3 m	6 m	9 m	1 y	3 y	
Control	2.30 (0.54)	2.10 (0.41)	2.39 (0.56)	2.25 (0.27)	2.21 (0.47)	p = 0.1078 (NS)
Test	2.57 (0.40)	2.39 (0.29)	2.24 (0.78)	2.51 (0.64)	2.39 (0.45)	

Data are expressed as mean (SD); Kruskal-Wallis test, *: $p < 0.05$; NS = non significant ($p > 0.05$).

Table 3 - Comparison of keratinized mucosa width (KMW) measurements of the implant at three and nine months and at one and three years after prosthesis installation.

Group	Keratinized mucosa width (mm)				p
	Periods				
	3 m	9 m	1 y	3 y	
Control	1.43 (0.21)	1.51 (0.34)	1.50 (0.64)	1.51 (0.47)	p = 0.1987 (NS)
Test	1.54 (0.40)	1.54 (0.55)	2.03 (0.85)	1.56 (0.51)	

Data are expressed as mean (SD); Kruskal-Wallis test, *: $p < 0.05$; NS = non significant ($p > 0.05$).

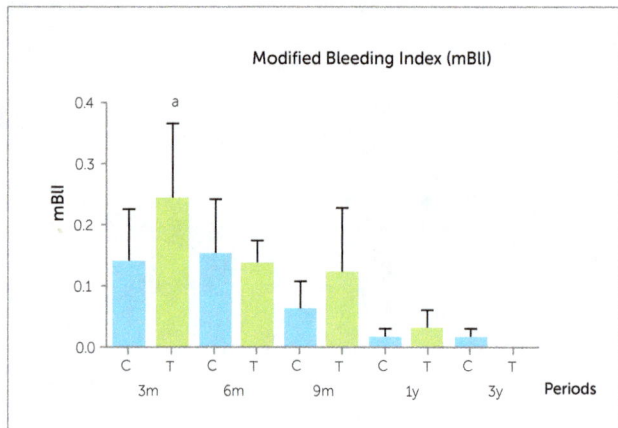

Figure 5 - Comparison of the modified bleeding index (mBlI) for all implants at 3, 6 and 9 months and at 1 and 3 years after prosthesis installation.

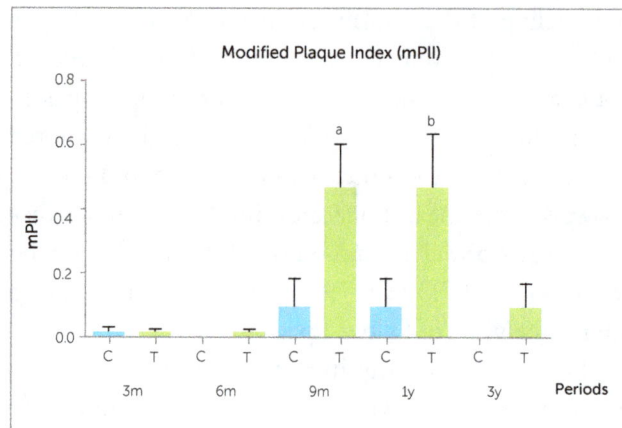

Figure 6 - Comparison of the modified plaque index (mPlI) for all implants at 3, 6 and 9 months and at 1 and 3 years after prosthesis installation.

Table 4 - Comparison of the modified bleeding index (mBlI) for all implants at 3, 6 and 9 months and at 1 and 3 years after prosthesis installation.

Modified bleeding index						
Group	Periods					p
	3 m	6 m	9 m	1 y	3 y	
Control	0.13 (0.29)	0.15 (0.29)	0.06 (0.15)	0.01 (0.05)	0.01 (0.05)	0.017
Test	0.24 (0.40)	0.13 (0.12)	0.12 (0.35)	0.03 (0.10)	0.0 (0.0)	

Data are expressed as mean (SD); Kruskal-Wallis test: * = $p < 0.05$; superscript a = $p < 0.05$, for T3m group *versus* T3y group; NS = non significant ($p > 0.05$).

Table 5 - Comparison of the modified plaque index (mPlI) for all implants at 3, 6 and 9 months and at 1 and 3 years after prosthesis installation.

Modified plaque index						
Group	Periods					p
	3 m	6 m	9 m	1 y	3 y	
Control	0.01 (0.05)	0.0 (0.0)	0.09 (0.30)	0.09 (0.30)	0.0 (0.0)	$p < 0.0001$
Test	0.01 (0.04)	0.01 (0.04)	0.46 (0.49)[a]	0.46 (0.60)[b]	0.08 (0.27)	

Data are expressed as mean (SD). Kruskal-Wallis test: * = $p < 0.05$; superscript a = $p < 0.05$, for T9m group *versus* C6m and C3y groups; superscript b = $p < 0.05$, for T1y group *versus* C3m, T3m, C6m, T6m and C3y groups; NS = non significant: $p > 0.05$.

The mean mBlI values did not differ significantly between groups, with both groups maintaining healthy peri-implant tissues throughout the three years of follow-up after prosthesis implantation (Fig 5 and Table 4). However, the test group revealed a trend towards an increase ($p > 0.05$) three and nine months after prosthesis installation.

The mean mPlI values did not differ significantly between groups. By evaluating different periods of control and test groups, we observed an increase in the mean mPlI values in the test group at nine months and one year, compared to control at three, six months and three years, and test group at three and six months (Fig 6 and Table 5); thus, indicating that the test group presented significantly higher plaque formation on the peri-implant gingiva during the period orthodontic forces were applied to the implants.

The rate of implant success was 100%, according to the criteria proposed by Karoussis et al.[21] No implant showed radiographic changes in the bone-implant interface; no annual vertical bone loss exceeded 0.2 mm after the first year since installation, thereby indicating successful osseointegration of implants; and no implant mobility was observed.

DISCUSSION

Difficulty controlling anchorage is a significant aspect in Orthodontics. Standard anchorage devices, such as extraoral appliances and elastics, rely on patient's cooperation, which may compromise treatment results. The introduction of implants for orthodontic anchorage has decreased the need for patient's cooperation, compared to extraoral appliances, and has provided absolute anchorage biomechanics.[9,14,25]

In the present study, osseointegrated implants placed according to the method proposed by Branemark[19] were clinically successful, fulfilling the proposed outcome criteria. In addition, the implants kept direct bone anchorage throughout the study period, in agreement with the results reported by Roberts et al[26] and Higuchi and Slack.[8] In the test group, it was possible to perform dental movement with an implant as anchorage, without any reciprocal action on the remaining teeth. The amount of peri-implant bone resorption of this group was similar to control.

Orthodontic forces on implants not only all the implants remained firm, but also maintained gingival relationships. This study provides evidence that orthodontic anchorage can have a favorable effect on marginal peri-implant gingival situation. In the test group, a slight increase ($p > 0.05$) was detected in keratinized mucosa width during orthodontic force application on implants, followed by a trend towards the reduction of such after three years of follow-up.

After the application of orthodontic force, there was clinical and radiographic peri-implant stability, as illustrated in Figures 1-6 and Tables 1-5. Results showed a 100% success rate for implants subjected to orthodontic forces of 200 cN; thus, indicating that, after orthodontic treatment, these implants can receive a fixed prosthesis replacing the missing teeth, in addition to improving patient's dental occlusion. Similarly, Cravero et al[7] reported a 100% success rate and satisfactory occlusion with 93 implants placed in the maxilla and mandible.

In the present study, we observed that implants maintained direct bone anchorage throughout orthodontic treatment, in agreement with data reported by Roberts et al[26] and Higuchi and Slack.[8] Trisi et al[25] also used implants for orthodontic anchorage in 41 adult patients. The implants were placed in different areas, all continued to be stable and were osseointegrated 12 months after prosthesis placement. These studies demonstrated that it was possible to perform small tooth movements without a reciprocal action, and that the dental occlusion of orthodontically treated patients was significantly improved.

On the other hand, there have been no reports demonstrating the association between anchorage orthodontic and peri-implant conditions. Different time points of the test group showed an increase in the mean mPlI values after nine months and one year of prosthesis installation. This difference became more pronounced during the application of orthodontic forces. The results showed that the mean mPlI values in the test group with bonded orthodontic devices were higher in comparison to control group without orthodontic devices. The influence of impaired oral hygiene was considered; however, mPlI for the test group did not improve in spite of detailed oral hygiene instructions. The result of the mPlI reveals the difficulty performing oral hygiene for the test group during tooth movement. After completion of orthodontic treatment, the mean mPlI values became normal. Over a 3-year follow-up, peri-implant parameters were considered satisfactory in terms of gingival health. The reason for higher susceptibility to biological complications around implants may be discussed in the light of bacterial plaque accumulation in partially edentulous dentitions or the host response to the bacterial challenge. The microbiota associated with periodontitis and peri-implantitis has supported the concept that periodontal pathogens are important etiological factors of peri-implant infections.[20,27] It is, therefore, obvious that the status of peri-implant health is of utmost importance for the longevity of implants installed.

According to Werbein and Merz[28] and Pinho et al,[29] intraosseous titanium implants yield the best results for orthodontic use; thus, reducing treatment time.

Furthermore, osseointegrated implants have proved to resist displacement forces of 100 to 200 cN on all planes, and to function as a unit of orthodontic anchorage.[7,30] After orthodontic treatment, implants also served as abutment for permanent fixed prostheses in edentulous areas, which could not have been properly carried out without implant anchorage.

CONCLUSION

On the basis of the present results, we suggest that subjecting osseointegrated implants to orthodontic forces can be a safe technique for prosthetic rehabilitation and an alternative for the orthodontic treatment of partially edentulous patients, since there was no significant peri-implant bone loss after orthodontic activation. Additionally, there were no changes in peri-implant probing depth or in the gingiva, and no bleeding or presence of peri-implant plaque was observed during a 3-year follow-up after installation of implant-supported prosthesis.

Author contributions

Conception or design of the study: MCAB, LCM, AYT. Data acquisition, analysis or interpretation: BRM, SEP, MCAB, LCM, AYT. Writing the article: BRM, SEP, MCAB, LCM, AYT. Critical revision of the article: BRM, SEP, AYT. Final approval of the article: BRM, SEP, MCAB, LCM, AYT. Obtained funding: AYT. Overall responsibility: BRM, SEP, MCAB, LCM, AYT.

REFERENCES

1. Adell R, Lekholm U, Rockler B, Branemark PI. A 15-year study of osseointegrated implants in the treatment of the edentulous jaw. Int J Oral Surg. 1981;10(6):387-416.

2. Carrión JP, Barbosa IR, López JP. Osseointegrated implants as orthodontic anchorage and restorative abutments in the treatment of partially edentulous adult patients. Int J Periodontics Restorative Dent. 2009;29(3):33340.

3. Jones SD, Jones FR. Tissue integrated implants for the partially edentulous patient. J Prosthet Dent. 1988;60(3):34957.

4. Lekholm U, Gunne J, Henry P, Higuchi K, Linden U, Bergstrom C, et al. Survival of the branemark implant in partially edentulous jaws: a 10-year prospective multicenter study. Int J Oral Maxillofac . 1999;14(5):639-45.

5. Albrektsson T, Dahl E, Enbom L, Engevall S, Engquist B, Eriksson AR, et al. Osseointegrated oral implants: a Swedish multicenter study of 8139 consecutively inserted nobelpharma implants. J Periodontol. 1988;59(5):287-96.

6. Oldman J, Lekholm U, Kholm U, Jemt T, Branemark PI, Thilander B. Osseointegrated titanium implants: a new approach in orthodontic treatment. Eur J Orthod. 1988 May;10(2):98-105.

7. Cravero RM, Ibañez JC. Assessing double acid-etched implants submitted to orthodontic forces and used as prosthetic anchorages in partially edentulous patients. Open Dent J. 2008; 2: 30-7.

8. Higuchi KW, Slack JM. The use of titanium fixtures for intraoral anchorage: report of a case. Int J Oral Maxillofac Implants. 1991;6:338-44.

9. Block MS, Hoffman DR. A new device for absolute anchorage for orthodontics. Am J Orthod Dentofacial Orthop. 1995;107(3):251- 8.

10. Goto M, Jin-Nouchi S, Ihara K, Katsuki T. Longitudinal follow-up of osseointegrated implants in patients with resected jaws. Int J Oral Maxillofac Implants. 2002;17(2):225-30.

11. Roumanas ED, Freymiller EG, Chang TL, Aghaloo T, Beumer J. Implant-retained prostheses for facial defects: an up to 14-year follow-up report on the survival rates of implants at UCLA. Int J Prosthodont. 2002;15(4):325-32.

12. Liaw Yc, Kuang Sh, Chen Yw, Hung Kf, Tsai Hc, Kao Sy, et al. Multimodality treatment for rehabilitation of adult orthodontic patient with complicated dental condition and jaw relation. J Chin Med Assoc. 2008 Nov;71(11):594-600.

13. Cochran DL, Bosshardt DD, Grize L, Higginbottom FL, Jones AA, Jung RE, et al. Bone response to loaded implants with nonmatching implant abutment diameters in the canine mandible. J Periodontol. 2009;80(4):609 17.

14. Thilander B, Odman J, Lekholm U. Orthodontic aspects of the use of oral implants in adolescents: a 10-year follow-up study. Eur J Orthod. 2001;23(6):715-31.

15. Drago CJ. Use of osseointegrated implants in adult orthodontic treatment: a clinical report. J Prosthet Dent. 1999;82(5):504-9.

16. Willems G, Carels CE, Naert IE, Van Steenberghe D. Interdisciplinary treatment planning for orthodontic-prosthetic implant anchorage in a partially edentulous patient. Clin Oral Implants Res. 1999;10(4):331-7.

17. Goodacre CJ, Brown DT, Roberts WE, Jeiroudi MT. Prosthodontic considerations when using implants for orthodontic anchorage. J Prosthet Dent .1997;77(2):162-70.

18. Celenza F. Implant-enhanced tooth movement: indirect absolute anchorage. Int J Periodontics Restorative Dent. 2003;23(6):533-41.

19. Bränemark P-I. An experimental and clinical study of osseointegrated in treatment of the edentulous jaws. Experience from a 10-year period. Scand J Plast Reconstr Surg. 1977;16:11-8.

20. Mombelli A, Van Oosten MAC, Schurch E, Lang NP. The microbiota associated with successful or failing osseointegrated titanium implants. Oral Microbiol Immunol. 1987 Dec;2(4):145-51.

21. Karoussis IK, Salvi GE, Heitz-Mayfield LJ, Brägger U, Hämmerle CH, Lang NP. Long-termimplant prognosis in patients with and without a history of chronic periodontitis: a 10-year prospective cohort study of the ITIs Dental Implant System. Clin Oral Implants Res. 2003 Jun;14(3):329-39.

22. Karoussis IK, Müller S, Salvi GE, Heitz-Mayfield LJ, Brägger U, Lang NP. Association between periodontal and peri-implant conditions: a 10-year prospective study. Clin Oral Implants Res. 2004 Feb;15(1):1-7.

23. Smith DE, Zarb G. Criteria for success of osseointegrated endosseous implants. J Prosthet Dent. 1989 Nov;62(5):567-72.

24. Weber HP, Buser D, Donath K, Fiorellini JP, Doppalapudi V, Paquette DW, et al. Comparison of healed tissues adjacent to submerged and non-submerged unloaded titanium dental implants. A histometric study in beagle dogs. Clin Oral Implants Res. 1996 Mar;7(1):11-9.

25. Trisi P, Rebaudi A. Progressive bone adaptation of titanium implants during and after orthodontic load in humans. Int J Periodontics Restorative Dent. 2002 Feb;22(1):31-43.

26. Roberts WE, Engen DW, Schneider PM, Hohlt WF. Implant anchored orthodontics for partially edentulous malocclusions in children and adults. Am J Orthod Dentofacial Orthop. 2004 Sept;126(3):302-4.

27. Leonhardt A, Adolfsson B, Lekholm U, Wikström M, Dahlén G. Longitudinal microbiological study on osseointegrated titanium implants in partially edentulous patients. Clin Oral Implants Res. 1993 Sept;4(3):113-20.

28. Wehrbein H, Merz BR, Hammerle CH, Lang NP. Bone-to-implant contact of orthodontic implants in humans subjected to horizontal loading. Clin Oral Implants Res. 1998 Oct;9(5):348-53.

29. Pinho T, Neves M, Alves C. Multidisciplinary management including periodontics, orthodontics, implants, and prosthetics for an adult. Am J Orthod Dentofacial Orthop. 2012 Aug;142(2):235-45.

30. Palagi LM, Sabrosa CE, Gava EC, Baccetti T, Miguel JA. Long-term follow-up of dental single implants under immediate orthodontic load. Angle Orthod. 2010 Sept;80(5):807-11.

8

Comparison of topical and infiltration anesthesia for orthodontic mini-implant placement

Matheus Miotello Valieri[1], Karina Maria Salvatore de Freitas[2], Fabricio Pinelli Valarelli[3], Rodrigo Hermont Cançado[3]

Objective: To compare the acceptability and effectiveness of topical and infiltration anesthesia for placement of mini-implants used as temporary anchorage devices. **Methods:** The sample comprised 40 patients, 17 males and 23 females, whose mean age was 26 years old and who were all undergoing orthodontic treatment and in need for anchorage reinforcement. Mini-implants were bilaterally placed in the maxilla of all individuals, with infiltration anesthesia on one side and topical anesthesia on the other. These 40 patients completed two questionnaires, one before and another after mini-implant placement and pain was measured through a visual analog scale (VAS). The data collected were analyzed using descriptive statistics and the measurements of pain were compared by means of the non-parametric test of Mann-Whitney. **Results:** It was found that 60% of patients felt more comfortable with the use of topical anesthesia for mini-implant placement; 72.5% of patients described the occurrence of pressure during placement of the anchorage device as the most unpleasant sensation of the entire process; 62.5% of patients felt more pain with the use of topical anesthesia. **Conclusion:** It was concluded that patients had less pain with the use of infiltration anesthesia, and also preferred this type of anesthetic.
Keywords: Anesthetics. Orthodontics. Dental implants. Orthodontic anchorage procedures.

[1] MSc in Orthodontics, Ingá College (UNINGÁ).
[2] Coordinator of the Master's program in Orthodontics, Ingá University (UNINGÁ).
[3] Adjunct professor, Department of Orthodontics, Master's program, Ingá College (UNINGÁ).

Karina Maria Salvatore de Freitas
Rua Jamil Gebara, 1-25 – Apto 111 – Bauru/SP – Brazil — CEP: 17017-150
E-mail: kmsf@uol.com.br

» The authors report no commercial, proprietary or financial interest in the products or companies described in this article.

INTRODUCTION

According to Newton's third law, every action has a reaction of equal magnitude and towards its opposite direction. Therefore, when a force is applied with the purpose of achieving orthodontic movement, the teeth used as support (anchorage) will have a reaction with the same intensity towards the opposite direction, which, in most cases, may generate undesirable effects.

In order to avoid such undesirable effects in orthodontic mechanics, the clinician should carefully plan the anchorage to be employed during treatment. However, some types of anchorage directly depend on patient's compliance, which may compromise the final results.

With a view to solving the issues related to anchorage, dentists have had the possibility of using devices that enable skeletal support for tooth movement.

Mini-implants and mini-plates are among the skeletal anchorage devices most commonly used for orthodontic mechanics. The use of mini-plates and mini-implants enable dental movement to be safely performed, many times, without undesirable side effects, at the vertical, transverse, and anterior-posterior planes.[1]

The orthodontic loads of continue and unidirectional nature and of low magnitude are not capable of generating osteolytic activity on the bone interface of the implant.[2,3]

Assessment of patients' acceptance factors regarding the use of mini-implants during orthodontic treatment reveals that the need for infiltrative anesthesia is one of the factors that patients reject the most.[4] Additionally, the association with osseointegrated implants is another factor that contributes to increase the rejection and fear of patients with regard to the use of mini-implants. Several topical anesthetics are available to be used before minor dental procedures are performed and they are largely accepted by the patients.

The ideal topical anesthetic would promote complete anesthesia, with fast action onset and without any side effects. The agents currently available, however, are only close to this ideal.[5]

The possibility of placing mini-implants with the use of topical anesthetic only, has already been suggested in the literature.[4,6,7] Some authors have reported that mini-implants could be successfully and comfortably placed with the use of topical anesthetic, only.[8] Two types of topical anesthetics used for mini-implant placement have been compared, and one of them showed highly satisfactory results.[9] Additionally, it has been proved that 90% of patients undergoing mini-implant placement with the aid of topical anesthesia only, would accept to have mini-implants replaced , if necessary. In this study, 40% of patients reported not having felt any type of pain during placement of the mini-implant, while 20% reported mild pain.[10,11]

However, no study has been conducted to compare the acceptability and effectiveness of infiltrative and topical anesthetics. Thus, the aim of this study was to compare, by means of pre and post-operative questionnaires answered by the patients, the acceptability and discomfort of infiltrative and topical anesthetics used for placement of mini-implants as skeletal anchorage in Orthodontics.

MATERIAL AND METHODS
Sample

This study was approved by the Ingá School of Dentistry Institutional Review Board. Sample calculation was based on alpha error of 5% and beta error of 20%, so as to reach a power test of 80% in order to detect a significant difference of 1.00 cm in VAS scale, with a standard deviation of 1.5, resulting in 36 subjects required for each group.

The study sample comprised 40 patients, 17 males and 23 females, with mean age of 26 years old (not younger than 14, not older than 45 years old). All patients underwent orthodontic treatment and needed bilateral absolute anchorage through mini-implants in the maxilla.

This was a prospective study of which patients were treated in the Orthodontic Clinics of the Masters Course of the Ingá School of Dentistry, and required the placement of bilateral maxillary mini-implants while the study was being carried out, until the number of 40 subjects was obtained.

All patients had the mini-implants placed at the same appointment. The anesthetic was used alternately, that is, the topical anesthetic was applied on one side, while the infiltrative anesthetic was used on the other side. The anesthesia was applied by one examiner who had been previously trained by a Professor of the Masters Course in Orthodontics who, in turn, has extensive expertise in the mini-implant placement either with infiltrative or topical anesthesia.

Two questionnaires (one before and one after mini-implant placement) were given to each patient in order to compare the efficiency of each anesthetic.

Anesthetics

Patients underwent two different anesthetic procedures for mini-implant placement:

» Infiltrative - lidocaine hydrochloride+ epinephrine 1:100,000 (Alphacine 100, DFL Commerce and Industry, Jacarepaguá-RJ, Brazil) applied where the mini-implant was placed, with the aid of a 0.30 x 21 mm gingival needle (Terumo) in the mucosa area, only, with 1/5 of the tube being injected. Mini-implant placement was performed 2 minutes after the infiltrative anesthesia was applied.

» Topical: on the opposite side, topical anesthetic gel with 20% lidocaine (Relva Dermatological Pharmacy, Campo Grande-MS, Brazil) was applied for 7 minutes on the area of the mucosa that received the mini-implant. If the patient reported great pain during mini-implant placement with topical anesthetic, the procedure would be interrupted and the infiltrative anesthetic would be used.

Mini-implants

Self-drilling mini-implants 6 mm in length and 1.5 mm in diameter (Conexão, São Paulo, Brazil) were used in this study. To place the implants, a surgical kit with hand key (Conexão, São Paulo, Brazil) was used.

Mini-implant placement

All patients included in this study were submitted to the following protocol:

» The patient answered the pre-operative questionnaire.

» Drying with air jet and relative isolation was performed with cotton rolls to move the lip away from the area where the mini-implant would be placed under topical anesthetic.

» Topical anesthesia with 20% lidocaine gel was applied on a cotton pellet placed onto the mucosa where the mini-implant would be placed. The gel had to be kept on the mucosa for 7 minutes.

» Removal of excess gel with the aid of a gauze.

» Mini-implant placement.

» On the opposite side, infiltrative anesthesia with Alphacaine 100 (lidocaine hydrochloride+ epinephrine1:100,000) was applied in the area where the mini-implant would be placed.

» Mini-implant placement 2 minutes after anesthesia.

» The patient answered the post-operative questionnaire.

The type of anesthesia that was applied first should be alternated for every other patient. All mini-implants were placed without the need for previous perforation.

Questionnaires

The patients included in the sample were submitted to questionnaires comprised of objective questions before and after mini-implant placement. (Questionnaires are available at http://dpjo.dentalpresspub.com/editions/v19n2/076-083/).

The visual analogue scale (VAS),[12] which is largely used for pain quantification, was employed in question number 4 of the post-operative questionnaire.

Statistical analysis

A descriptive statistical analysis was performed. The comparison of the VAS results for topical and infiltrative anesthetics was performed by means of the Mann-Whitney non-parametric test.

To evaluate the sexual dimorphism of the responses of VAS, the Mann-Whitney non-parametric test was applied.

All tests were performed with the aid of Statistica software (Statistica for Windows, version 7.0, Statsoft, 2005). The level of significance was set at $P < 0.05$.

RESULTS
Pre-operative results

Out of the 40 patients comprising the sample, 65% answered that they calmly accepted the proposal for mini-implant placement (Fig 1). 67.5% of patients reported that their main concern about the procedure was with regards to pain (Fig 2).

When asked about the most worrying procedure, the responses "Mini-implant placement" and "Infiltrative anesthesia (needle)" were the most frequent ones with 37.5% and 35% respectively (Fig 3).

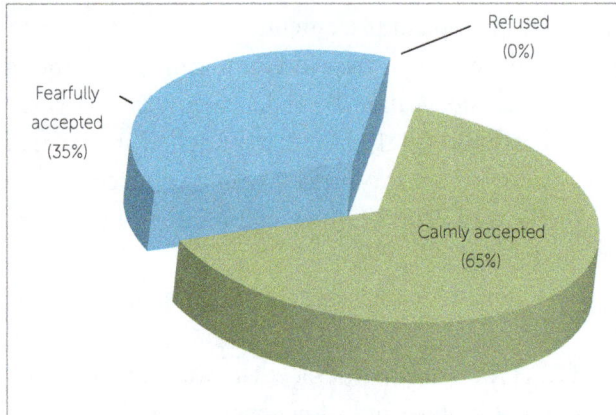

Figure 1 - Answers to question number one of the pre-operative question-naire: "When your orthodontist proposed mini-implant installation, how did you react?"

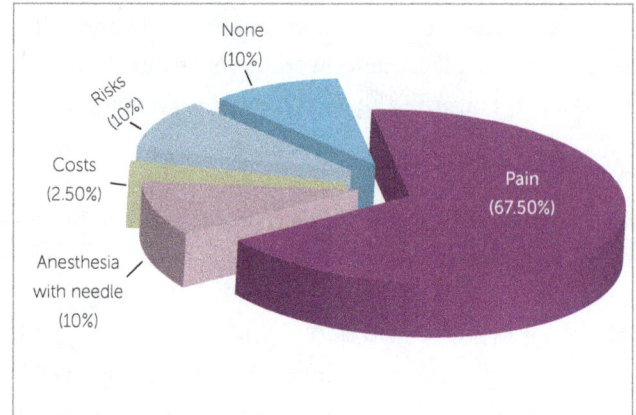

Figure 2 - Answers to question number two of the pre-operative question-naire: "After the dentist proposed mini-implant installation, which was your main doubt regarding the procedure?"

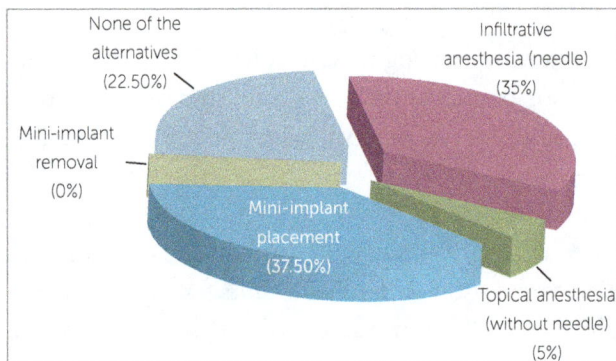

Figure 3 - Answers to question number three of the pre-operative question-naire: "Which of these procedures make you more fearful about installing the mini-implant?"

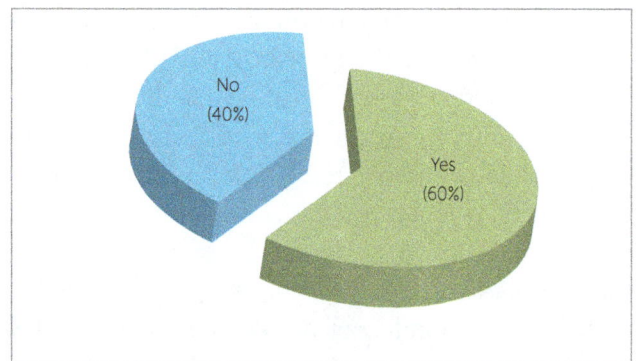

Figure 4 - Answers to question number four of the pre-operative question-naire: "Does the fact of using the topical anesthesia (without needle) make you more comfortable regarding the mini-implant installation?"

Sixty percent (60%) of patients claimed to feel more comfortable towards having mini-implants placed with topical anesthesia (Fig 4).

Post-operative results

Twenty-nine patients (72.5%) reported that pressure during mini-implant placement was the most unpleasant sensation they felt during treatment (Fig 5). When asked whether they felt pain at any moment during mini-implant placement, 65% of patients answered

affirmatively, while 35% claimed that they did not feel any pain (Fig 6). As for the type of anesthesia that caused the most severe pain, 62.5% of patients answered that pain was worse under topical anesthesia (Fig 7).

According to the responses obtained, the anesthetic of choice of the majority of patients was the infiltrative anesthetic (23 patients), while 13 patients preferred the topical anesthetic and 4 patients reported they did not have any preference regarding the anesthetic used (Fig 8).

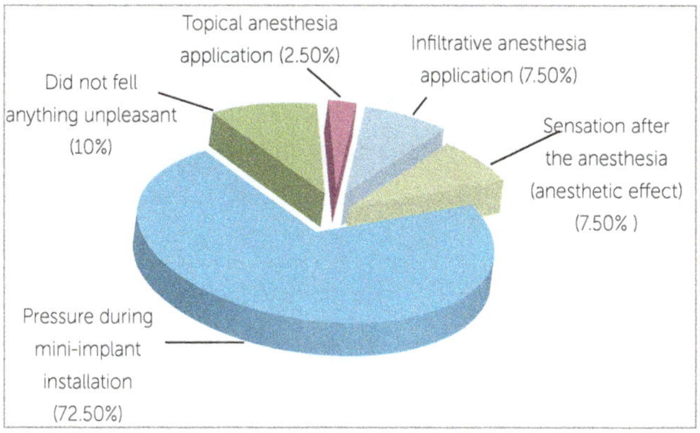

Figure 5 - Answers to question number one of the post-operative questionnaire: "Which was the most unpleasant sensation related to mini-implant installation?"

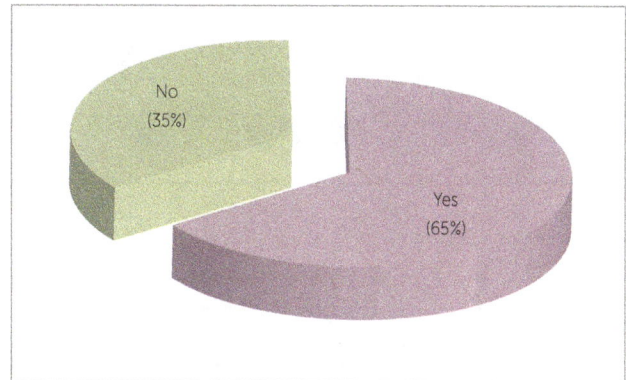

Figure 6 - Answers to question number two of the post-operative questionnaire: "Did you feel pain at any moment of the mini-implant installation?"

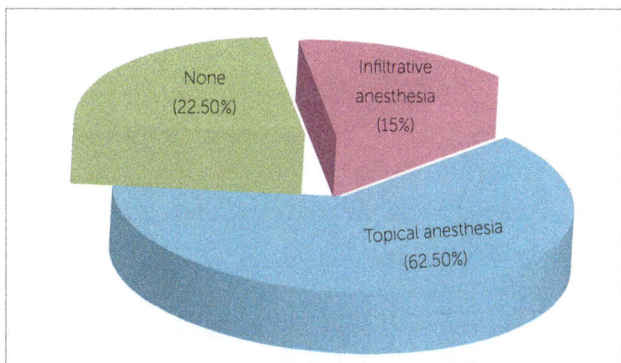

Figure 7 - Answers to question number three of the post-operative questionnaire: "With which type of anesthesia did you feel more painful sensation?"

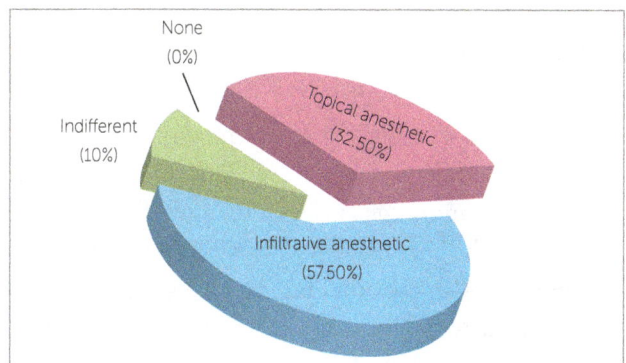

Figure 8 - Answers to question number five of the post-operative questionnaire: "By comparing topical and infiltrative anesthesia, which type did you prefer?"

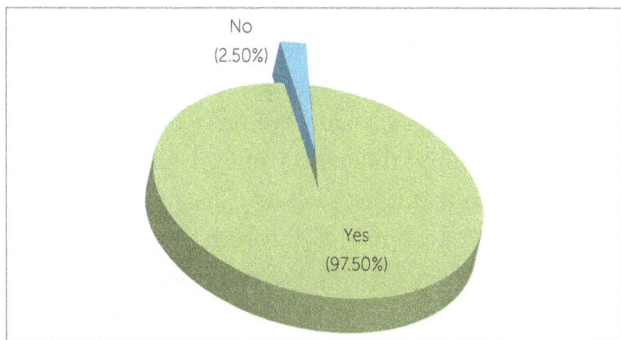

Figure 9 - Answers to question number six of the post-operative questionnaire: "If necessary, would you be submitted to mini-implant installation again?"

Only one patient claimed to refuse having mini-implant replaced, if necessary (Fig 9).

Mean values of pain were obtained by assessment of the visual analogue scale used in question 4 of the post-operative questionnaire. The infiltrative anesthetic obtained a mean value of 0.3125, while the topical anesthetic obtained a mean value of 3.0875. These data were compared through the Mann-Whitney non-parametric test, with statistically significant differences. As a result, mini-implants placed with topical anesthetic caused significantly more pain than those placed with topical anesthesia, as shown by the VAS scale (Table 1). When the sample was divided according to sex, the mean values obtained were 0.2647 with the infiltrative anesthesia and 3.6764 with the topical anesthesia in males; whereas females had mean values of 0.3478 with the infiltrative anesthesia and 2.6521 with the topical anesthesia. These data were also submitted to the Mann-Whitney non-parametric test, without statistically significant differences (Table 2).

Table 1 - Comparison of VAS results through the Mann-Whitney non-parametric test.

Variable	Infiltrative anesthesia (n = 40) Mean ± SD	Topical anesthesia (n = 40) Mean ± SD	p
VAS	0.31 ± 0.64	3.08 ± 2.54	0.000*

* Statistically significant for P < 0.05.

Table 2 - Sexual dimorphism assessment by comparison of VAS results through the Mann-Whitney non-parametric test.

Variable	Male (n = 17) Mean ± SD	Female (n = 23) Mean ± SD	p
Infiltrative	0.26 ± 0.66	0.34 ± 0.64	0.671
Topical	3.67 ± 2.29	2.65 ± 2.67	0.112

DISCUSSION

Discussion of the method

Many authors have suggested the possibility of using topical anesthetic for mini-implant placement with a view to obtaining the analgesia required for complete insertion of the anchorage device without blocking the sensibility of the surrounding structures, thus, reducing the chances of damages if the mini-implants reaches these structures.[4,6,11] In the present study, the use of topical gel anesthetic (20% lidocaine)[10,11] was chosen because it reaches good levels of analgesia, can be easily handled and does not cause tissue damage, as previously reported by the literature. The application protocol used in this study also followed the recommendations of a previous study,[10] that is, the gel was kept in contact with the mucosa for 7 minutes under relative isolation and care so that it did not surpass the area of interest.

With regard to the infiltrative anesthetic, lidocaine hydrochloride + epinephrine 1:100,000 (Alphacaine 100®) was used due to the fact that it is largely employed in Dentistry with low toxicity rates and enough anesthetic effect. The amount of anesthetic used was of 1/5 of the tube, injected in the area of the mucosa where the mini-implant would be placed so as to allow a satisfactory anesthesia and prevent the surrounding structures from being anesthetized, as suggested by the literature.[13,14]

Self-drilling mini-implants (Conexão®), 6 mm in length and 1.5 in diameter were used with the aid of a surgical kit (Conexão®). The sequence of insertion was carried out in turns: half of times infiltrative anesthesia was the first procedure, while half of times topical anesthesia was applied first. The sides of insertion were also alternated in order to avoid any potential influences over patients' responses.

The use of topical anesthetic is very common before infiltrative anesthesia so as to decrease the discomfort in the application of the latter. However, such procedure was not carried out in this study. Pain was assessed while the mini-implant was being placed and not during anesthesia application, whether topical or infiltrative.

The mini-implants were bilaterally placed in the area between pre-molars and molars, on both sides of the same patient, so that the insertion area would not influence patient's pain sensitivity. The alternate order of use of the anesthetics for mini-implant placement also enabled the differences in sensitivity of both types of anesthetics to follow a single pattern of influence over the results.

Other factor that could have influenced the results was the anatomical differences of each patient, as they could alter pain threshold. Notwithstanding, because mini-implants were placed with both anesthetics in the same patient, this factor was practically annulled.

The visual analogue scale was used to record pain rates. It was chosen due to its easy clinical applicability and great power of pain measurement.[12]

Discussion of results

In the present study, the acceptability of mini-implant placement was of 100% for all cases. However, 35% of patients answered they accepted with fear, while in another study 90% of patients answered "I immediately accepted because I totally trust my orthodontist". Nevertheless, this latter study comprised a considerably smaller sample (10 patients) and did not aim at evaluating different types of anesthesia, which could have influenced the data obtained.[4]

Infiltrative anesthesia was reported by 14 subjects as one of the most fearful procedures, followed by the fear of mini-implant placement, chosen by 15 patients. Sixty percent of patients reported that the use of topical anesthetic made them feel more comfortable with regard to the procedure, which proves that infiltrative anesthesia applied with the aid of a needle causes certain discomfort in a considerably number of patients,[15] leading some of them to refuse being submitted to procedures of anchorage device placement.

After mini-implant placement, patients reported that the most unpleasant sensation they felt during the entire procedure was the pressure during placement, which was also observed by another study,[4] but disagrees with what was found by Santos et al[11] who reported that patients did not feel anything unpleasant.

Twenty-five patients pointed out that topical anesthesia caused the most painful sensation, proving that infiltrative anesthesia resulted in greater anesthetic effect for the patients of the sample.

Mini-implant placement could not be completed in three patients who received topical anesthetic. These patients reported severe pain, and for this reason, the procedure was discontinued, following the methods of this study. Later on, these same patients underwent infiltrative anesthesia and in two of them, the mini-implants were placed under infiltrative anesthesia. The other case was initiated by topical anesthetic. In the study conducted by Reznik et al,[9] who compared two types of topical anesthetics, the failure rate (impossibility of finishing the installation under topical anesthesia) was of 71% (12 cases) when 20% benzocaine was used, whereas there was no failure when 20% lidocaine + 4% tetracaine + 2% phenylephrine anesthetic was used.

When patients were asked whether they would accept to have mini-implants replaced, 97.5% (39 patients) gave affirmative answers, while in the study conducted by Santos et al,[11] 10% of patients would not accept it, and according to Brandão and Mucha,[4] 10% of patients would not recommend this procedure to other patients.

The analysis of the data obtained with the visual analogue scale demonstrated that the mean values exhibited by the infiltrative anesthesia were minimum and significantly lower than those of the topical anesthesia (Table 1). Moreover, it could be observed that the discrepancy of pain values between both types of anesthetic was statistically significant. However, 42.5% of patients did not choose the infiltrative

anesthesia as their procedure of choice (Fig 8), which demonstrates the rejection of most patients in regard to anesthetic procedures performed with the aid of needles.

The results of the visual analogue scale divided by sex demonstrated lower mean values for females when topical anesthetic was used. However, when the Mann-Whitney non-parametric test was applied to verify sexual dimorphism, the values did not prove to be statistically significant (Table 2).

Clinical considerations

Failure was reported in three cases of mini-implant placement under topical anesthesia. Following the methods established for this study, infiltrative anesthesia was then applied and the anchorage device was installed. However, it was clear that, in all three cases of failure, the patients exhibited great anxiety while the procedure was being carried out, and after infiltrative anesthesia, they did not report any pain. The present study demonstrates that patients reported greater sensitivity in cases of mini-implant placement under topical anesthesia, without, however, reporting any discomfort during the anesthetic application. On the other hand, in cases of mini-implant placement carried out under infiltrative anesthesia, patients reported certain degree of discomfort during anesthetic application, but significant comfort during mini-implant placement, which must be assessed by both the dentist and the patient in the decision for which type of anesthetic should be employed.

Mini-implant placement under topical anesthesia seems to be a viable option in cases in which patients refuse to undergo infiltrative anesthesia in fear of the needle, especially in less anxious patients.

CONCLUSION

Based on the results of the present study, it is reasonable to conclude that:

» The use of topical anesthetic results in more comfort to patients undergoing mini-implant placement procedures;

» Patients considered pressure during mini-implant placement as the most unpleasant sensation;

» Pain sensitivity of mini-implant placement with topical anesthetic was significantly greater than that of infiltrative anesthesia;

» Most patients submitted to mini-implant placement preferred the procedure under infiltrative anesthesia.

REFERENCES

1. Faber J, Araújo TM. Ancoragem esquelética no início do século XXI. Rev Dental Press Ortod Ortop Facial. 2008;13(5):5.
2. Carano A, Velo S, Leone P, Siciliani G. Clinical applications of the Miniscrew Anchorage System. J Clin Orthod. 2005;39(1):9-24.
3. Lee JS, Park HS, Kyung HM. Micro-implant anchorage for lingual treatment of a skeletal Class II malocclusion. J Clin Orthod. 2001;35(10):643-7.
4. Brandão LBC, Mucha JN. Grau de aceitação de mini-implantes por pacientes em tratamento ortodôntico - estudo preliminar. Rev Dental Press Ortod Ortop Facial. 2008;13(5):118-27.
5. Friedman PM, Mafong EA, Friedman ES, Geronemus RG. Topical anesthetics update: EMLA and beyond. Dermatol Surg. 2001;27(12):1019-26.
6. Marassi C. Carlo Marassi responde (parte II) - Quais as principais aplicações clínicas e quais as chaves para o sucesso no uso dos miniimplantes em ortodontia? Rev Clín Ortod Dental Press. 2006;5(5):14-26.
7. Baumgaertel S, Razavi MR, Hans MG. Mini-implant anchorage for the orthodontic practitioner. Am J Orthod Dentofacial Orthop. 2008;133(4):621-7.
8. Kravitz ND, Kusnoto B. Placement of mini-implants with topical anesthetic. J Clin Orthod. 2006;40(10):602-4.
9. Reznik DS, Jeske AH, Chen JW, English J. Comparative efficacy of 2 topical anesthetics for the placement of orthodontic temporary anchorage devices. Anesth Prog. 2009;56(3):81-5.
10. Santos SHB. Avaliação da utilização de anestésico tópico para a instalação de mini-implantes ortodônticos [dissertação]. Maringá (PR): Faculdade Ingá; 2010.
11. Santos SHB, Freitas KMS, Valarelli FP, Cançado RH, Canuto LFG. Avaliação da utilização de anestésico tópico para instalação de mini-implantes ortodônticos. Ortodontia SPO. 2012;45(3):248-56.
12. Price DD, McGrath PA, Rafii A, Buckingham B. The validation of visual analogue scales as ratio scale measures for chronic and experimental pain. Pain. 1983;17(1):45-56.
13. Kyung HM, Park HS, Bae SM, Sung JH, Kim IB. Development of orthodontic micro-implants for intraoral anchorage. J Clin Orthod. 2003;37(6):321-8.
14. Marassi LA, Herdy JL. Miniimplantes como método de ancoragem em Ortodontia. In: Sakai E, editor. Nova visão em Ortodontia: Ortopedia Funcional dos Maxilares. 3ª ed. São Paulo: Ed. Santos; 2004.
15. Medeiros EPG, Bervique JA. O sentimento de vítima em pacientes da Odontologia. Odontol Mod. 1981;7(3):35-41.

9

Association between gingivitis and anterior gingival enlargement in subjects undergoing fixed orthodontic treatment

Fabricio Batistin Zanatta[1], Thiago Machado Ardenghi[1], Raquel Pippi Antoniazzi[2],
Tatiana Militz Perrone Pinto[2], Cassiano Kuchenbecker Rösing[3]

Objective: The aim of this study was to investigate the association among gingival enlargement (GE), periodontal conditions and socio-demographic characteristics in subjects undergoing fixed orthodontic treatment. **Methods:** A sample of 330 patients undergoing fixed orthodontic treatment for at least 6 months were examined by a single calibrated examiner for plaque and gingival indexes, probing pocket depth, clinical attachment loss and gingival enlargement. Socio-economic background, orthodontic treatment duration and use of dental floss were assessed by oral interviews. Associations were assessed by means of unadjusted and adjusted Poisson's regression models. **Results:** The presence of gingival bleeding (RR 1.01; 95% CI 1.00-1.01) and excess resin around brackets (RR 1.02; 95% CI 1.02-1.03) were associated with an increase in GE. No associations were found between socio-demographic characteristics and GE. **Conclusion:** Proximal anterior gingival bleeding and excess resin around brackets are associated with higher levels of anterior gingival enlargement in subjects under orthodontic treatment.

Keywords: Epidemiology. Orthodontics. Gingivitis. Gingival enlargement.

» The authors report no commercial, proprietary or financial interest in the products or companies described in this article.

[1] Associate professor, Department of Stomatology, Federal University of Santa Maria (UFSM).

[2] Assistant professor, Franciscano University Center (UNIFRA).

[3] Postdoc in Periodontics, Adjunct professor, Federal University of Rio Grande do Sul, (UFRGS).

Tatiana Militz Perrone Pinto
Rua Roberto Holtermann, 314 – Medianeira – Santa Maria/RS — Brazil.
CEP: 97.015-570 – E-mail: tatimilitz@hotmail.com

INTRODUCTION

The balance of health-disease processes in Periodontics depends on adequate supra and subgingival plaque control achieved by patient and professional's combined efforts. Accumulation of supragingival plaque results in inflammatory alterations of gingival tissues. However, interindividual differences might explain the different patterns of response and time needed for evident clinical responses. It is possible that these variations may be associated with different plaque growth patterns, local and systemic individual resistance or even a specific microbial challenge.[1,2]

Clinical studies suggest that orthodontic treatment may be associated with a decrease in periodontal health.[3,4,5] One of the adverse periodontal alterations is a hypertrophic form of gingivitis.[5,6,7] The exact mechanism for the development of gingival enlargement (GE) is not yet completely understood, but it probably involves increased production by fibroblasts of amorphous ground substance with a high level of glycosaminoglycans. Increases in mRNA expression of type I collagen and up-regulation of keratinocyte growth factor receptor could play an important role in excessive proliferation of epithelial cells and development of GE.[8] In some studies, poor oral hygiene increased GE.[9,10] Other clinical studies concluded that overall gingival changes during orthodontic treatment are transient with no permanent damage to the periodontal supporting tissues.[11,12]

The presence of orthodontic brackets also increases the skills and effort required to maintain good levels of oral hygiene, especially on the proximal surfaces.[11] Microbiological studies demonstrate that when fixed orthodontic appliances are placed, the potential for quantitative[13,14] and qualitative[15,16] changes in the microbial composition of these areas enhances. Thus, periodontal reaction might be elicited by a change in the microbiological environment.

To the best of our knowledge, there are no studies assessing GE and associated factors in individuals undergoing orthodontic therapy. Thus, this study aimed at assessing the prevalence of GE and associated factors in a group of orthodontic patients.

MATERIAL AND METHODS

This cross-sectional study examined subjects who were undergoing orthodontic treatment in an orthodontic graduate program in Santa Maria, Brazil. Ethical approval was obtained from the Franciscan University Center Institutional Review Board prior to the start of the study (protocol registration number 1246 in the National Ethics Committee). Subjects who agreed to participate signed an informed consent form. Patients diagnosed with oral pathological conditions were advised to seek consultation and treatment.

Eligibility criteria

To be eligible for the study, individuals should have been undergoing fixed orthodontic treatment for at least 6 months. Exclusion criteria comprised presence of diseases and conditions that could pose health risks to the participant or that could interfere in clinical examination, for instance, users of nifedipine, cyclosporine or phenytoin, contraceptive and decompensated diabetics. Individuals who had undergone antibiotic therapy within three months prior to examination were also excluded. Female subjects were excluded if they were pregnant or breastfeeding. Additionally, individuals who required a prophylactic regimen of antibiotics for clinical examination were excluded.

Study sample

The orthodontic dental clinic of Ingá College (UNINGÁ) was treating, during data collection period, an estimated population of seven hundred patients, six hundred of which were regularly under treatment and, therefore, were assessed for eligibility criteria. This process resulted in four hundred eligible individuals, 330 of which were assessed, resulting in a non-response rate of less than 20%. Clinical examinations were performed between September/2009 and July/2010.

Examinations

A single, calibrated examiner performed all clinical examinations with the aid of a dental assistant who took the records. All permanent and fully erupted teeth, except for third molars, were examined by means of a manual periodontal probe (Neumar®, São Paulo,SP, Brazil). Six sites (mesio-buccal, mid-buccal, disto-buccal, disto-lingual, mid-lingual, and mesio-lingual) were assessed for each tooth.

Teeth in each quadrant were washed with air and water spay as well as dried with air spray. Afterwards, Plaque Index (PlI),[17] Gingival Index (GI),[18] probing depth (PPD), attachment loss (CAL) and bleeding on probing were assessed. Thereafter, gingival enlargement[19] was assessed. The degree of gingival thickening in both labial and lingual aspects was scored as follows: 0 = normal; 1 = thickening up to 2 mm; 2 = thickening greater than 2 mm. The extent of gingival tissues encroachment onto the adjacent crowns was also graded, using 0, 1, 2 and 3 on the labial and lingual surfaces. The sum of both scores (thickening and gingival encroachment) resulted in an enlargement score for each gingival unit. The maximum score obtainable using this method is 5. Additionally, excess resin was dichotomously assessed by inspection with a probe around the bracket on the buccal surfaces of each bonded bracket. For this purpose, the buccal surface was divided into distal, mesial and cervical. Excess resin, located at less than 1 mm from the gingival margin was present.

After clinical examination, socioeconomic and demographic data were collected using a structured written questionnaire. Race was scored as white or non-white. Socioeconomic status was scored by the individual's level of education (≤ 11 years / > 11 years) which, in Brazil, corresponds to those who have completed high school or those educated beyond high school level. Household income information was measured in terms of the Brazilian minimum wage, which corresponded to approximately US$290 (US dollars) during the period of data collection. Income information was measured dichotomously (≤ 5 national minimum wages / > 5 national minimum wages). PII and GI were dichotomized as visible plaque (present / absent) and gingival bleeding[20](present / absent), respectively. The percentages of sites with visible plaque, gingival bleeding and bleeding on probing were calculated individually. The questionnaire also reported the declared frequency dental floss use. Regular interdental hygiene was defined as the use of dental floss at least once a day. Non-users of dental-floss were defined as subjects who did not use interdental oral hygiene devices every day or who did not perform interdental hygiene.

Measurement reproducibility

The examiner was trained and calibrated to perform the clinical measurements before the study started. Assessment of measurement reproducibility was conducted with 15 subjects who were divided into three groups of 5 subjects each. In each one of the groups,

replicate measurements were made by the examiner on two occasions, with a two-day interval. At the site level, reproducibility was assessed by means of the weighted Kappa (± 1 mm) and resulted in values of 0.73 for probing pocket depth and of 0.68 for clinical attachment loss. Gingival enlargement reproducibility was assessed by means of Intraclass Correlation coefficient at the site level in 15 subjects, resulting in an ICC of 0.86.

Data analysis

Most participants presented low mean values for PPD and CAL. Thus, these data were not used in the present analysis. For this exploratory analysis, data pattern distribution was analyzed and non-parametric (Mann-Whitney and Kruskal-Wallis) tests were used. After descriptive analysis, the frequencies of gingival enlargement scores (full mouth mean) were compared for differences between demographic characteristics, socioeconomic indicators and clinical status.

Unadjusted Poisson regression analysis with robust variance was performed to correlate the overall mean of the anterior gingival enlargement (AGE) score with each demographic, socioeconomic and clinical indicator. AGE was considered for anterior teeth located in esthetic regions, only. This region was chosen because a recent publication[21] emphasized the impact of AGE in oral health related quality of life (OHRQoL) in subjects undergoing fixed orthodontic treatment. In this analysis, the outcome was considered as continuous. Additionally, rate ratios (RR), which correspond to the quotient between average scores of each comparison group, and 95% confidence intervals (95% CI) were calculated. A multivariate model was then run with the covariates. These covariates were selected using a backward stepwise procedure. Only variables with p ≤ 0.20 or those that presented a conceptual association with the primary outcome were included in the model. In order to be retained in the final multivariate model, the variables should present p ≤ 0.05. The statistical software STATA 9.0 (Stata Corp, College Station, USA) was used for all analyses.

RESULTS

All subjects completed both the questionnaire and the clinical examination. The demographic characteristics, socioeconomic indicators and clinical status of the subjects are shown in Table 1. In the present investigation, the

Table 1 - Research subjects' clinical and socio-demographic characteristics.

Variables	n (%)
Demographic characteristics	
Sex	
Male	159 (48.1%)
Female	171 (51.8%)
Ethnicity	
White	263 (79.7%)
Non-White	67 (20.3%)
Age (years)	
14 - 19	162 (49.0%)
20 - 24	121 (36.6%)
25 - 30	47 (14.2%)
Socioeconomic status	
Household Income	
≤ 5	270 (81.8%)
> 5	60 (18.1%)
Educational level	
> 11 years	159 (48.1%)
≤ 11 years	171 (51.8%)
Clinical status	
TUFOT (Months)	
6 - 12	185 (56.06%)
> 12	145 (43.93%)
Dental floss	
Users	81 (24.5%)
Non-users	249 (75.5%)

TUFOT: Time under fixed orthodontic treatment.

study sample comprised 330 individuals aged between 14 and 30 years old, 171 (51.8%) female and 159 (48.2%) male, 263 (79.7%) white and 67 (20.3%) non-white. As for periodontal diagnosis, based on patient's age and periodontal data explored in another study[22] (2.06 mm ± 0.18 and 1.6 ± 0.11 for mean probing depth and clinical attachment levels in proximal sites, respectively) most patients had periodontal diagnosis of gingivitis, only.

The mean value for anterior gingival enlargement, percentage of whole mouth visible plaque and percentage of whole mouth gingival bleeding were 0.69, 47.38% and 58.72%, respectively. Table 2 shows the unadjusted analysis between demographic, socioeconomic and clinical variables related to different scores of gingival enlargement. Statistically significant differences were observed in each frequency of gingival enlargement for almost all covariates. Level of education was not associated with GE. When considering score 2 of GE, no association was detected with sex and for score 3 of GE, age was not associated.

The unadjusted Poisson regression assessment of associations revealed use of dental floss (RR 1.25; 95% CI 1.08-1.43), percentage of proximal anterior gingival bleeding (RR 1.01; 95% CI 1.0-1.01) and percentage of sites with excess resin around brackets (RR 1.02; 95% CI 1.02-1.03) as the main covariates associated with higher levels of anterior gingival enlargement. In the multivariate regression model, the percentage of proximal anterior gingival bleeding remained associated, in which higher frequencies of anterior gingival bleeding were associated with a 1.01 fold increase in average AGE scores (RR 1.01; 95% CI 1.0-1.01). Additionally, the percentage of sites with excess resin around brackets also remained associated, with higher frequencies of sites with excess resin around brackets being associated with a 1.02 fold increase in average AGE scores (RR 1.02; 95% CI 1.02-1.03).

DISCUSSION

The present study aimed at investigating potential associations among gingival enlargement, socio-demographic and clinical characteristics. When GE was assessed by frequency of scores, statistically significant differences between nearly all independent variables and frequencies of GE were observed. While the clinical relevance of these differences could be dubious for some of these variables, others such as household income, use of dental floss and time with orthodontic appliances presented substantial clinical differences for the prevalence of gingival enlargement score two. After regression analysis had been performed, proximal anterior gingival bleeding and excessive resin around brackets were revealed as independent variables associated with the level of anterior gingival enlargement.

Since hyperplasic gingival response is a common response to plaque accumulation in subjects undergoing fixed orthodontic therapy. this study used two indexes to assess gingival inflammatory status: color alteration and/or swelling and bleeding after marginal probing. Gingival bleeding IS shown by clinical and histological studies to be an earlier and more sensitive sign of gingival inflammation in comparison to cardinal signs such as redness and swelling, which may be rather subjective and not very reliable.[23,24] Furthermore, a single calibrated examiner, unaware of dental floss use habits, assessed all parameters. These methods probably increased the quality of data collection as well as results reliability.

Table 2 - Univariate analysis between socioeconomic factors and oral clinical conditions related to frequencies of different scores of gingival enlargement index.

Variables	N (%)	GE0 (%)	GE1 (%)	GE2 (%)	GE3 (%)
		Mean ± SD	Mean ± SD	Mean ± SD	Mean ± SD
Demographic characteristics					
Sex		p* = 0.010	p* = 0.010	p* = 0.120	p* < 0.001
Male	159 (48.1%)	58.10 ± 9.24	27.56 ± 4.55	12.52 ± 8.95	1.21 ± 3.43
Female	171 (51.8%)	58.15 ± 9.66	29.05 ± 5.53	10.48 ± 8.20	1.70 ± 2.67
Ethnics (%)		p* < 0.001	p* = 0.016	p* = 0.001	p* = 0.000
White	263 (79.7%)	59.17 ± 10.0	28.05 ± 5.04	11.17 ± 9.35	1.10 ± 3.19
Non-white	67 (20.3%)	54.04 ± 5.01	29.16 ± 5.23	13.0 ± 4.72	2.80 ± 2.21
Age (yrs)		p** = 0.037	p** < 0.001	p** < 0.001	p** = 0.083
14 - 19	162 (49.0%)	56.98 ± 10.15	27.59 ± 4.86	12.89 ± 9.19	1.88 ± 3.74
20 - 24	121 (36.6%)	59.88 ± 9.36	29.52 ± 5.30	8.91 ± 7.66	1.05 ± 2.51
24 - 30	47 (14.2%)	57.57 ± 5.79	27.46 ± 4.82	13.63 ± 7.51	0.95 ± 1.25
Socioeconomic status					
Household income (Wages)		p* < 0.001	p* < 0.001	p* < 0.001	p* < 0.001
≤ 5	270 (81.8%)	56.62 ± 8.72	27.55 ± 4.39	13.35 ± 8.25	1.77 ± 3.33
> 5	60 (18.1%)	64.88 ± 9.61	31.56 ± 6.60	3.36 ± 4.81	0.0 ± 0.0
Subject's education		p* = 0.055	p* < 0.001	p* = 0.011	p* < 0.001
≤ 11 years	159 (48.1%)	57.28 ± 9.91	27.51 ± 4.73	13.03 ± 9.11	1.46 ± 3.63
> 11 years	171 (51.8%)	59.41 ± 8.54	29.45 ± 5.41	9.28 ± 7.35	1.42 ± 2.03
Clinical status					
Dental floss users		p* = 0.018	p* < 0.001	p* < 0.001	p* = 0.031
Yes	81 (24.5%)	61.46 ± 8.28	31.25 ± 5.64	6.44 ± 6.66	0.45 ± 0.90
No	249 (75.5%)	57.04 ± 9.54	27.31 ± 4.51	13.2 ± 8.57	1.77 ± 3.46
TUFOT (Months)		p*<0.001	p*<0.001	p*<0.001	p*=0.016
6 a 12	185 (56.06%)	60.56 ± 6.40	29.26 ± 3.77	8.78 ± 3.66	0.81 ± 1.69
> 12	145 (43.93%)	55.02 ± 11.56	27.02 ± 6.18	15.02 ± 11.46	2.26 ± 4.13

Caption : GE0=Gingival enlargement score 0; GE1=Gingival enlargement score 1; GE2=Gingival enlargement score 2; GE3=Gingival enlargement score 3; TUFOT: Time under fixed orthodontic treatment; p*= Mann Whitney test; p**= Kruskall Wallis test

The use of dental floss was dichotomized into subjects who use it every day and individuals who do not have this habit. This cutoff was made based on evidence that demonstrates reduction in inflammatory parameters associated with gingivitis when flossing is performed every day.[25] The use of dental floss was not an independent predictor for AGE. There is no evidence in population basis evaluating the association between dental floss and GE. However, short-term clinical studies with subjects without orthodontic appliances have demonstrated a significant improvement in the interproximal gingival condition with the correct use of dental floss.[25,26,27] It is important to highlight that some studies conducted with highly motivated individuals who efficiently brush their teeth revealed that the incorporation of flossing in oral hygiene routines does not significantly contribute to improve interproximal gingival conditions.[28] Thus, the lack of association between dental floss and AGE may be due to the possibility of toothbrushing alone resulting in low levels of plaque accumulation in anterior segments. These results should be interpreted with care. Although no statistically significant differences were observed in AGE in users and non-users of dental floss, this habit is also recommended for other purposes, such as preventing attachment loss, halitosis, carious lesions, etc.

The positive correlation found between sites with excess resin around brackets and levels of AGE confirmed the hypothesis that oversight in the bonding of brackets might influence gingival enlargement. The standard of finishing/polishing techniques and surface roughness proved to be important factors for bacterial adhesion with different types of dental materials.[29,30] Thus, our results could hypothesize that excess resin causes greater adhesion of bacterial plaque and subsequent gingivitis formation. Moreover, poor oral hygiene proved to be an important causal factor of gingival enlargement.[9]

Table 3 - Unadjusted (RR) and Adjusted assessment (RR*) for association between socioeconomic factors and oral clinical conditions related to anterior gingival enlargement average. Robust poisson regression analysis.

Variables	n (%)	AGE Mean ± SD	AGE RR (95%IC)	AGE RR* (95% IC)
Demographic characteristics				
Sex			p = 0,142	**
Male	159 (48.1%)	0.72 ± 0.33	1.08 (0.97-1.20)	
Female	171 (51.8%)	0.66 ± 0.34	1	
Ethnics (%)			0.188	**
White	263 (79.7%)	0.7 ± 0.34	1	
Non-white	67 (20.3%)	0.64 ± 0.32	0.91 (0.79-1.04)	
Age (yrs)			p = 0.123	**
14-19	162 (49.0%)	0.73 ± 0.35	1.11 (0.96-1.29)	
20-24	121 (36.6%)	0.66 ± 0.34	1.00 (0.85-1.17)	
24-30	47 (14.2%)	0.65 ± 0.29	1	
Socioeconomic status				
Household income (Wages)			p = 0.213	**
≤ 5	270 (81.8%)	0.70 ± 0.33	1.10 (0.94-1.28)	
> 5	60 (18.1%)	0.64 ± 0.35	1	
Subject's education			p = 0.14	**
< 11 years	159 (48.1%)	0.73 ± 0.35	1.08 (0.97 – 1.20)	
≥ 11 years	171 (51.8%)	0.63 ± 0.31	1	
Clinical status				
Dental floss users (%)			p = 0.000	p = 0.239
Yes	81 (24.5%)	0.58 ± 0.34	1	1
No	249 (75.5%)	0.73 ± 0.33	1.25 (1.08-1.43)	1.07 (0.95-1.22)
TUFOT (Months)			p = 0.18	**
6 a 12	185 (56.06%)	0.64 ± 0.32	1	
> 12	145 (43.93%)	0.75 ± 0.35	0.91 (0.79-1.04)	
PAGB (%)	-		p = 0.000	p = 0.000
			1.01(1.0 – 1.01)	1.01 (1.00-1.01)
Excessive resin (% of sites)	-		p = 0.000	p = 0.000
			1.02 (1.02-1.03)	1.02 (1.02-1.03)

RR: Ratios rate; AGE: Anterior gingival Enlargement; TUFOT: Time under fixed orthodontic treatment; PAGB: Proximal anterior gingival bleeding. *Adjusted by sex, ethnics, age, Household income, subjects's education, TUFOT, dental floss, GAE and excessive resin ** Variables not included in the final multiple model after adjustment.

In this study, variables related to socio-demographic characteristics, such as sex, ethnicity, household income and subjects' level of education, were not associated with anterior gingival enlargement. However, it has been established that individuals from different socioeconomic backgrounds are exposed to different risk factors that affect oral health. Individuals with lower socioeconomic status are subjected to material deprivation which could influence their engaging in riskier behaviors, thereby resulting in worse oral health conditions.[31] Furthermore, low educational level may lead to reduced income, unemployment and poor occupational status, all of which could influence oral health.[31] Our contradictory results could be explained by one of the following hypotheses: First, in subjects with orthodontic appliances, socio-demographic characteristics may not influence gingival enlargement levels, differently to subjects without orthodontic appliances; second, the lack of extreme differences related to socioeconomic status in our sample may have influenced the results, i.e., individuals participating in this study were recruited at a private institution, presenting at least six years of education without a great disparity between educational levels.

Studies assessing the association between levels of anterior gingival enlargement and socioeconomic as well as clinical conditions in orthodontic subjects (using multiple regression analyses controlled for other socio-demographic and clinical variables which may act as confounders) are inexistent. From this perspective, the present study provides new information. In addition, Poisson regression with robust variance was used in order to provide PR estimates which are easier to interpret than odd ratios. In a situation of anterior gingival enlargement, with prevalence higher than 50%, odd ratios would strongly overestimate PRs.[32] It is important to highlight that this study had a cross-sectional design, which hypothesizes relations between the outcome and predictor variables without establishing causal relationships. This is a limitation of this study. However, conclusions from cross-sectional studies are important to identify indicators that may be included in longitudinal or, even, experimental studies. The present study comprised 330 orthodontic patients attending a private orthodontic specialist training program. This sample limited the extent to which these findings can be generalized to a larger population. Nevertheless, analyses were performed with sufficient power and the analytical results strengthen the hypotheses of this study.

Evidence shows that gingival enlargement is associated with esthetic impairment and, in more severe cases, with phonetic alterations and masticatory problems.[7] A recent publication[21] conducted with an orthodontic sample emphasized the impact of anterior gingival enlargement in oral health related quality of life (OHRQoL). Thus, prevention and/or treatment of gingival enlargement may contribute to improve the OHRQoL of orthodontic patients. According to our results, proximal anterior bleeding and excess resin around brackets were associated with higher levels of anterior gingival enlargement. However, further studies are required to understand whethwe it is possible that prevention and treatment of gingivitis and careful bonding of brackets may result in decrease in the prevalence or even the severity of GE in orthodontic subjects.

CONCLUSIONS

Anterior gingival enlargement is associated with gingival inflammation and excess resin around brackets.

Acknowledgements

The authors would like to thank all volunteers participating in the present research, as well as UNINGÁ for allowing us to use its dental clinics.

REFERENCES

1. Trombelli L, Scapoli C, Tatakis DN, Grassi L. Modulation of clinical expression of plaque-induced gingivitis: effects of personality traits, social support and stress. J Clin Periodontol. 2005;32(11):1143-50.

2. Antoniazzi RP, Miranda LA, Zanatta FB, Islabao AG, Gustafsson A, Chiapinotto GA, et al. Periodontal conditions of individuals with Sjogren's syndrome. J Periodontol. 2009;80(3):429-35.

3. Levin L, Samorodnitzky-Naveh GR, Machtei EE. The association of orthodontic treatment and fixed retainers with gingival health. J Periodontol. 2008;79(11):2087-92.

4. Polson AM, Subtelny JD, Meitner SW, Polson AP, Sommers EW, Iker HP, et al. Long-term periodontal status after orthodontic treatment. Am J Orthod Dentofacial Orthop. 1988;93(1):51-8.

5. Zachrisson S, Zachrisson BU. Gingival condition associated with orthodontic treatment. Angle Orthod. 1972;42(1):26-34.

6. Kloehn JS, Pfeifer JS. The effect of orthodontic treatment on the periodontium. Angle Orthod. 1974;44(2):127-34.

7. Kouraki E, Bissada NF, Palomo JM, Ficara AJ. Gingival enlargement and resolution during and after orthodontic treatment. N Y State Dent J. 2005;71(4):34-7.

8. Trackman PC, Kantarci A. Connective tissue metabolism and gingival overgrowth. Crit Rev Oral Biol Med. 2004;15(3):165-75.

9. Reali L, Zuliani E, Gabutti L, Schonholzer C, Marone C. Poor oral hygiene enhances gingival overgrowth caused by calcineurin inhibitors. J Clin Pharm Ther. 2009;34(3):255-60.

10. Somacarrera ML, Lucas M, Scully C, Barrios C. Effectiveness of periodontal treatments on cyclosporine-induced gingival overgrowth in transplant patients. Br Dent J. 1997;183(3):89-94.

11. Gomes SC, Varela CC, Veiga SL, Rosing CK, Oppermann RV. Periodontal conditions in subjects following orthodontic therapy. A preliminary study. Eur J Orthod. 2007;29(5):477-81.

12. Sadowsky C, Begole EA. Long-term effects of orthodontic treatment on periodontal health. Am J Orthod Dentofacial Orthop. 1981;80(2):156-72.

13. Diamanti-Kipioti A, Gusberti FA, Lang NP. Clinical and microbiological effects of fixed orthodontic appliances. J Clin Periodontol. 1987;14(6):326-33.

14. Paolantonio M, Festa F, di Placido G, D'Attilio M, Catamo G, Piccolomini R. Site-specific subgingival colonization by Actinobacillus actinomycetemcomitans in orthodontic patients. Am J Orthod Dentofacial Orthop. 1999;115(4):423-8.

15. Lee SM, Yoo SY, Kim HS, Kim KW, Yoon YJ, Lim SH, et al. Prevalence of putative periodontopathogens in subgingival dental plaques from gingivitis lesions in Korean orthodontic patients. J Microbiol. 2005;43(3):260-5.

16. Lo BA, Di Marco R, Milazzo I, Nicolosi D, Cali G, Rossetti B, et al. Microbiological and clinical periodontal effects of fixed orthodontic appliances in pediatric patients. New Microbiol. 2008;31(2):299-302.

17. Loe H, Silness J. Periodontal disease in pregnancy. I. Prevalence and severity. Acta Odontol Scand. 1963;21:533-51.

18. Loe H. The gingival index, the plaque index and the retention index systems. J Periodontol. 1967;38(6 Suppl.):s610-6.

19. Seymour RA, Smith DG, Turnbull DN. The effects of phenytoin and sodium valproate on the periodontal health of adult epileptic patients. J Clin Periodontol. 1985;12(6):413-9.

20. Ainamo J, Bay I. Problems and proposals for recording gingivitis and plaque. Int Dent J. 1975;25(4):229-35.

21. Zanatta FB, Ardenghi TM, Antoniazzi RP, Pinto TM, Rosing CK. Association between gingival bleeding and gingival enlargement and Oral health-related quality of life (OHRQoL) of subjects under fixed orthodontic treatment: a cross-sectional study. BMC Oral Health. 2012;12(1):53.

22. Zanatta FB, Moreira CH, Rosing CK. Association between dental floss use and gingival conditions in orthodontic patients. Am J Orthod Dentofacial Orthop. 2011;140(6):812-21.

23. Greenstein G, Caton J, Polson AM. Histologic characteristics associated with bleeding after probing and visual signs of inflammation. J Periodontol. 1981;52(8):420-5.

24. Polson AM, Greenstein G, Caton J. Relationships between epithelium and connective tissue in inflamed gingiva. J Periodontol. 1981;52(12):743-6.

25. Sharma NC, Charles CH, Qaqish JG, Galustians HJ, Zhao Q, Kumar LD. Comparative effectiveness of an essential oil mouthrinse and dental floss in controlling interproximal gingivitis and plaque. Am J Dent. 2002;15(6):351-5.

26. Finkelstein P, Grossman E. The effectiveness of dental floss in reducing gingival inflammation. J Dent Res. 1979;58(3):1034-9.

27. Lobene RR, Soparkar PM, Newman MB. Use of dental floss. Effect on plaque and gingivitis. Clin Prev Dent. 1982;4(1):5-8.

28. Reitman WR, Whiteley RT, Robertson PB. Proximal surface cleaning by dental floss. Clin Prev Dent. 1980;2(3):7-10.

29. Al-Marzok MI, Al-Azzawi HJ. The effect of the surface roughness of porcelain on the adhesion of oral Streptococcus mutans. J Contemp Dent Pract. 2009;10(6):E017-24.

30. Aykent F, Yondem I, Ozyesil AG, Gunal SK, Avunduk MC, Ozkan S. Effect of different finishing techniques for restorative materials on surface roughness and bacterial adhesion. J Prosthet Dent. 2010;103(4):221-7.

31. Sisson KL. Theoretical explanations for social inequalities in oral health. Community Dent Oral Epidemiol. 2007;35(2):81-8.

32. Barros AJ, Hirakata VN. Alternatives for logistic regression in cross-sectional studies: an empirical comparison of models that directly estimate the prevalence ratio. BMC Med Res Methodol. 2003;3:21.

10

Three-dimensional assessment of external apical root resorption after maxillary posterior teeth intrusion with miniscrews in anterior open bite patients

Bilal Al-Falahi[1], Ahmad Mohammad Hafez[1], Maher Fouda[1]

Objective: The objective of this study was to assess the external apical root resorption (EARR) of the maxillary posterior teeth after intrusion with miniscrews. **Methods:** Fifteen patients (13 females and 2 males) with age ranging from 14.5 to 22 years (mean 18.1 ±2.03 years) were selected to participate in this study. All patients presented with anterior open bite of 3 mm or more. An intrusion force of 300 g was applied on each side to intrude the maxillary posterior teeth. Cone beam computed tomography (CBCT) scans were taken pretreatment and post-intrusion and were analyzed to evaluate the EARR. **Results:** The maxillary posterior teeth were intruded in average 2.79 ± 0.46 mm ($p<0.001$) in 5.1 ± 1.3 months, and all examined roots showed statistically significant EARR ($p < 0.05$) with an average of 0.55 mm, except the distobuccal root of the left first permanent molars and both the palatal and buccal roots of left first premolars, which showed no statistically significant changes. **Conclusions:** The evaluated teeth presented statistically significant EARR, but clinically, due to the small magnitude, it was not considered significant. Moreover, the CBCT provided a good visualization of all roots in all three planes, and it was effective in detecting minimal degrees of EARR.

Keywords: Root resorption. Molar intrusion. Miniscrews. CBCT. Anterior open bite.

[1] Mansoura University, Faculty of Dentistry, Department of Orthodontics
(Mansoura, Egypt).

» The authors report no commercial, proprietary or financial interest in the products
or companies described in this article.

Bilal Al-Falahi
Orthodontics Department, Faculty of Dentistry, Mansoura University
Mansoura, Dakahlia, Egypt. E-mail: bilalm2004@yahoo.com

INTRODUCTION

Treatment of anterior open bite has been considered one of the most challenging orthodontic therapies. True molar intrusion is usually needed to correct the skeletal open bite without orthognathic surgery.[1,2]

In the last years, skeletal anchorage devices, including miniplates and miniscrews, gained more popularity due to their ability to provide stable anchorage throughout orthodontic treatment.[3-5] Orthodontic treatment may be the most common cause of EARR in the modern world. The treatment duration, magnitude of applied force, direction of tooth movement, amount of apical displacement, and method of force application are considered the most related risk factors to the EARR.[6] Furthermore, EARR is one of the most difficult procedure-related adverse events to predict in cases of orthodontic tooth movement (OTM), and may cause permanent loss of the dental structure at the root apex.[7] EARR is characterized by loss of the external surface layer of cells that protect the tooth roots by the action of clastic cells and hyalinization. Its prevalence is high and it depends on different factors, such as root shape, tooth groups, and measuring techniques.[8-10] However, Roscoe et al[11] found that there is a positive correlation between the amount of orthodontic force, treatment time and increased EARR.

Several studies[6,8,9,15-23] were conducted to evaluate the EARR of teeth. Research also suggested that individuals with skeletal anterior open bite were at a greater risk of developing EARR during orthodontic treatment than individuals with other types of malocclusion.[21] Orthodontic intrusion has been described as one of the worst types of OTM in relation to susceptibility to EARR.[22] Han et al[23] also concluded that teeth intrusion has four times more chances to cause EARR than extrusion.

Several studies[2,24,25] evaluated the EARR after intrusion. However, these studies had used conventional radiographic exams, such as the lateral cephalogram, panoramic and periapical films, to detect the presence of EARR. In addition, these studies were not accurate enough to evaluate the amount of resorption, due to the magnification errors, which might lead to underestimation or overestimation of the amount of root resorption.[26,27] Besides, due to the overlapping of images, not all roots could be examined, such as the palatal roots.

After the scientific and technological developments of medical imaging exams, CBCT was introduced to be a specific diagnostic tool for dentistry.[28,29] The accuracy of CBCT radiography has already been proved, providing more precise three-dimensional images of the teeth than conventional radiographs.[26,30-34]

As an examination tool, though, CBCT should be carefully used. The CBCT exposure dose might be 7 to 8 times lower than that of multi-slice CT, and 5 to 6 times higher than that associated with the conventional panoramic radiograph.[35,36]

To the best of our knowledge, no study has been performed to evaluate EARR in all posterior teeth in both right and left sides after intrusion with miniscrews in patients with anterior open bite. Therefore, the aim of this study was to evaluate the EARR after intrusion, using measurements based on CBCT.

MATERIAL AND METHODS

This study was approved by the Ethical Research Committee, Faculty of Dentistry, Mansoura University (Code No: 15020418).

The sample size was calculated for the difference in maxillary molar length based on a paired samples t-test using the software PS Power and Sample Size Calculations v. 3.1.2 (Department of Biostatistics, Vanderbilt University School of Medicine, Nashville, Tennessee, USA). The mean difference tested for was 0.71 mm. A more liberal standard deviation of the mean difference that was reported by Ari-Demirkaya et al[2] was used ($\sigma = 0.66$ mm), with type I error (alpha significance level) of 0.05 and power of 90%. The estimated sample size was 11 subjects.

A sample of fifteen patients was selected to participate in this prospective clinical trial. High angle patients with skeletal Class I, II or mild Class III relationship were enrolled in this study. Moderate to severe Class III skeletal relationship patients were excluded, as the molars intrusion would lead to increase the severity of Class III malocclusion. CBCT was used to evaluate 260 roots of 15 non-growing patients (13 female and 2 males), with age ranging from 14.5 to 22 years (mean age of 18.1 ±2.03 years).

The patients included in this study were selected according to the following criteria:

1. Patients with anterior open bite requiring maxillary posterior teeth intrusion as part of orthodontic treatment.

2. Long-face pattern, with anterior open bite equal to or greater than 3 mm.

3. Healthy adult patients.

4. No previous orthodontic treatment.

5. No evidence of either periodontal problems, gingival problems, or bruxism, at the beginning of orthodontic treatment.

6. No medical problems interfering with orthodontic treatment.

However, patients with a history of trauma and all teeth with endodontically treated roots or with big restoration were excluded from this study.

Orthodontic treatment progress

Orthodontic bands were cemented on maxillary first and second premolars and first and second permanent molars. Then leveling and alignment were started using sectional wires changed every two weeks, in the following sequence: 0.016-in NiTi, 0.018-in NiTi, 0.016 x 0.022-in NiTi, 0.016 x 0.022-in SS, and 0.017 x 0.025-in SS.

After leveling and alignment, an impression was taken with the bands on the teeth. Later, the bands were removed of the teeth and reseated on the impression. The impression was delivered to the laboratory for manufacture of the appliance (Fig 1).

The appliance was cemented and a self-drilling titanium alloy mini-screw (1.8 mm in diameter and 8 mm in length) was inserted into the buccal alveolar bone, between the second premolar and first permanent molar on each side. Loading of the miniscrews was initiated two days after insertion and continued until sufficient intrusion had been achieved. An intrusion force of about 300 g was applied on each side by using an elastomeric chain (Memory Power Chain, Ormco™, USA) (Fig 2). Follow-up visits were assigned every two weeks until the required intrusion was obtained. After that, post-intrusion records were taken and analyzed, to evaluate the EARR. However, the orthodontic treatment was continued, with upper and lower fixed appliances, for all cases included in the study (Fig 3).

The sectional CBCT scans were obtained at pre-treatment (T_1) and post-intrusion (T_2), by using i-CAT CBCT machine (Imaging Sciences International, Hatfield, PA). The CBCT machine specifications were as follows: 0.3-mm voxel size, 120 kV, 5 mA, 14.7 seconds exposure time, and 16-cm exposure field, to avoid the exposure to excessive radiation. A three-dimensional (3D) analysis was performed for all CBCT scans, using In Vivo software version 5.01 (Anatomage, San José, USA). After performing the reorientation of the 3D image, the examiner started locating the landmarks. To calculate the amount of molar intrusion performed, difference in the linear distance from the mesio-buccal cusp of maxillary first permanent molar to the palatal plane, between the pretreatment and post-intrusion CBCT records, was measured (Fig 4); while to calculate the amount of root resorption, each cusp tip or root apex was precisely detected in all three planes (sagittal, coronal and axial), for all teeth included in the study. The In Vivo software calculated the maximum linear distance between the two landmarks located by the examiner on both the cusp tip and root apex (Fig 5). The changes between pre and post-intrusion measurements were considered as root resorption.

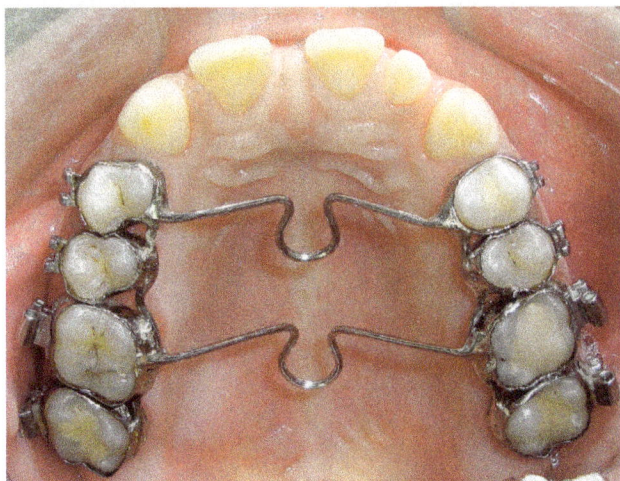

Figure 1 - Appliance used to intrude the maxillary posterior teeth.

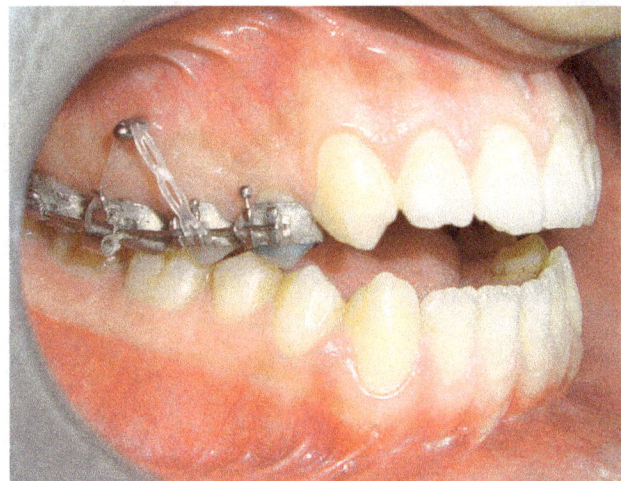

Figure 2 - Force application for intrusion.

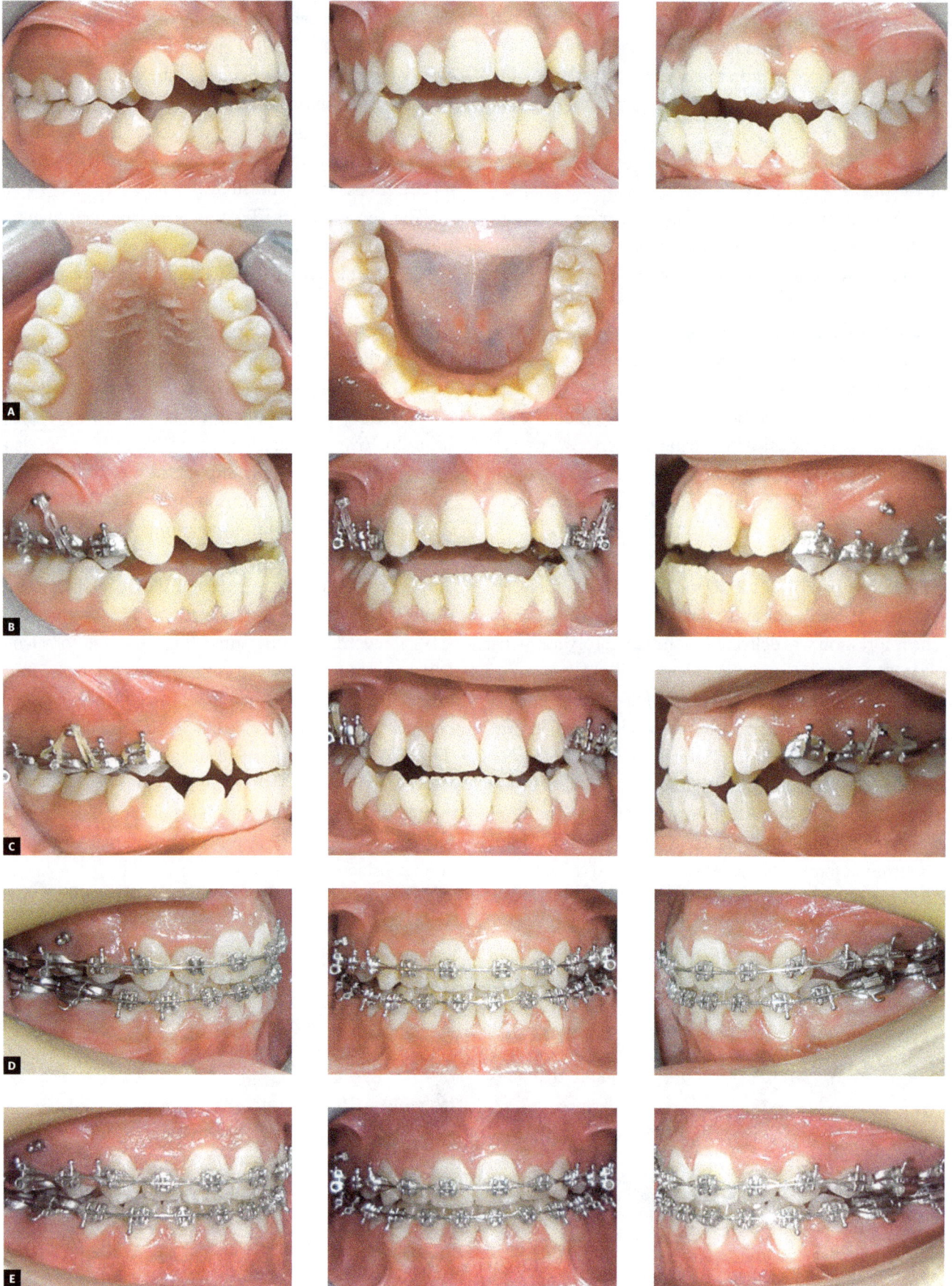

Figure 3 - Progress of treatment: **A)** pretreatment; **B)** pre-intrusion; **C)** after maxillary posterior teeth intrusion; **D, E)** progress of treatment with fixed appliance after intrusion.

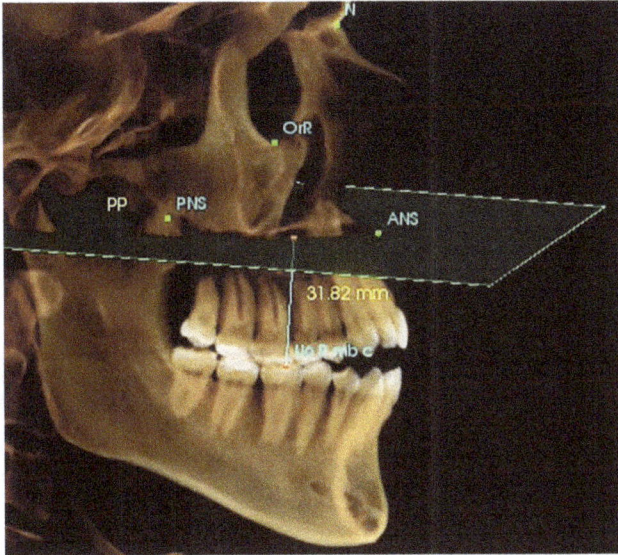

Figure 4 - Three-dimensional calculation of the linear distance between the mesio-buccal cusp of maxillary first permanent molar and the palatal plane. The palatal plane was defined as the plane passing through points ANS and PNS, and perpendicular to mid-Sagittal plane, which was constructed during reorientation of the volumetric image.

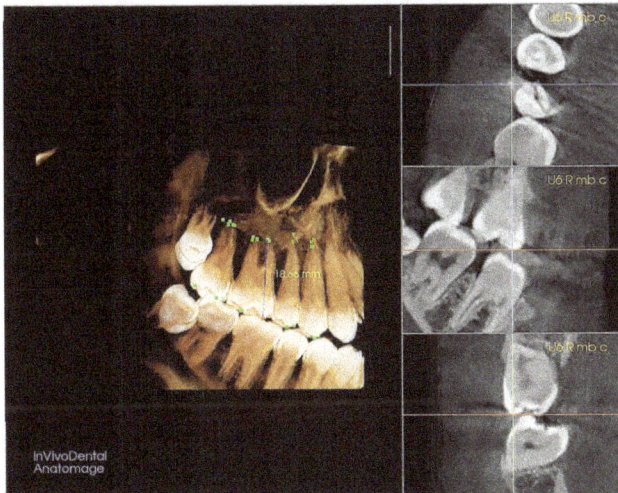

Figure 5 - The three-dimensional determination of mesio-buccal cusp landmark of permanent maxillary right first molar (U6 R mbc) on the CBCT volumetric image.

The following linear measurements were performed on the 3D volumetric images to all treated patients:

1. Tooth #27 mesiobuccal root: The linear distance between the mesiobuccal cusp and root apex of the mesiobuccal root of the maxillary left second molar.

2. Tooth #27 distobuccal root: The linear distance between the distobuccal cusp and root apex of the distobuccal root of the maxillary left second molar.

3. Tooth #27 palatal root: The linear distance between the palatal cusp and root apex of the palatal root of the maxillary left second molar.

4. Tooth #26 mesiobuccal root: The linear distance between the mesiobuccal cusp and root apex of the mesiobuccal root of the maxillary left first molar.

5. Tooth #26 distobuccal root: The linear distance between the distobuccal cusp and root apex of the distobuccal root of the maxillary left first molar.

6. Tooth #26 palatal root: The linear distance between the palatal cusp and root apex of the palatal root of the maxillary left first molar.

7. Tooth #25 buccal root: The linear distance between the buccal cusp and root apex of the buccal root of the maxillary left second premolar.

8. Tooth #24 palatal root: The linear distance between the palatal cusp and root apex of the palatal root of the maxillary left first premolar.

9. Tooth #24 buccal root: The linear distance between the buccal cusp and root apex of the buccal root of the maxillary left first premolar.

10. Tooth #17 mesiobuccal root: The linear distance between the mesiobuccal cusp and root apex of the mesiobuccal root of the maxillary right second molar.

11. Tooth #17 distobuccal root: The linear distance between the distobuccal cusp and root apex of the distobuccal root of the maxillary right second molar.

12. Tooth #17 palatal root: The linear distance between the palatal cusp and root apex of the palatal root of the maxillary right second molar.

13. Tooth #16 mesiobuccal root: The linear distance between the mesiobuccal cusp and root apex of the mesiobuccal root of the maxillary right first molar.

14. Tooth #16 distobuccal root: The linear distance between the distobuccal cusp and root apex of the distobuccal root of the maxillary right first molar.

15. Tooth #16 palatal root: The linear distance between the palatal cusp and root apex of the palatal root of the maxillary right first molar.

16. Tooth #15 buccal root: The linear distance between the buccal cusp and root apex of the buccal root of the maxillary right second premolar.

17. Tooth #14 palatal root: The linear distance between the palatal cusp and root apex of the palatal root of the maxillary right first premolar.

18. Tooth #14 buccal root: The linear distance between the buccal cusp and root apex of the buccal root of the maxillary right first premolar.

Methods error

The measurements of the present study were performed by one orthodontist, as the software needs a skilled operator to locate the landmarks. To assess the reliability of the method, the intraclass correlation coefficient (ICC) analysis was used. According to Roberts and Richmond,[37] reliability is excellent if ICC value is higher than 0.75; acceptable if it is between 0.4 and 0.75; and low if the ICC is smaller than 0.4.

In the present study, the ICC showed excellent intra-examiner reliability. The ICC for linear measurements showed an average of 92.6%, with a range from 0.827 to 0.995, and the used method presented high reproducibility.

Statistical analysis

The statistical analysis was performed with the software Statistical Package for the Social Sciences v. 24.0 (SPSS, Chicago, IL, USA). Data were explored for normality using Shapiro-Wilk test, showing normal distribution. A descriptive statistical analysis was used to present the data as mean and standard deviation (SD). Paired sample t-test was used to evaluate the significance of the difference in the pre- and post-intrusion data.

RESULTS

The maxillary posterior teeth were truly intruded, with an average of 2.79 ± 0.46 mm. The mean time for maxillary posterior teeth intrusion was 5.1 ± 1.3 months. Results of the present study revealed that all examined roots showed statistically significant ($p < 0.05$) EARR, which ranged from 0.34 to 0.74 mm, between pre- and post-intrusion measurements (Table 1).

DISCUSSION

The aim of the present study was to evaluate the EARR of maxillary posterior teeth after intrusion, by using CBCT. According to the literatures, there is no safe tooth movement with regard to EARR. Because intrusion is probably the most detrimental to the roots involved,[25,38] this study attempted to evaluate the effects on root structure caused by intrusion of posterior teeth with mini-implants.

The identification of the landmarks is considered the main source of error inherent in the measuring procedure. The conventional two-dimensional imaging methods show a high frequency and overestimate EARR after orthodontic treatment;[12,14-16] however, CBCT images provided a more accurate analysis of treatment results. By comparing the accuracy of CBCT to that of periapical radiographs with regard to detection of EARR, several studies showed that the three-dimensional method was more effective and reliable.[10,29-32,36]

Although a number of studies have already evaluated EARR using CBCT images, the present study allowed a total view of resorption (possible resorption in all roots submitted to orthodontic forces). In the present study, a specific CBCT software was used to obtain accurate linear measurements of teeth in millimeters. Crowns without metal restorations or fractures were included in the study to ensure good visualization of the images and to avoid image artifacts. Three-dimensional tracing of volumetric CBCT images allows an accurate detection of a specific landmark in all three planes, and minimizes limitations inherent to conventional two-dimensional radiographs, such as lack of standardized radiographic technique and overlapping of teeth. However, from the

Table 1 - Pre- and post-intrusion changes and significance.

Variables	Pre-intrusion		Post-intrusion		Difference		P-value	Significance[a]
	Mean	SD	Mean	SD	Mean	SD		
Maxillary second molars distobuccal root	18.60	1.30	18.07	1.28	0.53	0.40	0.004	**
Maxillary second molars mesiobuccal root	19.87	1.29	19.23	1.35	0.34	0.40	0.033	*
Maxillary second molars palatal root	20.32	1.43	19.57	1.71	0.74	0.63	0.008	**
Maxillary first molars mesiobuccal root	19.49	0.84	18.87	0.95	0.61	0.43	0.003	**
Maxillary first molars distobuccal root	18.71	0.92	18.09	1.00	0.62	0.45	0.003	**
Maxillary first molars palatal root	20.94	1.29	20.24	1.47	0.70	0.50	0.003	**
Maxillary second premolars buccal root	20.93	1.12	20.44	1.23	0.48	0.53	0.026	*
Maxillary first premolars buccal root	21.15	1.38	20.58	1.13	0.57	0.56	0.017	*
Maxillary first premolars palatal root	19.89	1.03	19.37	1.08	0.52	0.54	0.020	*

[a] NS= non-significant; * $p < 0.05$; ** $p < 0.01$; *** $p < 0.001$.

insignificantly small method error, it can be concluded that the CBCT images and the software used in this study have the ability to provide a clear 3D image that shows the small details of different anatomical landmarks of the teeth, thus minimizing the possible errors during measuring procedures.

In this study, the maxillary posterior teeth were effectively intruded a mean of 2.79 ± 0.46 mm in 5.1 ± 1.3 months. Results showed that all intruded teeth presented with statistically significant EARR, with a mean of 0.55 mm, ranging from 0.34 to 0.74 mm. This result is in harmony with the findings of Heravi et al,[24] of 0.3-0.4 mm of root length loss, and Li et al,[26] who reported statistically significant EARR. On the other hand, there were less EARR in this study than in the one reported by Dermaut and De Munck[25] (2.5mm), as they had evaluated the EARR in the maxillary incisors, where there was more occurrence of EARR with continuous forces.[14,15] Acar et al[39] indicated that the application of intermittent force results in less EARR than does the application of continuous force. Moreover, Ari-Demirkaya et al[2] reported higher EARR after intrusion of maxillary first molars (0.8 mm). This difference may be due to the longer duration of treatment (20 months), in comparison with 5.1 months in this study. In addition, they used panoramic radiographs to assess EARR, which can overestimate resorption amount.[12] On the contrary, there were less EARR in this study than in the one reported by Castro et al.[10] The difference in the type of tooth movements,[23,40] as they studied the EARR in patients with crowding treated with nonextraction strategy, might explain the different results.

The correlation between EARR and orthodontic treatment has been thoroughly studied, but the comparison of the results is difficult as a result of heterogeneity among different studies, regarding techniques of treatment, radiographic evaluation criteria, and imaging methods.[12,16,17,19] Although the results of the present study were statistically significant, it is still considered clinically non-significant. The relatively small amount of EARR may be due to the optimal level of force used (300 g), as the high force levels correlate to the EARR, in addition to the relatively small intrusion period (5.1 ± 1.3 months).[11,13,33]

This study evaluated the EARR of all maxillary posterior teeth in both sides after orthodontic intrusion, by using a 3D analysis software that helped to analyze a volumetric image by which the anatomical landmarks were located directly on the 3D image. So, all parts of the tooth structures were visualized without overlapping, in a very clear and accurate image.

CONCLUSIONS

» All evaluated teeth had statistically significant EARR; but, because of its small magnitude, it should be considered as clinically irrelevant.

» The CBCT provided a good visualization of all examined roots in all three planes of space, specially the palatal roots of posterior teeth, without overlapping or magnification errors.

Author's Contribution (ORCID ⓘ)

Bilal Al-Falahi (BAF): 0000-0001-5973-8761 ⓘ
Ahmad M. Hafez (AMH): 0000-0003-2048-5087 ⓘ
Maher Fouda (MF): 0000-0002-7248-8514 ⓘ

Conception or design of the study: BAF, MF. Data acquisition, analysis or interpretation: BAF, AMH, MF. Writing the article: BAF. Critical revision of the article: BAF, AMH, MF. Final approval of the article: BAF, AMH, MF.

REFERENCES

1. Buschang PH, Sankey W EJ. Early treatment of hyperdivergent open-bite malocclusions. Semin Orthod. 2002;8(4):130–40.

2. Ari-Demirkaya A, Al Masry M, Erverdi N. Apical root resorption of maxillary first molars after intrusion with zygomatic skeletal anchorage. Angle Orthod. 2005;75(5):761–7.

3. Creekmore TD, Eklund MK. The possibility of skeletal anchorage. J. Clin. Orthod. 1983;17(4):266–9.

4. Costa A, Raffainl M, Melsen B. Miniscrews as orthodontic anchorage: a preliminary report. Int J Adult Orthodon Orthognath Surg. 1998;13(3):201–9.

5. Sherwood KH, Burch JG, Thompson WJ. Closing anterior open bites by intruding molars with titanium miniplate anchorage. Am J Orthod Dentofacial Orthop. 2002;122(6):593–600.

6. Weltman B, Vig KW, Fields HW, Shanker S, Kaizar EE. Root resorption associated with orthodontic tooth movement: a systematic. Am J Orthod Dentofacial Orthop. 2010 Apr;137(4):462-76; discussion 12A.

7. Hikida T, Yamaguchi M, Shimizu M, Kikuta J, Yoshino T, Kasai K. Comparisons of orthodontic root resorption under heavy and jiggling reciprocating forces during experimental tooth movement in a rat model. Korean J Orthod. 2016;46(4):228–41.

8. Gunraj MN. Dental root resorption. Oral Surg. Oral Med Oral Pathol Oral Radiol Endod. 1999;88(6):647–53.

9. Fuss Z, Tsesis I, Lin S. Root resorption--diagnosis, classification and treatment choices based on stimulation factors. Dent Traumatol. 2003;19(4):175–82.

10. Castro IO, Alencar AHG, Valladares-Neto J, Estrela C. Apical root resorption due to orthodontic treatment detected by cone beam computed tomography. Angle Orthod. 2013;83(2):196–203.

11. Roscoe MG, Meira JBC, Cattaneo PM. Association of orthodontic force system and root resorption: a systematic review. Am J Orthod Dentofacial Orthop. 2015;147(5):610-26.

12. Sameshima GT, Asgarifar KO. Assessment of root resorption and root shape: periapical vs panoramic films. Angle Orthod. 2001;71(3):185–9.

13. Segal GR, Schiffman PH, Tuncay OC. Meta analysis of the treatment-related factors of external apical root resorption. Orthod Craniofac Res. 2004;7(2):71–8.

14. Apajalahti S, Peltola JS. Apical root resorption after orthodontic treatment -- a retrospective study. Eur J Orthod. 2007;29(4):408–12.

15. Malmgren O, Goldson L, Hill C, Orwin A, Petrini L, Lundberg M. Root resorption after orthodontic treatment of traumatized teeth. Am J Orthod. 1982;82(6):487–91.

16. Levander E, Malmgren O. Evaluation of the risk of root resorption during orthodontic treatment: a study of upper incisors. Eur J Orthod. 1988;10(1):30–8.

17. Janson GR, Canto GL, Martins DR, Henriques JF, Freitas MR. A radiographic comparison of apical root resorption after orthodontic treatment with 3 different fixed appliance techniques. Am J Orthod Dentofacial Orthop. 2000;118(3):262–73.

18. Sameshima GT, Sinclair PM. Predicting and preventing root resorption: Part II. Treatment factors. Am J Orthod Dentofacial Orthop. 2001;119(5):511–5.

19. Harris EF, Boggan BW, Wheeler DA. Apical root resorption in patients treated with comprehensive orthodontics. J Tenn Dent Assoc. 2001;81(1):30–3.

20. Maués CPR, Nascimento RR do, Vilella OV. Severe root resorption resulting from orthodontic treatment: Prevalence and risk factors. Dental Press J Orthod. 2015;20(1):52–8.

21. Harris EF, Butler ML. Patterns of incisor root resorption before and after orthodontic correction in cases with anterior open bites. Am J Orthod Dentofacial Orthop. 1992;101(2):112–9.

22. Harry MR, Sims MR. Root resorption in bicuspid intrusion. A scanning electron microscope study. Angle Orthod. 1982;52(3):235–58.

23. Han G, Huang S, Von den Hoff JW, Zeng X, Kuijpers-Jagtman AM. Root resorption after orthodontic intrusion and extrusion: an intraindividual study. Angle Orthod. 2005;75(6):912–8.

24. Heravi F, Bayani S, Madani AS, Radvar M, Anbiaee N. Intrusion of supra-erupted molars using miniscrews: clinical success and root resorption. Am J Orthod Dentofacial Orthop. 2011;139(4 Suppl):S170-5.

25. Dermaut LR, De Munck A. Apical root resorption of upper incisors caused by intrusive tooth movement: a radiographic study. Am J Orthod Dentofacial Orthop. 1986;90(4):321–6.

26. Li W, Chen F, Zhang F, Ding W, Ye Q, Shi J, et al. Volumetric measurement of root resorption following molar mini-screw implant intrusion using cone beam computed tomography. PLoS One. 2013 Apr 9;8(4):e60962.

27. Yu L, He S, Chen S. Diagnostic accuracy of orthopantomogram and periapical film in evaluating root resorption associated with orthodontic force. Hua Xi Kou Qiang Yi Xue Za Zhi. 2012 Apr;30(2):169-72.

28. Mozzo P, Procacci C, Tacconi A, Martini PT, Andreis IA. A new volumetric CT machine for dental imaging based on the cone-beam technique: preliminary results. Eur Radiol. 1998;8(9):1558–64.

29. Arai Y, Tammisalo E, Iwai K, Hashimoto K SK. Development of a compact computed apparatus for dental use. Dentomaxillofac Radiol. 1999 July;28(4):245-8.

30. Patel S, Dawood A, Wilson R, Horner K, Mannocci F. The detection and management of root resorption lesions using intraoral radiography and cone beam computed tomography - an in vivo investigation. Int Endod J. 2009 Sept;42(9):831-8.

31. Estrela C, Bueno MR, De Alencar AH, Mattar R, Valladares Neto J, Azevedo BC, et al. Method to Evaluate Inflammatory Root Resorption by Using Cone Beam Computed Tomography. J Endod. 2009 Nov;35(11):1491-7

32. Durack C, Patel S, Davies J, Wilson R, Mannocci F. Diagnostic accuracy of small volume cone beam computed tomography and intraoral periapical radiography for the detection of simulated external inflammatory root resorption. Int Endod J. 2011 Feb;44(2):136-47.

33. Lunardi D, Be´ cavin T, Gambiez A, Deveaux E. Orthodontically induced inflammatory root resorption: apical and cervical complications. J Dentofacial Anom Orthod. 2013;16:102.

34. Lima TF, Gamba TO, Zaia AA, Soares AJ. Evaluation of cone beam computed tomography and periapical radiography in the diagnosis of root resorption. Aust Dent J. 2016;61(4):425–31.

35. Silva MAG, Wolf U, Heinicke F, Bumann A, Visser H, Hirsch E. Cone-beam computed tomography for routine orthodontic treatment planning: a radiation dose evaluation. Am J Orthod Dentofacial Orthop. 2008;133(5):640.e1-5.

36. Dreiseidler T, Mischkowski RA, Neugebauer J, Ritter L, Zöller JE. Comparison of cone-beam imaging with orthopantomography and computerized tomography for assessment in presurgical implant dentistry. Int J Oral Maxillofac Implants. 2009 Mar-Apr;24(2):216-25.

37. Roberts CT, Richmond S. The design and analysis of reliability studies for the use of epidemiological and audit indices in orthodontics. Br J Orthod. 1997 May;24(2):139-47.

38. McFadden WM, Engstrom C, Engstrom H, Anholm JM. A study of the relationship between incisor intrusion and root shortening. Am J Orthod Dentofacial Orthop. 1989 Nov;96(5):390-6.

39. Acar A, Canyürek U, Kocaaga M, Erverdi N. Continuous vs. discontinuous force application and root resorption. Angle Orthod. 1999 Apr;69(2):159-63; discussion 163-4.

40. Harris DA, Jones AS, Darendeliler MA. Physical properties of root cementum: Part 8. Volumetric analysis of root resorption craters after application of controlled intrusive light and heavy orthodontic forces: A microcomputed tomography scan study. Am J Orthod Dentofacial Orthop. 2006 Nov;130(5):639-47.

11

Effectiveness of orofacial myofunctional therapy in orthodontic patients

Márcio Alexandre Homem[1], Raquel Gonçalves Vieira-Andrade[2], Saulo Gabriel Moreira Falci[3], Maria Letícia Ramos-Jorge[4], Leandro Silva Marques[2]

Objective: The aim of the present systematic review was to determine the existence of scientific evidence demonstrating the effectiveness of orofacial myofunctional therapy (OMT) as an adjuvant to orthodontic treatment in individuals with orofacial disorders. A further aim was to assess the methodological quality of the studies included in the review. **Methods:** An electronic search was performed in eight databases (Medline, BBO, LILACS, Web of Science, EMBASE, BIREME, Cochrane Library and SciELO) for papers published between January 1965 and March 2011, with no language restrictions. Selection of articles and data extraction were performed by two independent researchers. The quality of the selected articles was also assessed. **Results:** Search strategy resulted in the retrieval of 355 publications, only four of which fulfilled the eligibility criteria and qualified for final analysis. All papers selected had a high risk of bias. **Conclusions:** The findings of the present systematic review demonstrate the scarcity of consistent studies and scientific evidence supporting the use of OMT in combination with orthodontic treatment to achieve better results in the correction of dentofacial disorders in individuals with orofacial abnormalities.

Keywords: Myofunctional therapy. Orthodontics. Malocclusion.

[1] MSc in Dentistry, Federal University of the Jequitinhonha and Mucuri Valleys (UFVJM).

[2] PhD Resident in Dentistry, Federal University of Minas Gerais (UFMG).

[3] Visiting professor, Federal University of the Jequitinhonha and Mucuri Valleys (UFVJM).

[4] Adjunct professor, Department of Dentistry, Federal University of the Jequitinhonha and Mucuri Valleys (UFVJM).

» The authors report no commercial, proprietary or financial interest in the products or companies described in this article.

Saulo Gabriel Moreira Falci
Rua Tiradentes, 195E – Vila Operária – Diamantina/MG — Brazil
CEP: 39100-000 - E-mail: saulofalci@hotmail.com

INTRODUCTION

Orofacial myofunctional therapy (OMT) techniques and principles can be used either alone or in combination with other forms of therapy.[1-7] In combination with Orthodontics, OMT has been reported to be effective in the treatment of myofunctional disorders.[2,5-11] According to a number of studies, this combination leads to improvements in myofunctional capacity, allows satisfactory growth and development of the maxilla and assists in the adaptation of dentition to the new occlusal pattern.[8,12,13] However, a critical literature analysis reveals that most studies on this topic have striking methodological differences, heterogeneous samples and a lack of representativity.[3] Such limitations have led to divergent results and compromise the quality of evidence, thereby hindering interpretation and clinical application of findings.

OMT generally involves exercising the facial and cervical muscles to improve proprioception, tone and mobility.[1,14-18] The main objectives are the treatment of disorders of the stomatognathic system, such as orofacial abnormalities, mouth-breathing pattern, lip incompetence, tongue thrust habit, mandibular deviation and improper joint patterns during speech; chewing and swallowing, as well as assistance in the correction of parafunctional oral habits, such as thumb-sucking and bruxism.[1,14-24] In some cases, OMT may also assist in improving body posture, thereby contributing to overall health.[1,14-18]

Since orofacial disorders increase the degree of difficulty of orthodontic treatment and contribute to the relapse of dentofacial abnormalities,[8,9,11] OMT may be favorable to orthodontic treatment. Although the literature reports the combination of these therapies to be fundamental to achieve a satisfactory outcome in orthodontic treatment, there have been no systematic reviews carried out to investigate whether this combination is truly capable of achieving better results regarding dentofacial disorders in individuals with orofacial abnormalities.

The aim of the present systematic review was to determine scientific evidence that confirms the effectiveness of OMT as a complement to orthodontic treatment in individuals with orofacial disorders. A further aim was to assess the methodological quality of the studies included in the review.

MATERIAL AND METHODS

Eligibility criteria were defined by the authors prior to beginning the study. *In vivo* prospective, longitudinal studies and randomized and/or controlled clinical trials that evaluated the effectiveness of OMT combined with orthodontic treatment in healthy patients with dentofacial deformities were included in the review. Case reports, case series, review articles, opinions and *in vitro* studies were excluded. No restrictions were made with regard to language.

Type of intervention

Orthodontic treatment combined with OMT in patients with malocclusions and/or deficiencies in the vertical, sagittal and transverse directions and/or orofacial dyskinesia.

Search strategy

Searches were performed in the following electronic databases:

» BIREME – Latin American and Caribbean Center of Health Sciences (www.bireme.br).
» LILACS – Latin American and Caribbean Literature on Health Sciences.
» MEDLINE –Medical Literature Analysis and Retrieval System Online.
» Web of Science – Referential database with abstracts in the fields of science, social science, arts and humanities.
» Cochrane Library (http://cochrane.bvsalud.org) – database of papers with a high degree of scientific evidence, including systematic reviews, controlled clinical trials, etc.
» BBO – Brazilian Library of Dentistry.
» SciELO – Online Electronic Scientific Library.

A search was performed for articles published between January 1965 and March 2011, suing the following keywords: "myofunctional therapy", "oral myofunctional therapy", "orofacial myofunctional therapy", "myofunctional therapy effectiveness", "orthodontic treatment and therapy myofunctional", "myofunctional therapy and orthodontics". All these keywords were used in all the aforementioned databases.

Selection criteria and data extraction

Three selection phases were carried out by two independent researchers, with differences in opinion settled by consensus. Initially, all titles were analyzed to eliminate irrelevant publications, review articles, studies involving animals and *in vitro* studies. All abstracts of the publications selected in the first phase were then analyzed and only those referring to prospective, longitudinal studies and randomized clinical trials were included. The full texts of the articles selected in the second phase were read and eligibility was based on the evaluation of effectiveness of OMT in combination with orthodontic treatment.

A table was constructed with data from all studies and the findings were discussed. The following data were recorded: author, year of publication, study design, study groups, sample, age, methods/measures and assessment of results. A high level of agreement between the two researchers was achieved in this phase.

Quality assessment

Methodological quality of studies was assessed with a combination of criteria established by Moose[25] and

Prisma.[26] The risk of bias was considered low when all the following criteria were reported: 1) randomized sample selection; 2) definition of inclusion and exclusion criteria for the sample; 3) declaration of losses during follow-up; 4) use of validated measures; and 5) adequate statistical analysis. When one of these criteria was absent, the risk of bias was considered moderate. When two or more criteria were absent, the risk of bias was considered high.

RESULTS

Search strategy resulted in 355 articles. Respecting all selection phases based on the eligibility criteria, four articles qualified for final analysis. Figure 1 displays the different steps of the selection process. Table 1 offers a detailed analysis of each article selected for the present systematic review.

Quality of studies

All articles included in this review had a high risk of bias (Table 2). None of the papers selected presented information on randomized selection of the sample or definition of the inclusion and exclusion criteria.

DISCUSSION

The present findings should be interpreted with caution, as only four papers met the eligibility criteria established and none exhibited a high degree of scientific evidence.[2,5,6,7] Thus, while the studies selected indicated the efficacy of OMT in the correction of dentofacial disorders when combined with orthodontic treatment, the scarcity of consistent studies underscores the lack of scientific evidence on the actual effectiveness of OMT as a complement to orthodontic treatment.

From a methodological standpoint, all papers employed adequate statistical tests for data analysis.[2,5,6,7] However, the considerable diversity of tests, together with the low number of studies included in the present review, impede carrying out a meta-analysis. Comparisons with other studies are also limited due to differences in study design, sample selection and sample size.

Two studies included in the present systematic review[5,7] were carried out to determine the effectiveness of OMT alone (control group) and in combination with

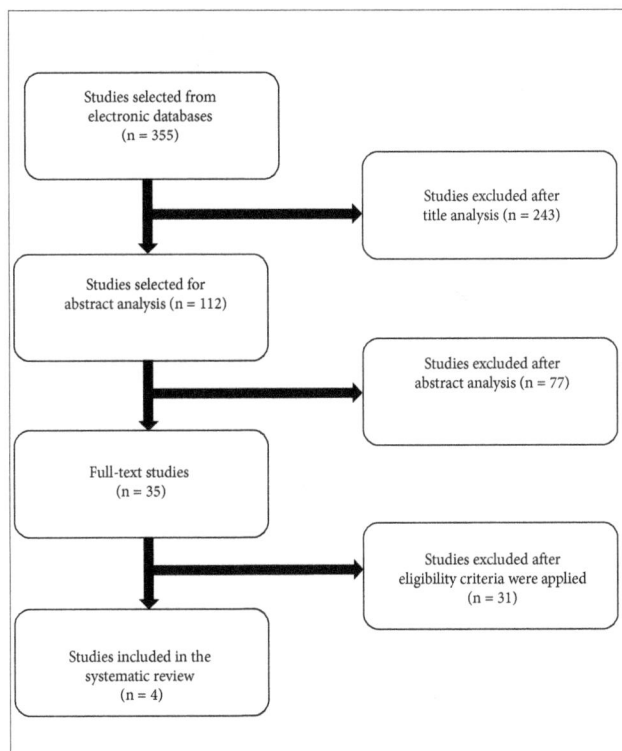

Figure 1 - Flowchart of article selection process.

Table 1 - Characteristics of studies selected.

Author (year)	Study design	Study groups	Sample	Age	Methods/ Measures	Assessment of results
Trawitzki et al[6]	LS	Experimental group: *P1 (before surgery): patients with Class III malocclusion *P3 (same patients 3 years and 3 years and 8 months after surgery): Finalization of orthodontic treatment and OMT Control group: Individuals without morphological facial abnormalities	13 15	21/42	Ultrasound of masseter muscle at rest and occlusion Linear regression test	Significantly greater (P < 0.01) masseter muscle thickness (cm) in P3 group
Smithpeter and Covell Jr[2]	LS	Patients with anterior open bite Experimental cohort group: Individuals who received orthodontic treatment or retreatment and OMT Control cohort group: Individuals with history of orthodontic treatment with relapse of open bite	27 49	8/41	T-test Analysis of covariance Linear regression Correlation coefficient	- Relapse was 0.5 mm in experimental group and 3.4 mm in control group (significant difference) - OMT combined with orthodontic treatment was more effective in closure and maintenance of closure of anterior open bite in comparison to orthodontic treatment alone
Daglio et al[5]	CCT, LS	Patients with malocclusions, deficiencies in vertical, sagittal and transverse dimensions and orofacial dyskinesis Control group (A): Treated with OMT alone Experimental group (B): treated with combined OMT and orthodontic appliance	13 15	8/17	Statistical homogeneity Payne test Frequency analysis	- Group A: Reduction in overjet from 3.5 to 2.6 mm; angle of base of mandible reduced from 30° to 28.31°; ANB angle reduced from 4.4° to 2.7°; statistically significant changes; better results with correction of overbite, which was normalized from a mean of -2.46 to 3.06 mm - Group B: Reduction in overjet from 6.6 to 2.6 mm; overbite improved from mean of -1.2 to +2.9 mm; angle of base of mandible reduced from 31.2° to 27.8°; ANB angle reduced from 7.3° to 3.7°
Daglio et al[7]	CCT, LS	Patients with orofacial dyskinensia and anterior open bite Experimental group: OMT + orthodontic treatment Control group: OMT alone	75	6/22	Payne test Homogeneity test Cephalometric analysis Correlation analysis Frequency analysis	Combination of OMT and orthodontic treatment was more successful in correction of resting lip posture than OMT alone

LS – Longitudinal Study, CCT – Controlled Clinical Trial.

Table 2 - Quality assessment of studies selected.

Quality criteria	Trawitzki et al[6]	Smithpeter and Covell Jr[2]	Daglio et al[5]	Daglio et al[7]
Randomized sample selection	No	No	No	No
Definition of inclusion and exclusion criteria	No	No	No	No
Declaration of losses during follow-up	No	Yes	No	No
Use of validated measures	Yes	Yes	No	No
Adequate statistical analysis	Yes	Yes	Yes	Yes
Estimated potential risk of bias	High	High	High	High

orthodontic treatment (experimental group). In one of these studies,[5] the authors assessed patients with malocclusions, deficiencies in the vertical, sagittal and transverse dimensions and orofacial dyskinesia. Based on the findings, the authors report that patients with dyskinesia and malocclusions can be treated with both forms of therapy. In the other study involving only patients with orofacial dyskinesis and anterior open bite,[7] the researchers found that the combination of OMT and orthodontic treatment was more successful in correcting lip incompetence than OMT alone. While their findings favor a combined therapeutic approach, the authors report that the decision regarding the use of OMT alone or in combination with orthodontic treatment is not conclusive and better planned studies are needed. Moreover, both studies have a high risk of bias and a substantial limitation, namely, that only one group was submitted to orthodontic treatment. Thus, the difference between groups is mainly related to the administration of orthodontic treatment.

Another article analyzed herein[2] assessed the effectiveness of OMT as a complement to maintaining closure of anterior open bite following orthodontic treatment or retreatment. The main conclusion was that the relapse of open bite in the experimental group treated with both orthodontics and OMT (0.48 ± 0.8 mm) was significantly less than that in the control group treated with orthodontics alone (3.38 ± 1.3 mm) (P < 0.0001). Therefore, the authors indicate the combination of these two forms of therapy for anterior open bite and stress the importance of documenting the oral and functional habits of each patient, along with the traditional orthodontic records, in any study aimed at assessing the efficacy of treatment for open bite. Such an investigation would allow one to determine what kind of patients would benefit from the combination of OMT and orthodontic treatment and what kind of patients would have a good prognosis with the use of orthodontic appliances alone.

The most recent paper selected for this review[6] assessed the effect of integrated treatment combining orthodontics, orthognathic surgery and OMT on the thickness of the masseter muscles in patients with Class III deformity. Although the study included orthognathic surgery as part of orthodontic treatment, the authors found that combined treatment with OMT and orthodontics led to an improvement in masseter muscle thickness in patients following orthognathic surgery in comparison to baseline and the control group. However, these findings should be interpreted with caution considering the high risk of bias as well as the fact that the difference between groups may have been related to the surgery itself, which was likely the main reason for the improvement in muscle thickness.

To reiterate, while the studies selected for the present systematic review indicate effectiveness of OMT in correcting dentofacial deformities when combined with orthodontic treatment, a number of limitations are found, especially with regard to the number and quality of the studies analyzed. Moreover, the papers investigated specific occlusal problems, such as anterior open bite, orofacial dyskinesia and masseter muscle thickness, which make the results quite particular to specific conditions. As one third of the population requires orthodontic treatment,[27] further studies with more rigorous methods, such as randomized, controlled clinical trials, should be carried out to determine the actual effectiveness of OMT as a complement to orthodontic treatment.

CONCLUSION

The findings of the present systematic review demonstrate a scarcity of consistent studies and scientific evidence supporting the use of OMT in combination with orthodontic treatment to achieve better results in the correction of dentofacial disorders in individuals with orofacial abnormalities. Studies with a high standard of quality and better study design are needed to establish strong scientific evidence that supports the indication of this form of combined therapy.

REFERENCES

1. Benkert KK. The effectiveness of orofacial myofunctional therapy in improving dental occlusion. Int J Orofacial Myology. 1997;23:35-46.

2. Smithpeter J, Covell D Jr. Relapse of anterior open bites treated with orthodontic appliances with and without orofacial myofunctional therapy. Am J Orthod Dentofacial Orthop. 2010;137(5):605-14.

3. Takahashi O, Iwasawa T, Takahashi M. Integrating orthodontics and oral myofunctional therapy for patients with oral myofunctional disorders. Int J Orofacial Myology. 1995;21:66-72.

4. Yamaguchi H, Sebata M. Changes in oral functions and posture at rest following surgical orthodontic treatment and myofunctional therapy. Evaluation by means of video recording. Int J Orofacial Myology. 1995;21:29-32.

5. Daglio S, Schwitzer R, Wüthrich J. Orthodontic changes in oral dyskinesia and malocclusion under the influence of myofunctional therapy. Int J Ororfacial Myology. 1993;19:15-24.

Orthodontics: Diagnosis and Treatment

7. Daglio SD, Schwitzer R, Wüthrich J, Kallivroussis G. Treating orofacial dyskinesia with functional physiotherapy in the case of frontal open bite. Int J Ororfacial Myology. 1993;19:11-4.

8. Klocke A, Korbmacher H, Kahl-Nieke B. Influence of orthodontic appliances on myofunctional therapy. J Orofac Orthop. 2000;61(6):414-20.

9. Ohono T, Yogosawa F, Nakamura K. An approach to open bite cases with tongue thrusting habits with reference to habit appliances and myofunctional therapy as viewed from an orthodontic standpoint. Int J Orofacial Myology. 1982;7:3-10.

10. Freitas KMS, Freitas MR, Janson G, Henriques JFC, Pinzan A. Avaliação pelo índice PAR dos resultados do tratamento ortodôntico da má oclusão de Classe I tratada com extrações. Rev Dental Press Ortop Facial. 2009;13(2):94-104.

11. Toronto AS. Long-term effectiveness of oral myotherapy. Int J Oral Myol. 1975;1(4):132-6.

12. Tartaglia GM, Grandi G, Mian F, Sforza C, Ferrario VF. Non-invasive 3D facial analysis and surface electromyography during functional pre-orthodontic therapy: a preliminary report. J Appl Oral Sci. 2009;17(5):487-94.

13. Yagci A, Uysal T, Kara S, OkkeYes S. The effects of myofunctional appliance treatment on the perioral and masticatory muscles in class II, division I patients. World J Orthod. 2010;11(2):117-22.

14. Das UM, Beena JP. Effectiveness of circumoral muscle exercises in the developing dentofacial morphology in adenotonsillectomized children: an ultrasonographic evaluation. J Indian Soc Pedod Prev Dent. 2009;27(2):94-103.

15. Felicio CM, Melchior MO, Ferreira CL, Silva MA. Otologic symptoms of temporomandibular disorder and effect of orofacial myofunctional therapy. Cranio. 2008;26(2):118-25.

16. Ruscello DM. Nonspeech oral motor treatment issues related to children with developmental speech sound disorders. Lang Speech Hear Serv Sch. 2008;39(3):380-91.

17. Kumar TV, Kuriakose S. Ultrasonographic evaluation of effectiveness of circumoral muscle exercises in adenotonsillectomized children. J Clin Pediatr Dent. 2004;29(1):49-55.

18. Ray J. Orofacial myofunctional therapy in dysarthria: a study on speech intelligibility. Int J Ororfacial Myology. 2002;28:39-48.

19. Mason, RM. A retrospective and prospective view of orofacial mycology. Int J Orofacial Myology. 2008;34:5-14.

20. Degan VV, Puppin-Rontani RM. Removal of sucking habits and myofunctional therapy: establishing swallowing and tongue rest position. Pro Fono. 2005;17(3):375-82.

21. Korbmacher HM, Schwan M, Berndsen S, Berndsen S, Bull J, Kahl-Nieke B. Evaluation of a new concept of myofunctional therapy in children. Int J Orofacial Myology. 2004;30:39-52.

22. Magnusson T, Syrén M. Therapeutic jaw exercises and interocclusal appliance therapy. A comparison between two common treatments of temporomandibular disorders. Swed Dent J. 1999;23(1):27-37.

23. Tallgren A, Christiansen RL, Ash M Jr, Miller RL. Effects of a myofunctional appliance on orofacial muscle activity and structures. Angle Orthod. 1998;68(3):249-58.

24. Umberger FG, Johnston RG. The efficacy of oral myofunctional and coarticulation therapy. Int J Orofacial Myology. 1997;23:3-9.

25. Stroup DF, Berlin JA, Morton SC, Olkin I, Williamson GD, Rennie D, et al. Meta-analysis of observational studies in epidemiology: a proposal for reporting. Meta-analysisof Observational Studies in Epidemiology (MOOSE) group. J Am Med Assoc. 2000;283(15):2008-12.

26. Liberati A, Altman DG, Tetzlaff J, Mulrow C, Gotzsche PC, Ioannidis JPA, et al. The PRISMA statment for reporting systematic reviews and meta-analysis os studies that evaluate health care interventions: explanation and elaboration J Clin Epidemiol. 2009;62(10):e1-34.

27. Dias PF, Gleiser R. Orthodontic treatment need in a group of 9-12-year-old Brazilian schoolchildren. Braz Oral Res. 2009;23(2):182-9.

12

Effect of vertical placement angle on the insertion torque of mini-implants in human alveolar bone

Rafael Ribeiro Maya[1], Célia Regina Maio Pinzan-Vercelino[2], Julio de Araujo Gurgel[2]

Objective: The aim of the present *ex-vivo* study was to evaluate the effect of the vertical placement angle of mini-implants on primary stability by analyzing maximum insertion torque (MIT). **Methods:** Mini-implants were placed in 30 human cadavers, inserted at either a 90° or 60° angle to the buccal surface of the maxillary first molar. Out of 60 self-drilling mini-implants used, half were of the cylindrical type and half were of the conical type. Primary stability was assessed by means of measuring the MIT. Data were subjected to analysis of variance (ANOVA) and Newman-Keuls tests. A significance level of 5% was adopted. **Results:** The MIT was higher for both mini-implant types when they were placed at a 90° angle (17.27 and 14.40 Ncm) compared with those placed at a 60° angle (14.13 and 11.40 Ncm). **Conclusions:** MIT values were differed according to the vertical mini-implant placement angle in the maxillary posterior area. Regardless of the type of mini-implant used, placement at a 90° angle resulted in a higher MIT.

Keywords: Anchorage. Torque. Orthodontics.

» The authors report no commercial, proprietary or financial interest in the products or companies described in this article.

[1] MSc in Orthodontics, Universidade Ceuma (UNICEUMA), São Luís, Maranhão, Brazil.

[2] Professor, Universidade Ceuma (UNICEUMA), Masters Program in Dentistry, São Luis, Maranhão, Brazil.

Julio de Araujo Gurgel
Rua Cel José Braz, 480 , Marilia, São Paulo 17501570, Brazil
E-mail: gurgelja@hotmail.com

INTRODUCTION

Insertion and removal torques of mini-implants are numerical representations of the quality of primary stability achieved; therefore, such measures are important factors in the success of orthodontic anchorage by means of mini-implants.[1] Primary stability of mini-implants mainly relies on the device dimension and type, thickness of patient's cortical bone and the insertion technique used.[2,3,4] Among several factors related to mini-implant success, cortical bone thickness has been reported as a factor that affects the placement angle.[5] The current trend is to use mini-implants measuring between 1.4 and 2.0 mm because of the improved primary stability that results from placement into the inter-radicular space, as well as the improved mechanical characteristics of the interface between the mini-implant and the maxillary and mandibular cortical bone.[6,7] Although reducing the placement angle has been proven to increase the contact area between the screw and the cortical bone, angle reductions are not believed to provide greater mini-implant retention.[8]

The recommended insertion technique for mini-implants is placement at an angle relative to the long axis of teeth to help the screw reach the uppermost portion of the alveolar crest, which avoids proximity to the dental roots while placing the mini-implant in an area with more bone contact available because of the conical shape of dental roots. This angle provides adequate mechanical stability without damaging tooth roots.[1, 8-11]

The amount of maximum insertion torque (MIT) represents the quality of primary stability achieved. It is not the only factor related to the success of mini-implants, but it is a measure that can be compared; however, it is important to study the variables that influence MIT. Cortical thickness and age seem to be the patient-related factors that most influence the amount of MIT. For self-tapering mini-implants, MIT has been reported to be between 5 and 10 Ncm. Because partial osseointegration should occur for mini-implants, the MIT value represents not only primary stability, but also the numerical quantification of mini-implant stability.[3]

Technical difficulties in measuring the amount of accumulated stress and cortical bone tissue regeneration in humans has led to different types of in vitro studies. Studies of artificial bone, finite elements, animals and cadavers have shown that increased mini-implant placement angle improves stability.[12-16]

It is at present unclear how the placement angle influences the MIT.[17] However, more numerical evidence will help understanding the insertion torque variability for different insertion angles in human cortical bone.

The aim of the present ex vivo study was to evaluate the primary stability of two types of mini-implants (cylindrical and conical) by means of measuring the MIT for their placement at 90° and 60° angulation relative to the buccal surface of the maxillary first molar.

MATERIAL AND METHODS

A total of 60 self-drilling mini-implants were used with different diameters, but with the same length (Table 1). Thirty of them had a cylindrical body of 1.6 × 9 mm, while the other 30 had a conical body with dimensions of 1.8 × 9 mm. Mini-implants were placed by a single operator in 30 human cadavers (23 males and 7 females) aged between 21 and 39 years old (mean age: 29.4 years), with the posterior maxillary bone and dentition preserved. This study received approval from the institutional review board of UNICEUMA (protocol #2011/0544). The sample was divided into groups according to mini-implant type (1.8-mm conical or 1.6-mm cylindrical) and placement angle, as follows: Group 1, cylindrical mini-implants placed at a 90° angle; Group 2, cylindrical mini-implants placed at a 60° angle; Group 3, conical mini-implants placed at a 90° angle; and Group 4, conical mini-implants placed at a 60° angle (Table 1).

Because of the split-mouth design of this study, all mini-implants were placed manually on both sides of the maxilla of the same cadaver without pilot drilling. The insertion point was standardised by a millimeter probe used to measure the height at 7 mm from the gingiva margin or the tip of the papilla between the second premolar and maxillary first molar.[18] MIT values were measured with the aid of a digital torque meter (Lutron TQ-8800, Taipei, Taiwan) and a manual screwdriver suitable for every type of mini-implant. The peak placement torque value obtained during the final turn of the screwdriver during mini-implant placement was recorded for analysis. The 60° and 90° angles were standardised with a protractor positioned laterally to the maxilla. The base of the protractor touched the photograph retractor used to expose the maxillary first molar area. The manual driver tip was positioned beside the flat surface of the protractor over

Table 1 - Mini-implant specifications and codes.

Code	Group	Type	Diameter	Length	Angle	Manufacturer
CL 90	1	Cylindrical	1.6 mm	9 mm	90°	Dewimed (Germany)
CL 60	2	Cylindrical	1.6 mm	9 mm	60°	Dewimed (Germany)
CN 90	3	Conical	1.8 mm	9 mm	90°	Conexão (Brazil)
CN 60	4	Conical	1.8 mm	9 mm	60°	Conexão (Brazil)

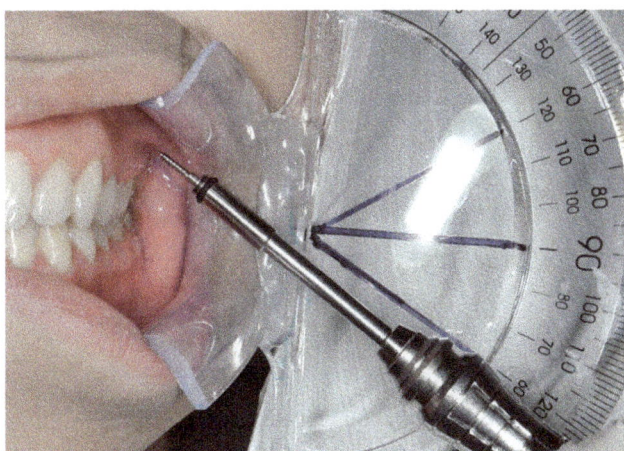

Figure 1 - The manual driver tip positioned beside the flat surface of the protractor over the 60° angle.

Table 2 - Means and standard deviation (SD) of MITs (Ncm) for two types of mini-implants and placement angles (n = 15).

Diameter	Angle	Torque (Ncm)	
		Mean	SD
1.6 mm	60°	14.13[b]	3.93
	90°	17.27[a]	3.22
1.8 mm	60°	11.40[c]	1.99
	90°	14.40[b]	2.06

Different superscript letters indicate significant differences between groups.

Table 3 - Newman-Keuls test for placement angle comparisons for each type of mini-implant.

Comparison	p value
(CL 60 vs. CL 90)	0.013 *
(CN 60 vs. CN 90)	0.018 *

* significant difference (p < 0.05).

the 60° or 90° lines that run from the protractor base line (Fig 1). Mini-implants of the same type were then placed into the same cadaver at a 90° angle on one side and a 60° angle on the other side.

To evaluate the hypothesis that the vertical placement angle would influence MIT, the values obtained for screws with the same diameter were compared. Two-way fixed-effects analysis of variance (ANOVA) and Newman-Keuls tests were used to compare MIT values. All calculations were performed by means of Statistica software Version 10.0 (StatSoft Inc., Tulsa, OK, USA). A significance level of $p < 0.05$ was adopted.

RESULTS

The mean MIT values differed among groups and varied between 11.40 and 17.27 Ncm. The mean MIT values for cylindrical mini-implants were 14.13 Ncm for the 60° angle and 17.27 Ncm for the 90° angle. The mean MIT values for the conical mini-implants were 11.40 Ncm for the 60° angle and 14.40 Ncm for the 90° angle (Table 2).

Evaluating the relationship of MIT values with the placement angles in the axial plane, we observed significant differences between Groups 1 and 2 ($p = 0.013$) and Groups 3 and 4 ($p = 0.018$). Mini-implants placed at 90° in the cortical bone exhibited greater insertion torque than those placed at 60° relative to the cortical bone (Tables 2 and 3).

DISCUSSION

In order to add information to evaluate the variables that affect mini-implant stability, this research focused on insertion torque to study angle effect as a surgery-related factor for stability. The present study reveals that the vertical placement angle of mini-implants might interfere in the amount of MIT. *Ex vivo* placing of orthodontic mini-implants at a 90° angle resulted in increased MIT. It needs to be emphasized that our results are related to human maxillary alveolar bone, and not to all maxillomandibular areas. For example, for the posterior mandibular area, the vertical placement angle seems necessary to increase the contact area between the screw and the cortical bone.[8]

The literature reports that axial angles from 45° to 70° are the most appropriate for preventing the screw from contacting the dental roots and increasing the amount of bone surrounding the screw.[1,9] However, such angles seem to compromise screw insertion depth and cortical bone integrity, despite providing better contact with the bone of the inter-radicular space compared with greater angles. In other words, it was not related to the 90° insertion angle. Therefore, in our study, the comparison between 90° and 60° angles was proposed because a 60° angle represents a mean point of the rate for vertical angle placement recommended in the literature, which is between 45° to 70°.[1,9] Another study in human alveolar bone did not find any influence regarding placement angle; nevertheless, this clinical study was performed in multiple maxillomandibular areas with three different types of screw.[2]

The placement area between the second premolar and maxillary first molar was chosen because it provides the widest maxillary inter-radicular space and it is, therefore, a safe space for mini-implant placement.[8,18-22] The standardization of insertion height at 7 mm away from the interdental papilla made it possible to place mini-implants in the attached gingiva, and also to have a sufficient inter-radicular space.[18,19,21,23,24]

Although routinely used in dental studies, human cadavers present some restrictions in clinical applications. There was some concern regarding variability in the post-mortem interval among cadavers; therefore, the experiment used newly deceased cadavers (up to 24 hours post-mortem), so that the cortical bone density of the sample components could be compared.[24,25] For greater reliability of the obtained results and to reduce standard deviation, we used more cadavers than the average commonly reported in the literature for this type of study.[14,26-31]

Similarly to our findings, studies using several experimental models have shown that a mini-implant angle of 90° relative to the cortical bone is advantageous compared with other angles indicated for technical advantages.[13] Placing orthodontic mini-implants to the alveolar process bone surface at angles less than 90° did not offer force anchorage resistance advantages.[14]

The 1.6-mm screws placed at a 90° angle displayed the greatest insertion torque, suggesting that the increased mini-implant diameter had a significant effect on insertion torque. Greater structural preservation of the cortical bone may have resulted from the lower pressure of the smaller-diameter mini-implant because larger-diameter mini-implants and greater cortical bone thickness require more insertion force.[1,9,12]

Therefore, variations in screw design and diameter lead to changes in the MIT value.[12] However, in this study, it was found that 1.6-mm mini-implants exhibited a MIT value higher than 1.8 mm for the same insertion angle. In addition, the commercial brands used in our study had different diameters and types, which did not allow statistical analysis between the types of mini-implant. Nevertheless, we were able to compare the influence of placement angle for mini-implants of the same type. Variation in placement angle may lead to reduced strain on the cortical bone, thus overcoming the increased tendency towards damage associated with increased mini-implant diameter.[13]

The insertion torque values found were similar to those observed in human cadavers[28] and in another clinical study.[3] Thus, the variations found when placement angles were compared represent changes that may also occur in patients. Furthermore, when two brands of mini-implants with different designs and diameters were used, the values differed according to whether they were placed at 60° or 90°. Regardless of the type of mini-implant used, the MIT value was higher when the implants were placed at 90°. This finding means that, for self-drilling mini-implants, placement at a 90° angle should be prioritized to reduce stress on the cortical bone.

The cylindrical mini-implant (1.6 mm) exhibited a higher MIT value, probably in regard to the cylindrical design of the screws and not as a consequence of the diameter. This reinforces a previous report in the literature, in which conical mini-implants induced more microdamage than the cylindrical ones.[12] In another study, the range for MIT in human bone was from 5 to 10 Ncm.[3] The self-drilling mini-implant used in our study exhibited higher MIT values; thus, the high MIT is related to the drill-free system insertion technique.[17,32]

Conflicting findings concerning factors that influence MIT values have yielded no evidence to suggest that specific MIT levels result in higher success rates for mini-implants.[17] Therefore, it is not possible to understand the high torque values obtained here as overload of the cortical bone. Furthermore, our results obtained in human cortical bone will help to provide better association and quantitative records to identify a specific relationship with mini-implant primary stability. In previous human studies, the mini-implant system used increased MIT values with self-drilling insertion when compared with self-tapping.[32,33] Also, variations in the MIT value for human cortical bone have been presented, possibly as a consequence of the different devices (mechanical and digital) used to record torque during mini-implant placement.[34] In our research, we used a digital instead of mechanical torquimeter to provide more accurate values.[17,35]

Histological studies have shown that mini-implant design affects the amount of damage caused to the cortical bone and may be useful in clarifying the types of changes in the area of contact between the mini-implant and the cortical bone associated with MIT.[29,36]

The quantity and quality of cortical bone on the failure force of mini-implants have been shown when comparing maxillae and mandibles. In our study, we analyzed the mini-implant/cortical bone interface related to the posterior maxillary alveolar region.

The same results should not be extrapolated to other areas, such as the posterior mandibular cortical bone. Cortical bone thickness and bone hardness of mandibles are different when compared with maxillae, mainly in the posterior region.[1,7,11]

An *in vitro* study, which did not take into consideration different cortical bone thickness, reported that angled insertion provides greater MIT as a consequence of increased contact in the mini-implant–cortical bone interface.[37] The results of this present study suggest that the characteristics of the alveolar cortical bone should be taken into consideration when determining a suitable placement angle for mini-implant insertion.

Future studies should analyze whether damage to the cortical bone surface and/or reduced screw insertion depth are associated with the vertical placement angle of the mini-implant. Additionally, further research should be conducted to investigate mini-implant placement in other sites, especially those with different buccal cortical bone thicknesses.

CONCLUSION

Based on the results of this *ex vivo* study, MIT values differed according to the vertical mini-implant placement angle in the maxillary posterior area. Regardless of the type of mini-implant used, placement at a 90° angle resulted in higher MITs.

REFERENCES

1. Watanabe H, Deguchi T, Hasegawa M, Ito M, Kim S, Takano-Yamamoto T. Orthodontic miniscrew failure rate and root proximity, insertion angle, bone contact length, and bone density. Orthod Craniofac Res. 2013 Feb;16(1):44-55.

2. Park HS, Jeong SH, Kwon OW. Factors affecting the clinical success of screw implants used as orthodontic anchorage. Am J Orthod Dentofacial Orthop. 2006 July;130(1):18-25.

3. Motoyoshi M, Yoshida T, Ono A, Shimizu N. Effect of cortical bone thickness and implant placement torque on stability of orthodontic mini-implants. Int J Oral Maxillofac Implants. 2007 Sept-Oct;22(5):779-84.

4. Chen YJ, Chang HH, Huang CY, Hung HC, Lai EH, Yao CC. A retrospective analysis of the failure rate of three different orthodontic skeletal anchorage systems. Clin Oral Implants Res. 2007 Dec;18(6):768-75.

5. Santos RF, Ruellas ACO, Fernandes DJ, Elias CN. Insertion torque versus mechanical resistance of mini-implants inserted in different cortical thickness. Dental Press J Orthod. 2014 May-June;19(3):90-4.

6. Motoyoshi M, Uemura M, Ono A, Okazaki K, Shigeeda T, Shimizu N. Factors affecting the long-term stability of orthodontic mini-implants. Am J Orthod Dentofacial Orthop. 2010 May;137(5):588.e1-5; discussion 588-9.

7. Monnerat-Aylmer C, Restle L, Mucha JN. Tomographic mapping of mandibular interradicular spaces for placement of orthodontic mini-implants. Am J Orthod Dentofacial Orthop. 2009 Apr;135(4):428-37.

8. Lim JE, Lee SJ, Kim YJ, Lim WH, Chun YS. Comparison of cortical bone thickness and root proximity at maxillary and mandibular interradicular sites for orthodontic mini-implant placement. Orthod Craniofac Res. 2009 Nov;12(4):299-304.

9. Wilmes B, Su YY, Drescher D. Insertion angle impact on primary stability of orthodontic mini-implants. Angle Orthod. 2008 Nov;78(6):1065-70.

10. Poggio PM, Incorvati C, Velo S, Carano A. "Safe zones": a guide for miniscrew positioning in the maxillary and mandibular arch. Angle Orthod. 2006 Mar;76(2):191-7.

11. Baumgaertel S, Hans MG. Buccal cortical bone thickness for mini-implant placement. Am J Orthod Dentofacial Orthop. 2009 Aug;136(2):230-5.

12. Lim SA, Cha JY, Hwang CJ. Insertion torque of orthodontic miniscrews according to changes in shape, diameter and length. Angle Orthod. 2008 Mar;78(2):234-40.

13. Petrey JS, Saunders MM, Kluemper GT, Cunningham LL, Beeman CS. Temporary anchorage device insertion variables: effects on retention. Angle Orthod. 2010 July;80(4):446-53.

14. Woodall N, Tadepalli SC, Qian F, Grosland NM, Marshall SD, Southard TE. Effect of miniscrew angulation on anchorage resistance. Am J Orthod Dentofacial Orthop. 2011 Feb;139(2):e147-52.

15. Jasmine MI, Yezdani AA, Tajir F, Venu RM. Analysis of stress in bone and microimplants during en-masse retraction of maxillary and mandibular anterior teeth with different insertion angulations: a 3-dimensional finite element analysis study. Am J Orthod Dentofacial Orthop. 2012 Jan;141(1):71-80.

16. Lee SJ, Jang SY, Chun YS, Lim WH. Three-dimensional analysis of tooth movement after intrusion of a supraerupted molar using a mini-implant with partial-fixed orthodontic appliances. Angle Orthod. 2013 Mar;83(2):274-9.

17. Meursinge Reynders RA, Ronchi L, Ladu L, van Etten-Jamaludin F, Bipat S. Insertion torque and success of orthodontic mini-implants: a systematic review. Am J Orthod Dentofacial Orthop. 2012 Nov;142(5):596-614.e5.

18. Park J, Cho HJ. Three-dimensional evaluation of interradicular spaces and cortical bone thickness for the placement and initial stability of microimplants in adults. Am J Orthod Dentofacial Orthop. 2009 Sept;136(3):314.e1-12; discussion 314-5.

19. Silvestrini Biavati A, Tecco S, Migliorati M, Festa F, Marzo G, Gherlone E, et al. Three-dimensional tomographic mapping related to primary stability and structural miniscrew characteristics. Orthod Craniofac Res. 2011 May;14(2):88-99.

20. Kim HJ, Yun HS, Park HD, Kim DH, Park YC. Soft-tissue and cortical-bone thickness at orthodontic implant sites. Am J Orthod Dentofacial Orthop. 2006 Aug;130(2):177-82.

21. Santiago RC, de Paula FO, Fraga MR, Picorelli Assis NM, Vitral RW. Correlation between miniscrew stability and bone mineral density in orthodontic patients. Am J Orthod Dentofacial Orthop. 2009 Aug;136(2):243-50.

22. Martinelli FL, Luiz RR, Faria M, Nojima LI. Anatomic variability in alveolar sites for skeletal anchorage. Am J Orthod Dentofacial Orthop. 2010 Sept;138(3):252.e1-9.

23. Kuroda S, Sugawara Y, Deguchi T, Kyung HM, Takano-Yamamoto T. Clinical use of miniscrew implants as orthodontic anchorage: success rates and postoperative discomfort. Am J Orthod Dentofacial Orthop. 2007 Jan;131(1):9-15.

24. Choi JH, Park CH, Yi SW, Lim HJ, Hwang HS. Bone density measurement in interdental areas with simulated placement of orthodontic miniscrew implants. Am J Orthod Dentofacial Orthop. 2009 Dec;136(6):766.e1-12; discussion 766-7.

25. Kribbs PJ. Comparison of mandibular bone in normal and osteoporotic women. J Prosthet Dent. 1990 Feb;63(2):218-22.

26. Kingsmill VJ, Boyde A. Variation in the apparent density of human mandibular bone with age and dental status. J Anat. 1998 Feb; 192 (Pt 2):233-44.

27. Friberg B, Sennerby L, Roos J, Lekholm U. Identification of bone quality in conjunction with insertion of titanium implants. A pilot study in jaw autopsy specimens. Clin Oral Implants Res. 1995 Dec;6(4):213-9.

28. Brettin BT, Grosland NM, Qian F, Southard KA, Stuntz TD, Morgan TA, et al. Bicortical vs monocortical orthodontic skeletal anchorage. Am J Orthod Dentofacial Orthop. 2008 Nov;134(5):625-35.

29. Pickard MB, Dechow P, Rossouw PE, Buschang PH. Effects of miniscrew orientation on implant stability and resistance to failure. Am J Orthod Dentofacial Orthop. 2010 Jan;137(1):91-9.

30. Suzuki EY, Suzuki B, Aramrattana A, Harnsiriwattanakit K, Kowanich N. Assessment of miniscrew implant stability by resonance frequency analysis: a study in human cadavers. J Oral Maxillofac Surg. 2010 Nov;68(11):2682-9.

31. Lemieux G, Hart A, Cheretakis C, Goodmurphy C, Trexler S, McGary C, et al. Computed tomographic characterization of mini-implant placement pattern and maximum anchorage force in human cadavers. Am J Orthod Dentofacial Orthop. 2011 Sept;140(3):356-65.

32. Suzuki EY, Suzuki B. Placement and removal torque values of orthodontic miniscrew implants. Am J Orthod Dentofacial Orthop. 2011 May;139(5):669-78.

33. Chaddad K, Ferreira AF, Geurs N, Reddy MS. Influence of surface characteristics on survival rates of mini-implants. Angle Orthod. 2008 Jan;78(1):107-13.

34. Schätzle M, Golland D, Roos M, Stawarczyk B. Accuracy of mechanical torque-limiting gauges for mini-screw placement. Clin Oral Implants Res. 2010 Aug;21(8):781-8.

35. Crismani AG, Bertl MH, Celar AG, Bantleon HP, Burstone CJ. Miniscrews in orthodontic treatment: review and analysis of published clinical trials. Am J Orthod Dentofacial Orthop. 2010 Jan;137(1):108-13.

36. Lee NK, Baek SH. Effects of the diameter and shape of orthodontic mini-implants on microdamage to the cortical bone. Am J Orthod Dentofacial Orthop. 2010 July;138(1):8.e1-8; discussion 8-9.

37. Meira TM, Tanaka OM, Ronsani MM, Maruo IT, Guariza-Filho O, Camargo ES, et al. Insertion torque, pull-out strength and cortical bone thickness in contact with orthodontic mini-implants at different insertion angles. Eur J Orthod. 2013 Dec;35(6):766-71

13

Comparative study of the soft tissue of young Japanese-Brazilian, Caucasian and Mongoloid patients

Thais Maria Freire Fernandes[1], Arnaldo Pinzan[2], Renata Sathler[3], Marcos Roberto de Freitas[4], Guilherme Janson[4], Fabiano Paiva Vieira[5]

Objective: To determine the normality mean values in the soft tissue cephalometric measurements of young Japanese-Brazilian, with normal occlusion and compare the results of the variables with compatible samples of young Caucasians and Mongoloids. **Methods:** Forty radiographs of young Caucasians, 32 of Japanese-Brazilians and 33 of Mongoloids were used. The three samples presented individuals with normal occlusion and well-balanced face. The samples were divided by gender due to the soft tissue characteristics and to facilitate comparison. The following statistical tests were performed: Analysis of variance (ANOVA) and analysis of covariance (ANCOVA) with $p < 0.05$. **Results:** The Japanese-Brazilian sample of females showed thinner soft tissues in the nasion region and smaller nose when compared to the Caucasians. The Mongoloid sample showed thinner tissues in the supramentonian and pogonion regions. In males, the Japanese-Brazilians had thinner tissues in the nasion region; thicker lower lip and supramentonian region in comparison to the Caucasian sample. For the Mongoloid, soft tissue was thicker in the glabella and ANS-Sn regions. **Conclusion:** It is necessary to use specific soft tissue standards for this mixed race.

Keywords: Ethnic groups. Reference values. Orthodontics.

[1] PhD and Postdoc in Orthodontics, Bauru Dental School - University of São Paulo (FOB-USP).

[2] Associate Professor, Department of Pediatric Dentistry, Orthodontics and Public Health, Bauru Dental School, FOB-USP.

[3] MSc in Orthodontics, USP.

[4] Head Professor, Department of Pediatric Dentistry, Orthodontics and Public Health, FOB-USP.

[5] Head Professor, Department of Pediatric Dentistry, Orthodontics and Public Health, FOB-USP.

» The author reports no commercial, proprietary or financial interest in the products or companies described in this article.

Thais Maria Freire Fernandes
Alameda Octávio Pinheiro Brisolla, 9-75 – Bauru/SP – Brazil
CEP: 17.012-901 – E-mail: thaismaria@hotmail.com

INTRODUCTION

Orthodontics has the cephalometric analysis as a great diagnostic aid. Since the advent of the cephalostat, many authors have focused on establishing analyses that facilitate orthodontic planning. These studies were initially conducted in Caucasians, but it has been shown that different races have different[12] cephalometric standards, thus making it necessary to establish normative values for the different racial and ethnical groups.

In multicultural societies such as Brazil, the racial differences have assumed great importance.[12] The Brazilian population is presented today with a lot of intermingled people, making it necessary to recognize that the best esthetic and functional results cannot be found when using as a guide another race or ethnicity.[22] Although many studies are found in the scientific literature about the soft tissue profile, there is no research on this subject comparing young Japanese-Brazilians with other races. Brazil is currently considered the country with the largest number of Japanese outside Japan and has different generations of nipponic origin,[27] and a lot of miscegenation, thus it is believed that a more specific study is necessary for this ethnic group.

This study aimed to determine the normality of mean values in the soft tissue profile of young Japanese-Brazilians, with normal occlusion, as well as Brazilians and Japanese descendants comparing these results with samples of young Caucasian Brazilians and young Mongoloid Brazilians.

MATERIAL AND METHODS

Material

The sample consisted of 105 radiographs of young Japanese-Brazilians, Caucasians and Mongoloids, with normal occlusion and balanced face. The Japanese-Brazilian sample was selected by 3 researchers in different schools of Bauru (Brazil), and the other two samples were collected from files of the Department of Orthodontics of the Bauru Dental School - University of São Paulo. The total study sample included 40 young Caucasians (20 of each gender), 32 young Japanese-Brazilian adults (17 females and 15 males) and 33 young Mongoloid adults (17 females and 16 males). The means and standard deviations of patients' ages are shown in Table 1.

All individuals had the upper and lower permanent teeth in occlusion, with or without second and third

molars; showing a balanced growth pattern; harmonic profile, satisfactory occlusion or Angle Class I malocclusion with dental casts showing a discrepancy of up to 2 mm in the lower anterior region. None of them went through prior orthodontic treatment.

The Caucasian group consisted of Mediterranean descendents and the Mongoloid group of individuals with Japanese ancestries. These two samples did not include individuals of mixed heritage. For the Japanese-Brazilian group, the individuals should be children or grandchildren resulting from the union of Caucasian Brazilians and Japanese (Fig 1), not including individuals from the island of Okinawa, since it was colonized by Chinese people.

Methods

Cephalometric radiographs were taken from all sample individuals in maximum intercuspation (MHI), as it is known that the differences between this mandibular position and centric relation (CR) are minimal at this age, and they minimally interfere in the cephalometric results, especially in cases of normal occlusion.[30]

The cephalogram tracings and measurements were made by the same researcher. The images were scanned through a flatbed Numonics, AccuGrid A30TL (Numonics Corporation, Montgomeryville, PA, USA) connected to a PC with 700MHz Intel P3 processor, to obtain the cephalometric measurements, and subsequent data transfer to the Dentofacial Planner 7.02 software (Dentofacial Planner Software Inc., Toronto, Ontario, Canada). The correction of the magnification factor due to the use of different radiographic equipment (6% for the Caucasian sample, 9.8% for Japanese-Brazilian, and from 7% to 8% for the Mongoloid sample) was performed by the software itself.

After obtaining the lateral cephalometric radiographs, the anatomic design and location of classic cephalometric points was performed. To determine the linear horizontal measurements,[9,11,13] representing the soft tissue thickness, some measurements were made perpendicular to the N-perp line, taking the points of the soft tissue facial profile and their respective points in the dentoskeletal structures (Table 2, Fig 2).

Method error

Thirty days after the end of this stage, 20 radiographs were randomly selected and re-traced, manually and digitally, to determine result reliability. For each

Table 1 - Number of individuals (n) in each group, the distribution by gender, sample mean age and standard deviations (SD).

Groups	Total	Females	Males	Mean age	SD
Caucasian	40	20	20	13.64	0.97
Japanese-Brazilian	32	17	15	13.96	1.28
Mongoloid	33	17	16	15.61	2.44

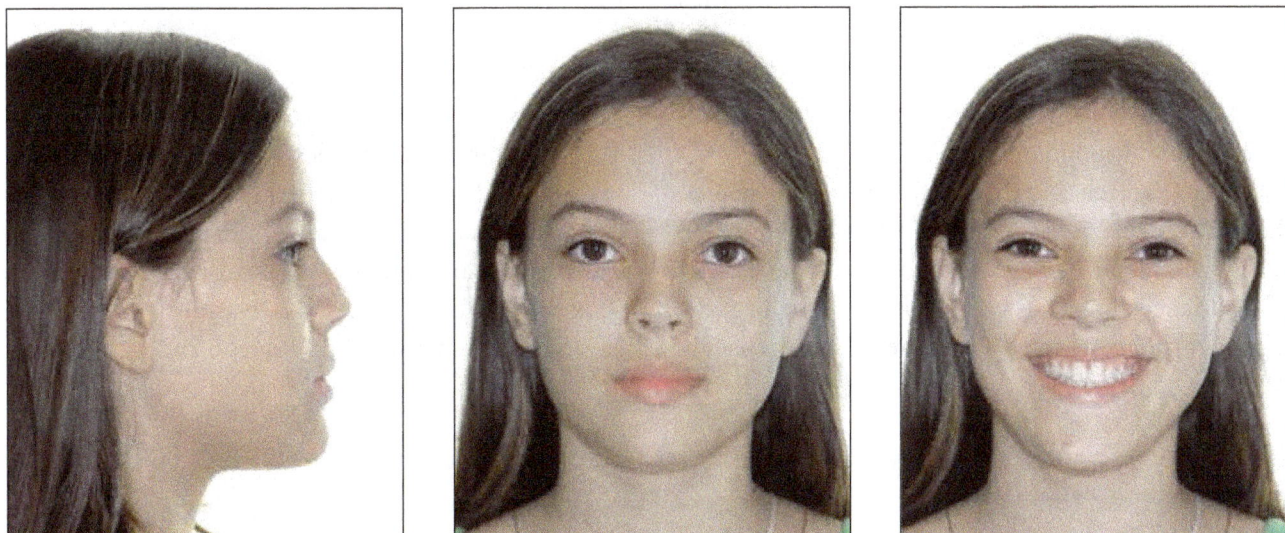

Figure 1 - Extraoral photographs of young Japanese-Brazilian female.

Table 2 - Linear horizontal measurements.

Nº	Name (Abbreviation)	Definition
1	Thickness of the glabella soft tissue (Gl-GL')	Distance between the hard tissue and the soft tissue glabella points
2	Nasion soft tissue thickness (N-N ')	Distance between the hard tissue and the soft tissue nasion points
3	Nasal thickness (Prn-Nperp)	Distance between the pronasal point and its perpendicular projection to the N-perp line
4	Nasal projection (Sn-Prn)	Horizontal distance between the subnasale and pronasale points
5	Thickness of the subnasale region (ANS-Sn)	Distance between the anterior nasal spine and subnasale points
6	Soft tissue thickness of the anterior maxillary region (A-A')	Distance between points A and A'
7	Upper lip thickness (ULp-UL)	Distance between the UL point and its projection on the upper incisor[11]
8	Lower lip thickness (LLp-LL)	Distance between LL point and its projection on the lower incisor[11]
9	Thickness of the mentolabial sulcus (B-B')	Distance between points B and B'
10	Anterior thickness of the soft tissue mentum (Pog-Pog')	Distance between the hard tissue and the soft tissue pogonion points

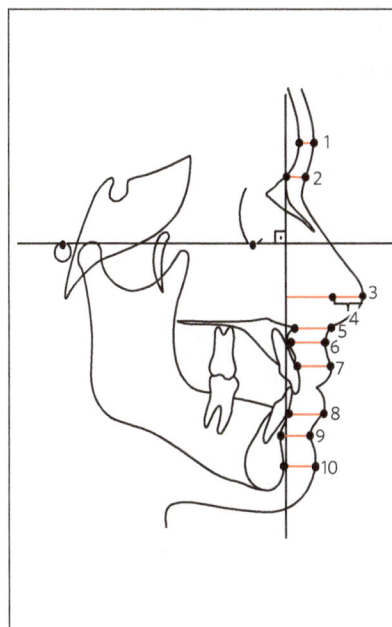

Figure 2 - Horizontal linear measurements.

one of the cephalometric measurements, the systematic and random errors were evaluated, independently. The *t* test was used to calculate the dependent systematic error at a significance level of 5%. To estimate the random error, the formula proposed by Dahlberg ($Se^2 = \Sigma d^2/2n$) was applied, where Se^2 is the error variation, d is the difference between the first and second measurement and n is the number of double measurements.

Statistical analysis

Descriptive statistics was used (mean and standard deviation). The Kolmogorov-Smirnov test demonstrated normal distribution for all variables allowing the use of parametric tests. Thus, for comparative statistical analysis of the data, the following parametric tests were used: ANOVA, analysis of variance with a criterion for comparison of ages, and Ancova, analysis of covariance for comparison of cephalometric variables between the samples (Caucasian, Japanese-Brazilian and Mongoloid).

Due to the lack of age compatibility in the samples, the analysis of covariance (ANCOVA) was used to verify the influence of age on the results. The analysis of covariance aims to assess the effect of one or more explanatory factors rated in nature (in this research, the race) in a given variable, excluding the influence of possible quantitative factors (in this case, the age) that may influence the variables. The results were considered statistically significant for $p < 0.05$. The tests were performed using the Statistica software for Windows 6.0 (Statistica for Windows 6.0, Copyright StatSoft, Inc. Tulsa, USA).

RESULTS

The systematic and random errors are shown in Table 3. Only two variables showed a systematic error and for the random error all variables showed acceptable values of less than 1 mm (Table 3). There were significant differences regarding age for both genders (Table 4) and for this reason the analysis of covariance was performed (Tables 5 and 6).

Table 3 - Evaluation of systematic and random errors by dependent t test and Dahlberg's formula.

Variable	1st tracing		2nd tracing		p	Dahlberg
	Mean	SD	Mean	SD		
Soft tissue thickness (mm)						
Upper face						
GI-GL'	5.93	0.96	5.90	0.93	0.746	0.31
N-N'	5.56	1.47	5.38	1.40	0.273	0.43
Midface						
Prn-Nperp	26.98	2.64	26.86	2.57	0.729	0.97
Sn-Prn	12.05	1.37	12.11	1.38	0.245	0.32
ANS-Sn	10.31	3.51	9.95	2.98	0.384	0.96
Lower face						
A-A'	13.98	2.88	14.97	2.88	0.098	0.89
ULp-UL	14.39	2.21	13.78	1.98	0.032*	0.84
LLp-LL	14.66	1.72	14.23	1.57	0.039*	0.62
B-B'	12.17	1.59	12.35	1.61	0.294	0.45
Pog-Pog'	11.71	1.41	11.69	1.37	0.946	0.47

* Statistically significant at $p < 0.05$.

Table 4 - Comparison of mean ages between the different races, in males and females included in the samples, by analysis of variance (ANOVA).

Gender	Caucasian			Japanese-Brazilian			Mongoloid			p
	n	Mean	SD	n	Mean	SD	n	Mean	SD	
Female	20	13.70[a]	0.87	17	13.22[a]	1.04	17	15.65[b]	2.44	0.000*
Male	20	13.57[a]	1.03	15	14.79[a,b]	1.01	16	15.56[b]	2.51	0.002*
Total	40	13.63[a]	0.97	32	13.96[a]	1.29	33	15.61[b]	2.44	0.000*

* Statistically significant at $p < 0.05$
Different letters show significant differences between means by Tukey test.

Table 5 - Comparison of variables between the female samples (ANCOVA and Tukey's test).

Variable	Caucasian (n = 20)		Japanese-Brazilian (n = 17)		Mongoloid (n = 17)		p Age	p
	Mean	SD	Mean	SD	Mean	SD		
Soft tissue thickness (mm)								
Upper face								
Gl-GL'	5.87	0.49	6.01	0.68	5.94	0.87	0.196	0.652
N-N'	7.01[a]	0.88	6.14[b]	1.19	5.87[b]	1.01	0.744	0.005*
Midface								
Prn-Nperp	28.83[a]	3.75	26.35[a,b]	2.52	24.90[b]	3.29	0.939	0.005*
Sn-Prn	14.52[a]	1.45	12.01[b]	1.48	11.73[b]	1.66	0.128	0.000*
ANS-Sn	10.07	1.93	9.64	1.48	8.84	1.96	0.504	0.115
Lower face								
A-A'	14.38[a]	1.92	13.10[a,b]	1.58	12.65[b]	1.45	0.941	0.010*
ULp-UL	12.80	1.35	13.50	1.85	12.66	1.86	1.000	0.386
LLp-LL	13.82	1.09	13.79	1.19	14.11	1.63	0.555	0.944
B-B'	11.23[a]	1.49	10.71[a]	0.63	13.02[b]	1.84	0.475	0.002*
Pog-Pog'	11.47[a]	1.26	11.22[a]	1.36	12.25[b]	2.20	0.002*	0.003*

Different letters show significant differences between means by Tukey test.
* Statistically significant at p < 0.05.

Table 6 - Comparison of variables between the male samples (ANCOVA and Tukey's test).

Variable	Caucasian (n = 20)		Japanese-Brazilian (n = 15)		Mongoloid (n = 16)		p Age	p
	Mean	SD	Mean	SD	Mean	SD		
Soft tissue thickness (mm)								
Upper face								
Gl-GL'	5.91[a,b]	1.04	6.54[a]	0.81	5.69[b]	0.65	0.478	0.026*
N-N'	7.93[a]	1.00	6.56[b]	1.09	6.08[b]	1.12	0.455	0.000*
Midface								
Prn-Nperp	28.50	3.38	29.56	3.18	26.72	3.13	0.304	0.090
Sn-Prn	13.02	2.44	13.43	2.05	13.32	1.54	0.432	0.938
ANS-Sn	11.37[a]	2.27	11.17[a]	2.26	9.52[b]	2.21	0.369	0.033*
Lower face								
A-A'	15.60	1.95	15.76	2.02	14.58	1.49	0.936	0.268
ULp-UL	14.24	1.78	15.06	1.66	14.17	2.34	0.071	0.298
LLp-LL	14.88[a]	1.21	16.60[b]	1.74	16.77[b]	2.17	0.745	0.008*
B-B'	11.23[a]	1.07	12.68[b]	1.30	13.68[b]	1.49	0.142	0.000*
Pog-Pog'	12.18	1.69	12.95	1.49	12.64	2.14	0.277	0.252

Different letters show significant differences between means by Tukey test.
* Statistically significant at p < 0.05.

DISCUSSION

The same appearance is not always appropriate for all races and ethnic groups, however, normative studies of cephalometric variables are important for precisely determining the variations of what is normal.[22] There are some studies about soft tissue in Caucasians and Mongoloids, but no specific study about Japanese-Brazilians and the comparison of these three groups.

Besides, it is difficult to compare cephalometric studies in different races due to sample characteristics, statistical methods, geographic distribution and racial definitions. The groups that were used in this study met the same inclusion criteria, especially regarding race, which was strictly evaluated.

Some studies explained that when analyzing the soft tissue profile, it is necessary to differentiate the variables for men and women.[4,17] The subdivision by gender and racial group has received support in other studies,[14,22] that emphasized that the accurate use of cephalometrics, should consider these aspects. In this study, the genders were analyzed separately for better comparison of soft tissue profile.

Thickness alterations on the soft tissue profile vary with age and gender.[29] Besides this fact, the dento-skeletal changes can directly influence the desired esthetics. The soft tissue may also vary in thickness, length and position, which makes the study of the outline of these tissues necessary, in order to achieve a total facial harmony.[8] According to Arnett et al,[4] the thickness measurements of the upper lip, lower lip, point B region, pogonion, and chin alter the facial profile. As well as the variation of lip thickness, especially during retraction or dental protraction.[8] Differences found in the soft tissue profile in this study can be seen in the pictures of the mean profile of the three samples (Figs 3A and B).

Only the variables that showed statistically significant difference after comparison with a sample of Caucasian and Mongoloid, will be discussed (Tables 5 and 6). These magnitudes were grouped according to their representation and to facilitate the understanding, divided into upper, middle and lower face. The results are discussed focusing on the Japanese-Brazilian sample and their differences to the Mongoloid and Caucasian samples.

Upper face

Considering the upper face a difference was observed in the thinnest region of the nasion (N-N') for the Mongoloid (female 5.87 mm, female 6.08) and Japanese-Brazilian groups (female 6.14 mm, 6 male, 56 mm) when compared to the Caucasian sample (female 7.01 mm, 7.93 mm female). This may be related to the fact that the soft tissues of the Japanese individuals in these regions are more firmly attached and have

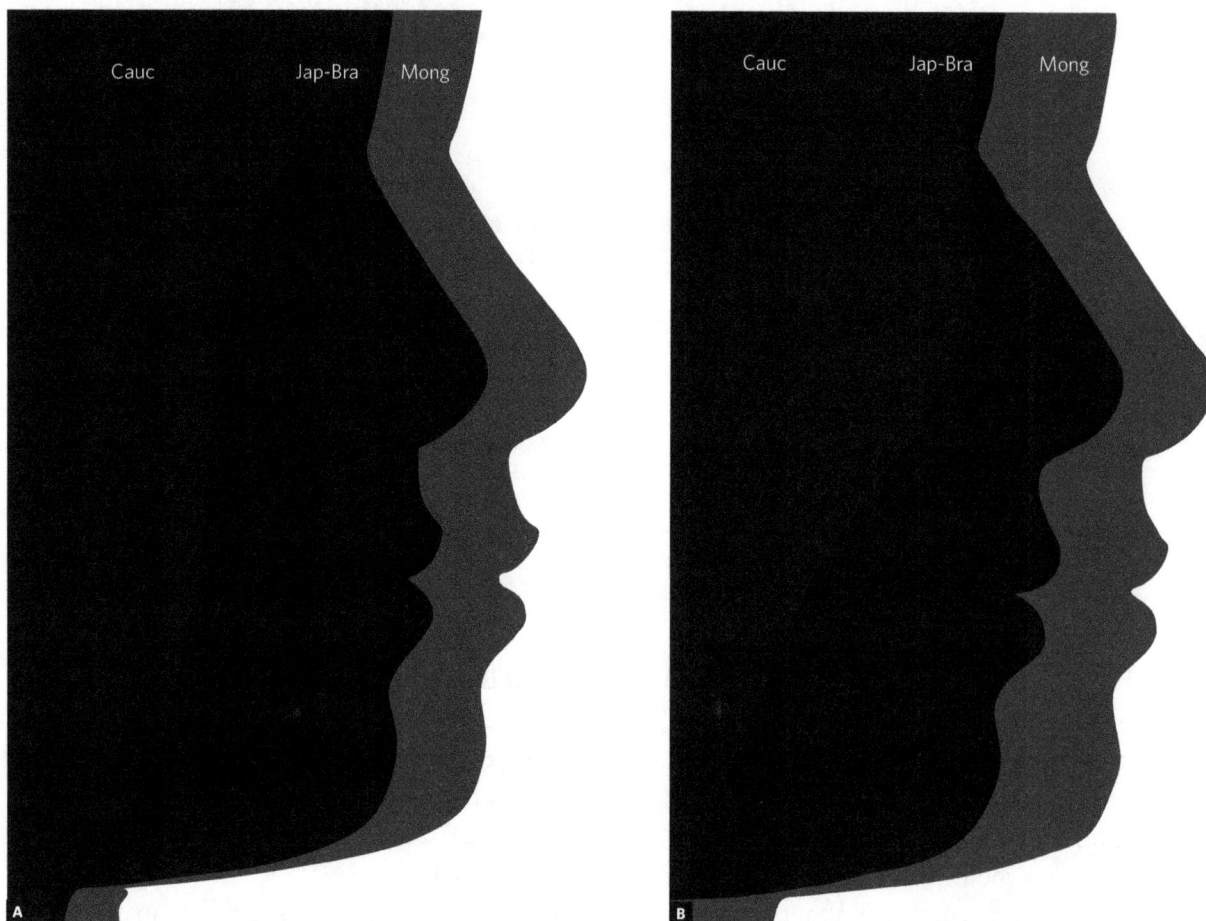

Figure 3 - Illustrative comparison of the profile means between Caucasian, Japanese-Brazilian and Mongoloid groups: (A) female, (B) male.

more subtle growth when compared to the Caucasian sample.[29] The expectation that Japanese descendents have a flatter area in the region of the nasion and this appearance can be associated to a thinner soft tissue is, therefore, confirmed.

Also regarding the upper face, males of the Japanese-Brazilian sample showed statistically higher values of soft tissue thickness (6.54 mm) in the glabella region (Gl-Gl') when compared to the Mongoloid sample (5.69 mm). This increased thickness emphasizes even more the flattening found for Japanese-Brazilians in the region of nasion (N-N'). This variable quantifies the thickness in the nasion region and presented particular characteristics regarding the ethnicity for both genders. In most cases, the thickness in the nasion region is greater in men than in women and in both genders, the thickness of this area tends to remain constant or decrease slightly with age.[25,29]

Although the upper face area is not an area of direct action for the orthodontist and it will not be changed with orthodontic treatment itself, the practitioner must be aware of the general profile aspect.

Midface

As for the thickness of soft tissues in this region in females, it was observed that the Japanese-Brazilian sample showed intermediate values for variables Sn-Prn and Prn-Nperp. When compared to Caucasians (14.52 mm), statistically lower values for the size of the nose (Prn-Sn) were found in the Japanese-Brazilian sample (12.01 mm) and Mongoloids (11.73 mm), which can be confirmed by previous findings that Asians have smaller noses when compared to other populations.[1] Corroborating with these findings, the smallest nose size was also evidenced by the variable Prn-Nperp in the Mongoloid sample (24.90 mm) when compared to Caucasians (28.83 mm).

The only variable for males that showed a significant difference in this region of the face was the ANS-Sn which showed intermediate values for Japanese-Brazilians (11.17 mm) but similar to the values found for the Caucasians (11.37 mm). This variable is also related to the nose and confirmed the trend of Mongoloids having smaller noses (9.52 mm) when compared to other races.[1,24] As the amount of increase in nasal projection (Prn-Nperp and Sn-Prn) in boys occurs in older ages,[6,8] it is speculated that this is the reason for the lack of dif-

ference for this gender in this research, since Japanese individuals, even older, show a smaller nose (26.72 mm) when compared to other samples.

Angle, in his book published in 1907, stated that the amount of nose development may influence the final treatment result, and correction of isolated dental disharmonies can often detract the profile.[13] Thus, the nose size is a factor that should be evaluated in terms of treatment[25] because irreversible procedures such as extractions and retractions may affect facial profile esthetics.

Lower face

The lower face is the actual area of orthodontic action and this requires strict evaluation, which justifies the fact that most of the variables in this study are related to this region.

Subspinale region (A-A')

The thickness of the subspinale region (A-A') directly affects the shape of the soft tissue profile and only females showed significant differences between the races. The Caucasian sample showed the highest value (14.38 mm) and it is known that the increased thickness of soft tissues in this region, may mask a dental protrusion.[9] In this Japanese-Brazilian sample, the thickness was numerically intermediate (13.10 mm) and the lowest value was found in the Mongoloid sample (12.65 mm) which, associated to the small nose in this group, may evidence even more a lip protrusion in Japanese descendents.

According to Subtelny[25] the thickness of this region grows on average 5 mm, from 3 to 18 years old, and comparatively, there is more soft tissue covering point A region then there is covering the nasion and pogonion regions. This was also found in this study for all samples, in both genders. Thus, the soft profile tends to change more in the direction of increased thickness than in the reduction of facial convexity. This may partly explain why the soft tissue, without the inclusion of the nose, tends to get progressively less convex over the age, as occurs in the skeletal profile.[25]

Lower lip (LLp-LL)

Assessing the region of the lower face in males (Table 6), attention is drawn to the thickness of the lower lip (LLp-LL), which was higher in Japanese-Brazilians (16.60 mm) and Mongoloids (16.77 mm). This thickness probably also contributes to the appearance of a more convex profile in the Asian descents.[28] The increased thickness of the lower lip can mask a Class II relation and promote a more straight profile, bringing at least esthetic benefits to Asian descendants with malocclusions such as these.

Over the years, the lips suffer a redirection that causes a wilted appearance. The decrease in thickness is compensated with a proportional increase in height of the lips, allowing the volume to remain the same.[15] Based on this, fact, orthodontic planning can be established more thoroughly in young patients with gingival smile, considering these changes during growth.

The thickness, height and position of the lips, particular characteristics of the individuals, can influence the response of the soft tissue to retraction movement. Patients with thicker lips respond differently to orthodontic treatment than patients with thinner lips.[20] Patients with thinner lips have a higher correlation between changes in hard tissue and these changes' reflect in the soft tissue. It is important to note that orthodontists should be aware of the thickness of the lips in the treatment plan, not to overestimate the changes that may occur in soft tissue.

Supramentonian region (B-B')
and pogonion (Pog-Pog')

Japanese-Brazilian girls had less thickness in the supramentonian region (10.71 mm) and the Mongoloid sample had more thickness (13.02 mm) in this region. In this aspect, the girls had similar characteristics to the Caucasians. Unlike males, the supramentonian region (B-B') showed greater thickness in Japanese-Brazilians (12.68 mm) and Mongoloids (13.68 mm), which contributes to a straighter mentolabial sulcus. For these races, the greater thickness of the lower lip and mentolabial sulcus features, emphasize the care that the orthodontist should have with relapses, since it is known that muscle behavior, depending on the intensity, has a greater chance of recurrence[7] and more stretched muscles tend to act even more.

The pogonion region for girls was statistically significant, both for the race factor as for the age factor, suggesting the need for attention to this variable, because the difference occurs even for the same ages. A smaller thickness of this region for the Japanese-Brazilians (11.22 mm) and greater for the Mongoloid

sample (12.25 mm) was found, which is also the sample of older people. Thus, the greater thickness of this area, may be related to higher mean age of Japanese women (15.65 years), since the tendency is that the pogonion thickness increases with age, when evaluating only the thickness itself.[5,21]

The previous aspects clearly show that soft tissues do not form a layer of uniform thickness that simply molds to the configuration of the underlying dento-skeletal structures. Therefore, it must be considered that individual variability on the thickness of soft tissues may reflect greatly on facial profile harmony, making the evaluation of this factor necessary during the diagnosis and planning of orthodontic treatment.[8]

FINAL CONSIDERATIONS

When performing comparisons such as the one performed in this study, it is emphasized that people should not be obsessed with numbers, but should observe the characteristics of each person. It is known that the period and environment in which people live has a direct influence on the concept of beauty. Alcalde et al[2] reported that Japanese living in Japan, have different expectations regarding the treatment of those living in other regions of the world, due to their social differences and cultural influences. Still, Miyajima et al[19] reported the revival of a sense of ethnic pride, especially in big cities. Besides, patient demands have increased in the search of an exclusive orthodontic treatment, which is based on standards derived from their race or specific ethnic group.[16]

Given the anthropological differences of facial and dental standards, Miura, Inoue and Suzuki[18] concluded that, besides having different values, the treatment target for the Japanese should also be different from the Caucasian. Although respecting the patient's expectations, it is important to make them aware of the effects that certain changes may bring. Many times, what is normal for a race may not be so for another race, and this has to be considered. In clinical terms, it is known that besides the labial biprotrusion, it is normal for the Asian descendants to show dental double protrusion[1,16,23,26] Thus, a combination of different individualized brackets prescriptions[10] could allow a satisfactory final result for this race, because the requirements for Class II malocclusion cases have more buccal torque for the lower incisors and those used for Class III malocclusion have greater buccal torque for the upper incisors.[10]

Recognizing that racial influences and characteristics have an important role in guiding the goals of orthodontic treatment and their esthetic results is critical to understand the value and necessity of individualized orthodontic treatment and the study of specific standards for each ethnic group. Thus, common sense should prevail, since it is often not possible to achieve the "ideal standard". The amount of tooth movement, tissue damage and increased risk of recurrence may contraindicate an action that seeks only the rigorous esthetic imposed by social environment. It is necessary to safeguard the conditions of muscle balance and notice what is acceptable for each individual.

CONCLUSION

Based on the methodology and results of this research, it can be concluded that the mixed race sample of Japanese-Brazilians has its own characteristics, such as:

» Females:
• Reduced thickness in the nasion and lower nose regions in relation to Caucasians.
• Reduced thickness in the supramentonian and pogonion regions compared to Mongoloids.
» Males:
• Reduced thickness in the nasion region, greater thickness of the lower lip and the supramentonian regions in relation to Caucasians.
• Greater thickness in the glabella and the ANS-Sn regions compared to Mongoloids.

REFERENCES

1. Alcalde RE, Jinno T, Orsini MG, Sasaki A, Sugiyama RM, Matsumura T. Soft tissue cephalometric norms in Japanese adults. Am J Orthod Dentofacial Orthop. 2000;118(1):84-9.

2. Alcalde RE, Jinno T, Pogrel MA, Matsumura T. Cephalometric norms in Japanese adults. J Oral Maxillofac Surg. 1998;56(2):129-34.

3. Angle EH. Treatment of malocclusion of the teeth. Angle's system. Phipadelphia: Angle; 1907.

4. Arnett GW, Jelic JS, Kim J, Cummings DR, Beress A, Worley CM Jr, et al. Soft tissue cephalometric analysis: diagnosis and treatment planning of dentofacial deformity. Am J Orthod Dentofacial Orthop. 1999;116(3):239-53.

5. Behrents RG. An atlas of growth in the aging craniofacial skeleton [monograph]. Arbor: Center for Human Growth and Development; 1985.

6. Bishara SE, Hession TJ, Peterson LC. Longitudinal soft-tissue profile changes: a study of three analyses. Am J Orthod. 1985;88(3):209-23.

7. Brock RA 2nd, Taylor RW, Buschang PH, Behrents RG. Ethnic differences in upper lip response to incisor retraction. Am J Orthod Dentofacial Orthop. 2005;127(6):683-91; quiz 755.

8. Burstone CJ. The integumental profile. Am J Orthod Dentofacial Orthop. 1958;44(1):1-25.

9. Burstone CJ. Integumental contour and extension patterns. Angle Orthod. 1959;29(2):93-104.

10. Capelozza Filho L, Silva Filho O, Ozawa TE, Cavassan A. Individualização de braquetes na técnica de straight-wire: revisão de conceitos e sugestão de indicações para uso. Rev Dental Press Ortod Ortop Facial. 1999;4(4):87-106.

11. Dainesi EA. A influência dos padrões extremos de crescimento da face sobre o perfil tegumentar, analisada cefalometricamente em jovens leucodermas brasileiros [tese]. Bauru (SP): Universidade de São Paulo; 1998.

12. Freitas LM, Pinzan A, Janson G, Freitas KM, Freitas MR, Henriques JF. Facial height comparison in young white and black Brazilian subjects with normal occlusion. Am J Orthod Dentofacial Orthop. 2007;131(6):706.e1-6.

13. Holdaway RA. A soft-tissue cephalometric analysis and its use in orthodontic treatment planning. Part I. Am J Orthod. 1983;84(1):1-28.

14. Huang WJ, Taylor RW, Dasanayake AP. Determining cephalometric norms for Caucasians and African Americans in Birmingham. Angle Orthod. 1998;68(6):503-11; discussion 512.

15. Iblher N. Changes in the aging upper lip — a photomorphometric and MRI-based study (on a quest to find the right rejuvenation approach). J Plast Reconstr Aesthet Surg. 2008;61(10):1170-6.

16. Ioi H, Nakata S, Nakasima A, Counts A. Effect of facial convexity on anteroposterior lip positions of the most favored Japanese facial profiles. Angle Orthod. 2005;75(3):326-32.

17. Kalha AS, Latif A, Govardhan SN. Soft-tissue cephalometric norms in a South Indian ethnic population. Am J Orthod Dentofacial Orthop. 2008;133(6):876-81.

18. Miura F, Inoue N, Suzuki K. Cephalometric standards for Japanese according to the Steiner analysis. Am J Orthod. 1965;51:288-95.

19. Miyajima K, McNamara JA Jr, Kimura T, Murata S, Iizuka T. Craniofacial structure of Japanese and European-American adults with normal occlusions and well-balanced faces. Am J Orthod Dentofacial Orthop. 1996;110(4):431-8.

20. Oliver BM. The influence of lip thickness and strain on upper lip response to incisor retraction. Am J Orthod. 1982;82(2):141-9.

21. Pecora NG, Baccetti T, McNamara JA Jr. The aging craniofacial complex: a longitudinal cephalometric study from late adolescence to late adulthood. Am J Orthod Dentofacial Orthop. 2008;134(4):496-505.

22. Pinzan A. "Upgrade" nos conceitos da interpretação das medidas cefalométricas. In: Sakai E, Cotrim-Ferreira FA, Martins NS. Nova visão em ortodontia, ortopedia funcional dos maxilares. São Paulo: Ed. Santos; 2006. p. 41-9.

23. Sathler RC. Estudo comparativo do padrão cefalométrico de jovens mestiços nipo-brasileiros: grandezas dentárias e esqueléticas [dissertação]. Bauru (SP): Universidade de São Paulo; 2009.

24. Scavone H Jr, Trevisan H Jr, Garib DG, Ferreira FV. Facial profile evaluation in Japanese-Brazilian adults with normal occlusions and well-balanced faces. Am J Orthod Dentofacial Orthop. 2006;129(6):721.e1-5.

25. Subtelny JD. A longitudinal study of soft-tissue facial structures and their profile characteristics defined in relation to underlying skeletal structures. Am J Orthod Dentofacial Orthop. 1959;45(7):481-507.

26. Takahashi R. Padrão cefalométrico FOB-USP para jovens nipo-brasileiros com oclusão normal [dissertação]. Bauru (SP): Universidade de São Paulo; 1998.

27. Tomita NE, Chinellato LEM, Franco LJ, Iunes M, Freitas JAS, Lopes ES. Condições de saúde bucal e diabetes mellitus na população nipo-brasileira de Bauru-SP. J Appl Oral Sci. 2003;11(1):15-20.

28. Utsuno H, Kageyama T, Deguchi T, Umemura Y, Yoshino M, Nakamura H, et al. Facial soft tissue thickness in skeletal type I Japanese children. Forensic Sci Int. 2007;172(2-3):137-43.

29. Utsuno H, Kageyama T, Uchida K, Yoshino M, Miyazawa H, Inoue K. Facial soft tissue thickness in Japanese female children. Forensic Sci Int. 2010;199(1-3):109.e1-6.

30. Williamson EH, Caves SA, Edenfield RJ, Morse PK. Cephalometric analysis: comparisons between maximum intercuspation and centric relation. Am J Orthod. 1978;74(6):672-7.

14

Reliability of Bolton analysis evaluation in tridimensional virtual models

Marianna Mendonca Brandão[1], Marcio Costal Sobral[2], Carlos Jorge Vogel[3]

Objective: The present study aimed at evaluating the reliability of Bolton analysis in tridimensional virtual models, comparing it with the manual method carried out with dental casts. **Methods:** The present investigation was performed using 56 pairs of dental casts produced from the dental arches of patients in perfect conditions and randomly selected from Universidade Federal da Bahia, School of Dentistry, Orthodontics Postgraduate Program. Manual measurements were obtained with the aid of a digital Cen-Tech 4"® caliper (Harpor Freight Tools, Calabasas, CA, USA). Subsequently, samples were digitized on 3Shape® R-700T scanner (Copenhagen, Denmark) and digital measures were obtained by Ortho Analyzer software. **Results:** Data were subject to statistical analysis and results revealed that there were no statistically significant differences between measurements with p-values equal to $p = 0.173$ and $p = 0.239$ for total and anterior proportions, respectively. **Conclusion:** Based on these findings, it is possible to deduce that Bolton analysis performed on tridimensional virtual models is as reliable as measurements obtained from dental casts with satisfactory agreement.

Keywords: Computer-assisted diagnosis. Dental casts. Tridimensional imaging.

[1] Postgraduate student in Orthodontics and Facial Orthopedics, Universidade Federal da Bahia (UFBA), Salvador, Bahia, Brazil.

[2] Professor, Universidade Federal da Bahia (UFBA), Postgraduate Program, Salvador, Bahia, Brazil.

[3] PhD in Orthodontics, Universidade de São Paulo (USP), São Paulo, São Paulo, Brazil.

» The authors report no commercial, proprietary or financial interest in the products or companies described in this article.

Marianna Mendonça Brandão
Rua da Paz, n 301, Graça, Salvador, BA, Brazil.
E-mail: mmb.orto@outlook.com

INTRODUCTION

When identifying patients' dental and bone problems, orthodontists rely on clinical findings, which are associated with radiographs, photographs and dental casts, to determine the most adequate treatment plan necessary to resolve each unique case.[1]

Dental casts allow malocclusions to be assessed tridimensionally and constitute one of the most important elements of diagnosis; thus, they are considered the "gold standard" in Orthodontics.[1-4] Dental casts reproductions have acceptable reliability and enable complete assessment of patient's malocclusion, including shape and symmetry of dental arches and palate, individual dental positions, curves of Spee and Wilson, relationship between molars and canines, axial tipping of teeth, Bolton analysis, overbite and overjet, among other features.[5,6]

Correct overbite and overjet, as well as an adequate relationship between molars and canines result from the ideal proportional sum of mesiodistal diameters of both maxillary and mandibular teeth, among other aspects. The importance of proportionality for the orthodontist is obvious during the final phases of treatment. Minor discrepancies are insignificant from a clinical point of view; however, major discrepancies result in additional treatment challenges, requiring additional corrective treatment and/or compensations that were initially unplanned.[5,7,8]

In this context, a variety of methods have been developed to analyze discrepancy. The method proposed by Bolton in 1958 has become one of the most reliable methods, mainly due to its ease of execution and application.[9,10] Bolton analysis is a valuable tool that is able to identify disagreement in tooth size between maxillary and mandibular teeth, which could negatively affect a correct dental relationship, highly desired during orthodontic treatment.[11]

When applying the formulas proposed by Bolton, if total proportion exceeds 91.3%, discrepancy corresponds to excess dental structure in the lower arch; whereas if proportion is lower than 91.3%, excess will be seen in the upper arch. If proportion in the anterior region exceeds 77.2%, excess dental structure will be in the lower arch; whereas if proportion is lower than 77.2%, it will be seen in the upper arch.[9]

Traditionally, Bolton indexes are measured manually with the aid of a bow divider or a caliper in dental casts.[7] Nevertheless, with significant technological development, many orthodontists use computers and digitized

orthodontic records to aid diagnosis and treatment planning.[4,12] The use of scanned dental casts was announced by the orthodontic industry as the newest component of totally digitized records.[13]

The motivation for using digital models arose from the disadvantages of using dental casts, including the following: need for proper storage places, resulting in greater need for space in the office; risk of breaking which would cause permanent destruction of patient's records; duplication of casts in order to communicate with other dentists and specialists; increased hours of laboratory work and associated costs.[1,4,6]

Digital models and tridimensional technology minimize many of the previously mentioned problems, while providing the orthodontist with standard routine data, such as tooth size, overbite, overjet, Bolton and cast discrepancy, symmetry and shape of arches, intensity of the curves of Spee and Wilson, among others.[12,14,15]

However, as it is the case of any new method, it is necessary to assess the reliability of measurements taken with digital models, and correlating those results with the traditional dental cast method. Thus, the aim of this study is to assess the reliability of Bolton analysis performed on tridimensional virtual models, and compare those findings with the traditional dental cast method.

MATERIAL AND METHODS

This is an experimental study that used dental casts taken from the dental arches of adult individuals. Initially, measurement taking was carried out by hand on dental casts, followed by digitization and digital measurement taking for comparison. The study was approved by Universidade Federal da Bahia Institutional Review Board (UFBA Protocol. #718.989/2014).

Initially, a total of 56 dental casts produced from the dental arches of patients treated and randomly selected from Universidade Federal da Bahia, School of Dentistry, Orthodontics Postgraduate Program were used. Dental casts were considered to have been perfectly preserved, with permanent teeth completely erupted and without the need for second and third molars.

Sample size calculation was performed by means of Epi Info software(version 6.0), using an expected difference of 0.09%, with test power of 80% and alpha level of 5%. Sample size (n) was determined at 56.

Direct measurements were taken on the dental casts (T_1), followed by digitization. They corresponded to the largest mesiodistal width of all permanent teeth: first molars, pre-molars, canines and incisors. Measurement taking was performed by a single operator, previously trained. After 15 and 30 days (T_2 and T_3), 20% of casts were measured again, so as to confirm reproducibility.

Analysis of dental casts by means of the traditional method was performed with the aid of a digital caliper Cen-Tech 4" (Harpor Freight Tools, Calabasas, CA, USA), with precision of 0.01 mm. The caliper was placed on the buccal surface of teeth, starting with first molars, followed by second pre-molars, first pre-molars, canines and incisors on both upper and lower arches. Anterior and total proportion of mesiodistal sizes was calculated by summing teeth size up and determining the matching index.

For computer analysis, the models were digitized with a 3Shape® R-700™ scanner (Copenhagen, Denmark) that uses a non-destructive scanning method. The scanner consists of a platform to support the model, a laser and two high-resolution digital cameras used to capture the images. To ensure complete coverage of the object shape, the platform can be manipulated, so as to allow a double image to be captured.

Before digitization, the scanner was calibrated once a day, following the manufacturer's recommendations. The process began by appropriately positioning the model to be digitized onto the machine platform, so that the laser beam could map the desired profile.

For the digitization process, images were processed by 3Shape® Ortho Impression™ software (Copenhagen, Denmark). After patient data had been recorded, digitization began. During this process, the laser captured images at specific dental cast locations, thereby producing a final virtual image. Image shape is a result of the organization of points in triangular shape. The image file was saved in DICOM format (Digital Imaging and Communications in Medicine).

Based on the digital images obtained, the digital models were manipulated by 3Shape® Ortho Analyzer™ software (Copenhagen, Denmark).

Digital measurements were taken by initially marking, from the buccal surface of teeth, the mesial and distal contact of first right maxillary molar, followed by second right maxillary pre-molar and all remaining teeth, until a complete set of measurements was obtained (Fig 1). The same approach was

repeated on the lower arch. Thus, the software automatically generated the mesiodistal size of each tooth and the result of Bolton analysis (Fig 2).

The values obtained by both manual and digital measurement techniques were compiled in a MS Excel spreadsheet and statistically assessed by SPPS v. 15 software and MedCalc 9. Kolmogorov-Smirnov statistical test was performed to assess normality of data, thereby confirming the hypothesis of normal distribution of data.

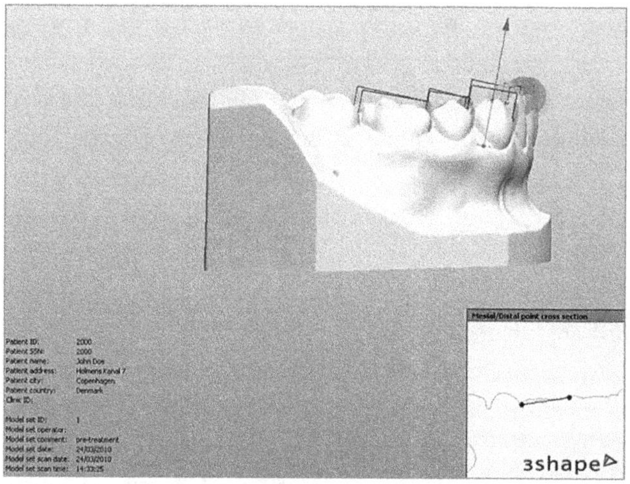

Figure 1 - Measurement of mesiodistal sizes by the digital method.

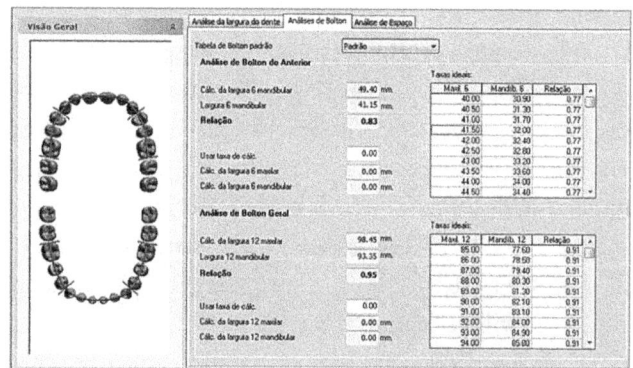

Figure 2 - Report of Bolton analysis by the digital method.

Descriptive analysis (mean and standard deviation) was performed. To investigate the reliability of measurements found by the different techniques, Students t-test for paired samples was implemented. Lin's concordance coefficient (r) was used to determine whether measurements deviated significantly from perfect agreement. Excellent agreement was determined as r > 0.90, whereas satisfactory r ranged between 0.60 and 0.9, and unsatisfactory r was < 0.6. Significance level was set at 95% and results were descriptively presented in comparative tables generated on MS Word.

RESULTS

The reproducibility of measurements obtained by means of the different methods were analyzed by Kappa test, with significance level set at 95%. No statistically significant differences were found between T_1, T_2 and T_3, with Kappa = 0.9.

Student's t-test for paired samples was used to assess whether or not measurements presented any significant differences. Confidence interval was 95%. There were no statistically significant differences between measurements for any measurement approach, with $p = 0.173$ and $p = 0.239$ for total and anterior proportions, respectively (Figs 3 and 4).

Measurement reproducibility assessed by means of Lin's concordance revealed that total proportion had r = 0.8715, with a confidence interval ranging from 0.7998 to 0.9187; whereas anterior proportion had r = 0.7785, with confidence interval ranging from 0.6506 to 0.8634 (Figs 5 and 6). According to Lin, those values suggest that the digital method had satisfactory agreement, both in total and e anterior proportions.[16]

DISCUSSION

With advances in technology, the use of digitized orthodontic records is becoming more and more common in clinical practice. Thus, it is necessary to test the effectiveness of this new digital method of which objective is to assist the orthodontist in

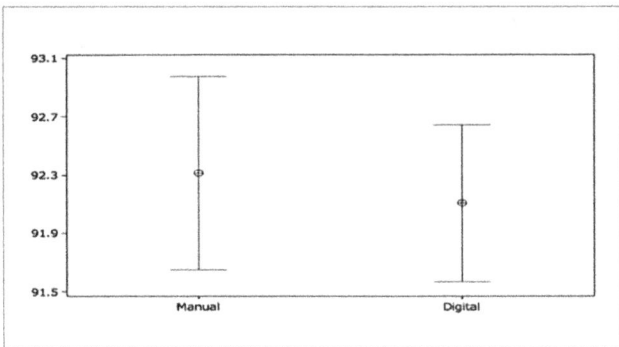

Figure 3 - Graphic comparing measurements of total proportion obtained by the manual and digital methods.

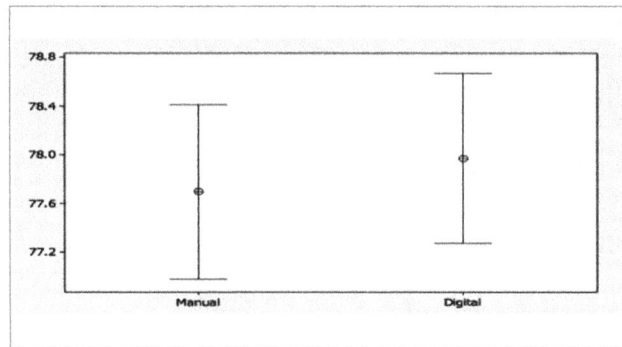

Figure 4 - Graphic comparing measurements of anterior proportion obtained with the manual and digital methods.

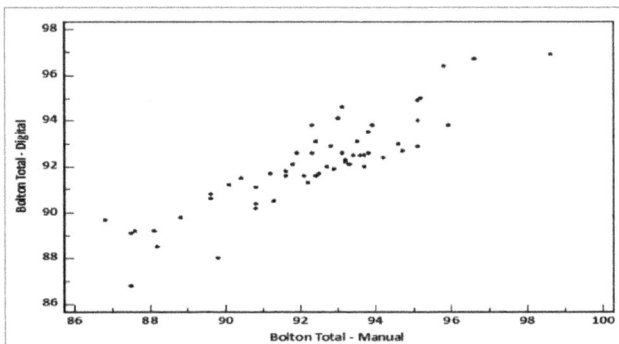

Figure 5 - Graphic of reproducibility of total proportion obtained with the manual and digital methods.

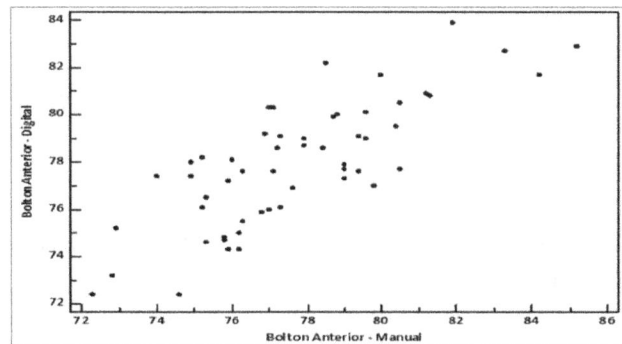

Figure 6 - Graphic of reproducibility of anterior proportion obtained with the manual and digital methods.

visualizing, measuring and analyzing models, as well as in reaching diagnosis and treatment plan.

The present study found no statistically significant differences when Student's t-test was performed for paired samples to compare digitally or manually-obtained measurement methods, with $p = 0.173$ and $p = 0.239$ for total and anterior proportions, respectively. These results are similar to those obtained by Tomasseti et al,[12] Paredes, Gandia and Cibrian,[17] Stevens et al[18] and Mullen et al[19] who compared the use of a digital caliper and the digital method by means of Bolton analysis. The authors did not find statistically significant differences between methods.

Other studies have also assessed the reliability of the digital method in relation to the manual one, namely: Oliveira et al,[4] Mayers et al,[20] Quimby et al,[1] Bell, Ayoub and Siebert,[21] Zilberman, Huggare and Parikakis,[22] Redlich et al,[23] Veenema et al,[24] Watanebe-Kanno et al.[25] Although measurements obtained by the present study were not identical to those of the previous studies, the authors of the latter did not report any statistically significant differences between manual and digital methods, thereby corroborating the observations presented herein.

Santoro et al[15] conducted a comparative study on the precision of measurements taken by the OrthoCAD system (Cadent, Carlstadt, NJ) on digital models and dental casts. Results showed that there were no statistically significant differences between measurements of overjet obtained by both methods, which agrees with the present study. However, there was statistically significant difference between methods, particularly with regard to teeth width and overbite. Bolton analysis requires teeth width measurements, which could affect total and anterior proportions. In the present study, there were no statistically significant differences for total or anterior proportion, which disagrees with Santoro et al.[15]

Bolton analysis did not result in excellent reproducibility, as demonstrated by Lin's concordance. One of the main reasons justifying the divergence between manual and digital methods is that points of reference may be challenging to locate and the opinion of the examiner regarding the exact location of a point can vary randomly.[26] While performing this study, it was found that measurements taken on the same tooth, with a minimum interlude time, presented minor divergences. This finding is similar to that reported by Shellhart et al[7] who concluded that Bolton analysis can vary in ± 2.2 mm when a bow divider is used. Tomassetti et al[12] found that 72.7% of measurements decreased within 1.0 mm from one to another (0 to 2.8 mm) when Bolton analysis was calculated three times with a digital caliper on dental casts.

Even though Bolton analysis is widely diffused and relatively easy to apply, many practitioners do not use it for clinical evaluation, since the method is somewhat time consuming when the necessary calculations are performed.[12] Digital measurements were easier to acquire than the manual ones, which is in agreement with studies by Abizadeh et al.[27] Tomasseti et al[12] concluded that the time spent by measuring casts with Quick-Ceph was 1.85 minutes, followed by Hamilton Arch Tooth System (HATS) at 3.4 minutes, OrthoCad at 5.37 minutes and caliper at 8.06 minutes. Mullen et al[19] also concluded that the digital method was faster than the manual one, thereby indicating an advantage in using the digital technique.

Additionally, computer programs assessing digital models, such as 3Shape® Ortho Analyzer™ (Copenhagen, Denmark), which was used in this study, offer additional information beyond Bolton analysis, including: teeth size, overbite, overjet, analysis of models, symmetry and dental arch shape, intensity of the curves of Spee and Wilson, manufacture of orthodontic setup, among others. This is in accordance with the studies by Redmond,[14] Santoro et al[15] and Tomassetti et al.[12] Quimby et al[1] suggest that easy storage, manipulation of models and reduced measurement time are features that make the digital method more attractive to orthodontists.

CONCLUSION

It is possible to conclude that Bolton analysis performed on tridimensional virtual models is as reliable as when it is performed on dental casts with satisfactory agreement.

REFERENCES

1. Quimby ML, Vig KWL, Rashid RG, Firestone AR. The accuracy and reliability of measurements made on computer-based digital models. Angle Orthod. 2004;74(3):298-3.

2. Hayashi K, Uechi J, Mizoguchi I. Three-dimensional analysis of dental casts based on a newly defined palatal reference plane. Angle Orthod. 2003;73(5):539-44.

3. Rheude B, Sadowsky PL, Ferreira A, Jacobson A. An evaluation of the use of digital study models in orthodontic diagnosis and treatment planning. Angle Orthod. 2005;75(3):292-96.

4. Oliveira DD, Ruellas ACO, Drummond MEL, Pantuzo MCG, Lanna AMQ. Confiabilidade do uso de modelos digitais tridimensionais como exame auxiliar ao diagnóstico ortodôntico: um estudo piloto. Rev Dental Press Ortod Ortop Facial. 2007;12(1):84-93.

5. Hou HM, Wong RWK, Hägg U. The uses of orthodontic study models in diagnosis and treatment planning. Hong Kong Dent J. 2006;3(2):107-15.

6. Peluso MJ, Josell SD, Levine SW, Lorei BJ. Digital Models: an introduction. Semin Orthod. 2004;10:226-38.

7. Shellhart WC, Lange DW, Kluemper GT, Hicks EP, Kaplan AL. Reliability of the Bolton tooth-size analysis when applied to crowded dentitions. Angle Orthod. 1995;65(5):327-34.

8. Araujo E, Souki M. Bolton anterior tooth size discrepancies among different malocclusion groups. Angle Orthod. 2003;73(3):307-13.

9. Bolton WA. Disharmony in tooth size and its relation to the analyses and treatment of malocclusion. Angle Orthod. 1958;28:113-30.

10. Crosby DR, Alexander CG. The occurrence of tooth size discrepancies among different malocclusion groups. Am J Orthod Dentofacial Orthop. 1989;95(6):457-61.

11. Bolton WA. The clinical application of a tooth-size analysis. Am J Orthod. 1962;48(7):504-29.

12. Tomassetti JJ, Taloumis LJ, Denny JM, Fischer JR. A comparison of 3 computerized Bolton tooth-size analyses with a commonly used method. Angle Orthod. 2001;71(5):351-7.

13. Motohashi N, Kuroda T. A 3D computer-aided design system applied to diagnosis and treatment planning in Orthodontics and Orthognathic Surgery. Eur J Orthod. 1999;21(3):263-74.

14. Redmond WR. Digital models: a new diagnostic tool. J Clin Orthod. 2001;35(6):386-87.

15. Santoro M, Galkin S, Teredesai M, Nicolay O, Cangialosi T. Comparison of measurements made on digital and plaster models. Am J Orthod Dentofacial Orthop. 2003;124(1):101-05.

16. Lin LI. A concordance correlation coefficient to evaluate reproducibility. Biometrics. 1989;45(1):255-68.

17. Paredes V, Gandia JL, Cibrian R. Determination of Bolton tooth-size ratios by digitization, and comparison with the traditional method. Eur J Orthod. 2006;28(2):120-5.

18. Stevens DR, Flores-Mir C, Nebbe B, Raboud DW, Heo G, Major PW. Validity, reliability, and reproducibility of plaster vs digital study models: comparison of peer assessment rating and Bolton analysis and their constituent measurements. Am J Orthod Dentofacial Orthop. 2006;129(6):794-03.

19. Mullen SR, Martin CA, Ngan P, Gladwin M. Accuracy of space analysis with e-models and plaster models. Am J Orthod Dentofacial Orthop. 2007;132(3):346-52.

20. Mayers M, Firestone AR, Rashid R, Vig KW. Comparison of peer assessment rating (PAR) index scores of plaster and computer-based digital models. Am J Orthod Dentofacial Orthop. 2005;128(4):431-4.

21. Bell A, Ayoub AF, Siebert P. Assessment of the accuracy of a three-dimensional imaging system for archiving dental study models. J Orthod. 2003;30(3):219-23.

22. Zilberman O, Huggare JAV, Parikakis KA. Evaluation of the validity of tooth size and arc width measurements using conventional and three-dimensional virtual orthodontic models. Angle Orthod. 2003;73(3):301-6.

23. Redlich M, Weinstock T, Abed Y, Schneor R, Holdstein Y, Fischer A. A new system for scanning, measuring and analyzing dental casts based on a 3D holographic sensor. Orthod Craniofac Res. 2008;11:90-5.

24. Veenema AC, Katsaros C, Boxum SC, Bronkhorst EM, Kuijpers-Jagtman AM. Index of complexity, outcome and need scored on plaster and digital models. Eur J Orthod. 2009;31(3):281-6.

25. Watanebe-Kanno GA, Abrão J, Miasiro J, Sánchez-Ayala A, Lagravère MO. Reproducibility, reliability and validity of measurements obtained from Cecile3 digital models. Braz Oral Res. 2009;23(3):288-95.

26. Sousa MVS, Vasconcelos EC, Janson G, Garib D, Pinzan A. Accuracy and reproducibility of 3-dimensional digital model measurements. Am J Orthod Dentofacial Orthop. 2012;142(2):269-73.

27. Abizadeh N, Moles DR, O'neill J, Noar JH. Digital versus plaster study models: how accurate and reproducible are they? J Orthod. 2012;39(3):151-9.

15

Perception of adults' smile esthetics among orthodontists, clinicians and laypeople

Enio Ribeiro Cotrim[1], Átila Valadares Vasconcelos Júnior[2], Ana Cristina Soares Santos Haddad[2], Sílvia Augusta Braga Reis[3]

Objective: Smile esthetics has become a major concern among patients and orthodontists. Therefore, the aim of this study was: (1) To highlight differences in perception of smile esthetics by clinicians, orthodontists and laypeople; (2) To assess factors such as lip thickness, smile height, color gradation, tooth size and crowding, and which are associated with smile unpleasantness. **Methods:** To this end, edited photographs emphasizing the lower third of the face of 41 subjects were assessed by three groups (orthodontists, laypeople and clinicians) who graded the smiles from 1 to 9, highlighting the markers that evince smile unpleasantness. Kruskall-Wallis test supplemented by Bonferroni test was used to assess differences among groups. Additionally, the prevailing factors in smile unpleasantness were also described. **Results:** There was no significant difference (P = 0.67) among groups rates. However, the groups highlighted different characteristics associated with smile unpleasantness. Orthodontists emphasized little gingival display, whereas laypeople emphasized disproportionate teeth and clinicians emphasized yellow teeth. **Conclusion:** Orthodontists, laypeople and clinicians similarly assess smile esthetics; however, noticing different characteristics. Thus, the orthodontist must be careful not to impose his own perception of smile esthetics.

Keywords: Orthodontics. Dental esthetics. Smile.

» The authors report no commercial, proprietary or financial interest in the products or companies described in this article.

[1] Specialist in Orthodontics, Sérgio Feitosa Institute for Health Studies and Management (IES).
[2] Assistant professor, IES.
[3] Assistant professor, UMESP.

Ana Cristina Soares Santos Haddad
Rua Penafiel, 420 – Anchieta – Belo Horizonte/MG — Brazil
E-mail: anacssantos@usp.br

INTRODUCTION

Smile esthetics has become a major concern among patients and orthodontists. It has been the main reason why patients seek orthodontic treatment.[1] The perception of beauty is associated with pleasure while seeing an object or a person, and while hearing a sound. For this reason, beauty is seen as a highly subjective feeling that results from individual factors such as sex, race, education and personal experiences, as well as social factors such as the environment and the media which has been increasingly responsible for globalizing the concept of beauty.[2] Assessing beauty is a highly subjective matter. Meanwhile, assessing patient's smile allows the clinician to see what needs to be done, what can be done and what should be accepted. Smile analysis includes assessing patient's smile arc, tooth and gingival display, presence of buccal corridor space (BCS), coincidence between facial and dental midlines, tooth proportionality, gingival esthetics, tooth color and occlusal plane inclination.[3]

A number of studies available in the literature have focused on smile geometric and objective analysis.[4-8] Nevertheless, different factors might influence esthetic patterns, including culture. Furthermore, perception of esthetics varies considerably among individuals and is influenced by personal experiences as well as by the social environment.[9]

Thus, in addition to assessing patient's smile in geometrical and objective terms, it is also necessary to scientifically understand smile pleasantness from the point of view of laypeople, orthodontists and clinicians. Rodrigues et al[10] used printed photographs to assess smile attractiveness according to variations in esthetic norms evaluated by 20 laypeople. The authors concluded that variations in esthetic norms do not necessarily hinder perception of smile attractiveness, whereas diastema exerts strong negative influence on smile esthetics.

Schabel et al[11] concluded that extremely unattractive smiles were characterized by great distance between the incisal edge of maxillary incisors and the lower lip, as well as by excessive smile height or insufficient smile width.

Sabherwal et al[12] compared the influence of skin and tooth color on smile attractiveness. The authors found that people with darker skin had lighter teeth in comparison to people with lighter skin; however, what most influenced the perception of white teeth was the color of gingiva and lips.

Dilalíbera et al[13] assessed the esthetic results of Class II patients subjected to corrective orthodontic therapy. Patients did not seem to be too concerned about the fact that facial angles and proportions did not coincide with what is mathematically proposed as esthetic, provided that these features were within the standards of normality accepted by them and established by society.

The literature has extensively covered the subject of smile in an objective manner; however, only a few studies have investigated the pleasant and unpleasant features of one's smile. With a view to discussing this issue and giving further contribution to the literature, this study aimed at:

» Highlighting the differences in perception of smile esthetics by clinicians, orthodontists and laypeople.
» Assessing factors such as lip thickness, smile height, color gradation, tooth size and crowding, which are associated with smile unpleasantness.

MATERIAL AND METHODS

A total of 41 photographs of Brazilian, Caucasian patients (16 males and 25 females) aged between 18 and 56 years old (mean age of 37 years old) and with permanent dentition were analyzed. The photographs were taken from SENAI (Brazilian National Service of Industrial Training) students and employees. All subjects included in the sample signed an informed consent form. The research project was approved by local Institutional Review Board (protocol 2011/0199).

Image acquisition offered low risks to patients' well-being, since biosafety guidelines were strictly followed. Research volunteers were benefited from receiving orthodontic diagnosis and for being referred to treatment whenever necessary. Furthermore, the researcher was always willing to clarify potential doubts.

The following exclusion criteria were applied: Patients undergoing orthodontic treatment during data collection, and patients with craniofacial syndromes.

Standardized frontal facial photographs of patients' smile were used for analysis. All photographs were taken with Canon EOS Rebel XSI® camera, flash Macro Ring Lite MR-14EX, Macro 100 sigma® lens (Tokyo, Japan) and standardized with the same background. Patients were advised to keep natural head posture, remaining in the same posture they do in daily routine.

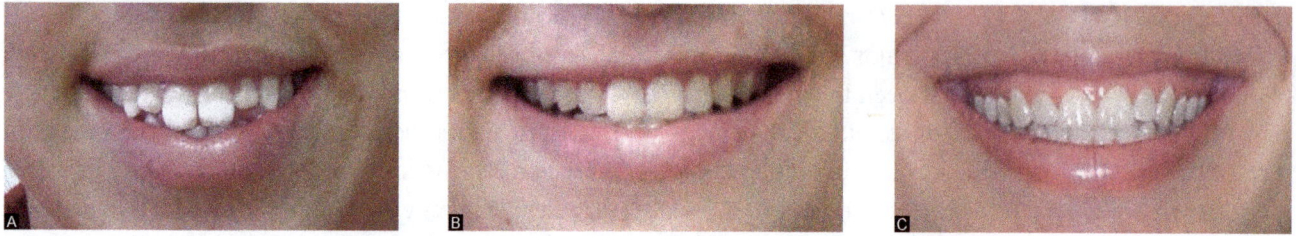

Figure 1 - Frontal smile photographs representing each category: (**A**) esthetically unpleasant, (**B**) esthetically acceptable and (**C**) esthetically pleasant.

In this research, patients were instructed to remain standing while looking ahead at the horizon. Photograph standardization was carried out in accordance with the parameters established by Reis et al.[14]

Frontal facial photographs of patients' smile were edited. In other words, they were cropped so as to evince the lower third of the face, particularly the smile. Examiners were asked to classify the photographs using scores from 1 to 9, as follows: esthetically unpleasant (scores 1, 2 or 3); esthetically acceptable (scores 4, 5 or 6) or esthetically pleasant (scores 7, 8 or 9) (Fig 1). Assessment was carried out by 5 orthodontists, 5 clinicians and 5 laypeople who also filled out a questionnaire so as to establish an association between smile unpleasantness and factors such as lip thickness, smile height, color gradation, teeth size and crowding.

Data were collected for descriptive statistics, highlighting the prevalence of pleasant, acceptable and unpleasant smiles as well as the mean scores attributed by each evaluator.

The scores attributed by the three groups of evaluators (orthodontists, clinicians and laypeople) were also submitted to Kruskall-Wallis statistical test supplemented by Bonferroni test so as to assess potential differences among groups. Additionally, the prevailing factors in smile unpleasantness were also described.

With a view to assessing intrarater agreement, ten facial photographs in frontal view were randomly selected and reassessed with a 30-day interval in between. Paired Student's t-test was used to assess systematic error. No significant difference was found between the first and second scores. Significance level was set at 5% (P > 0.05).

RESULTS

Table 1 shows the values obtained by descriptive statistical analysis (mean, standard deviation and median) for subjective smile assessment.

Kruskall Wallis test did not reveal any difference among evaluators (orthodontists, laypeople and clinicians) (P = 0.67), whereas Bonferroni test found no significant differences between orthodontists and laypeople (P = 0.93), orthodontists and clinicians (P = 0.62) and between laypeople and clinicians (P = 0.29).

Figure 2 shows the most prevalent factors observed in terms of smile unpleasantness, revealing that each group highlighted different features as being responsible for smile unpleasantness. Orthodontists emphasized little gingival display, whereas laypeople emphasized disproportionate teeth and clinicians emphasized stained teeth.

DISCUSSION

In the present study, scores varied between 4 and 5. In other words, acceptable smiles were most prevalent in the sample studied. No differences were found among the scores attributed by each class of evaluators. However, each group assessed the sample from a different point of view, highlighting different features to classify the same smile as pleasant or unpleasant. Orthodontists emphasized the amount of gingival display and thin lips as the most prevalent features in unpleasant smile esthetics. Laypeople, on the other hand, emphasized stained, crowded, disproportional teeth as the features that most contribute to an unpleasant smile; whereas clinicians associated smile unpleasantness with stained, disproportional, small teeth.

Table 1 - Descriptive statistics for subjective smile esthetics assessment.

	Orthodontists	Laypeople	Clinicians
Mean	4.78	4.48	4.89
SD	1.91	1.93	1.54
Median	5	4	5

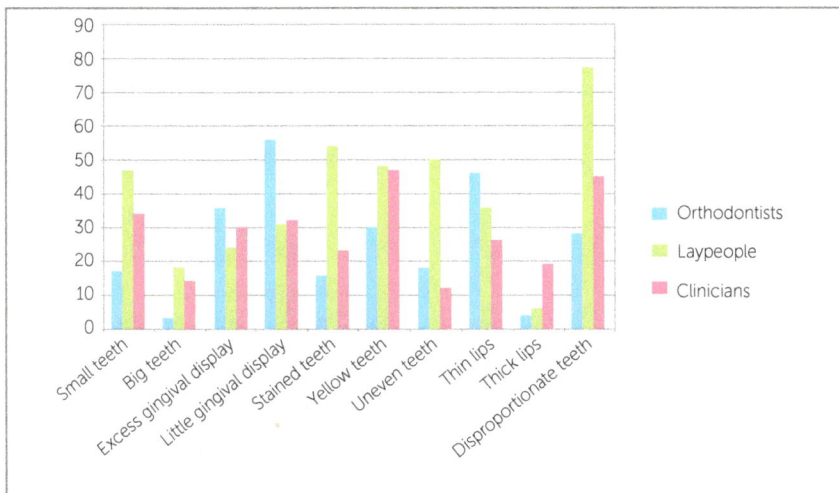

Figure 2 - Different features of smile unpleasantness assessed by orthodontists, laypeople and clinicians.

This means that beauty is subjective and, for this reason, establishing esthetic protocols for diagnosis and treatment planning based on orthodontists, clinicians and laypeople's perception might be a difficult task.

In all groups, thick lips and big teeth were less associated with smile unpleasantness (Fig 2), which suggests a cultural preference for proportionally big teeth and thick lips.

Only a few studies have been conducted to compare the opinion of different groups of evaluators about smile unpleasantness. Rodrigues et al[10] demonstrated that smile assessment by laypeople differs from objective esthetic norms. Additionally, according to Van der Geld et al,[8] smiles characterized by total exposure of clinical crowns and gingival display not greater than 1 mm are considered more esthetic. In the present study, orthodontists evinced little gingival display as the most unpleasant feature. In the study by Malkinson et al,[15] smile esthetics was assessed by clinicians who found that excess gingival display influenced smile attractiveness and affected patient's attraction, reliability, intelligence and self-confidence. Machado et al[16] assessed progressive tooth wear and consequent asymmetry of anterior teeth. Their results agree with the present study, as they evince that tooth size discrepancy contributes to smile unpleasantness.

The present study differs from other researches for identifying what characterizes smile unpleasantness instead of smile pleasantness.

The questionnaire applied in this study comprised pre-determined features of smile unpleasantness; however, other features could have been included, for instance, buccal corridor and curve of Spee. Ioi et al[17] found that narrow or intermediate buccal corridors are considered more esthetic. Nevertheless, these features were not included in the present research due to being difficult to understand by laypeople.

This study evinced the importance of assessing patient's chief complaint and clinician's requirements so as to guide treatment planning. The orthodontist must be careful not to impose his own perception of smile esthetics.

CONCLUSION

Based on the methods employed herein, it is reasonable to conclude that:

» The group conducting most strict smile assessment was that comprising laypeople, followed by orthodontists and clinicians. However, no statistical differences were found among groups.

» Laypeople were most concerned about disproportional teeth, whereas orthodontists evinced little gingival display and clinicians highlighted color gradation.

REFERENCES

1. Springer NC, Chang C, Fields HW, Beck FM, Firestone AR, Rosenstiel S, et al. Smile esthetics from the layperson's perspective. Am J Orthod Dentofacial Orthop. 2011;139(1):91-101.

2. Reis SAB, Abrão J, Capelozza FL, Claro CAA. Análise facial subjetiva. Rev Dental Press Ortod Ortop Facial. 2006;11(5):159-72.

3. Elham SJ, Alhaija ES, Shamsi AN, Khateeb SA. Perceptions of Jordanian laypersons and dental professionals to altered smile aesthetics. Eur J Orthod. 2011;33(4):450-6.

4. Ackerman MB, Brensinger C, Landis JR. An evaluation of dynamic lip-tooth characteristics during speech and smile in adolescents. Angle Orthod. 2004;74(1):43-50.

5. Câmara CALP. Estética em ortodontia: diagramas de referências dentárias (DRED) e faciais (DREF). Rev Dental Press Orthod Orthop Facial. 2006;11(6):130-56.

6. Lopes LVM, Staszak SR, Moro A, Bueno MR. Análise computadorizada do sorriso em ortodontia. Rev Sul-Bras Odontol. 2006;3(1):7-17.

7. Nikgoo A, Alavi K, Alavi K, Miefazaelian A. Assessment of the golden ratio in pleasing smiles. World J Orthod. 2009;10(3):224-8.

8. Van der Geld P, Oosterveld P, Schold J, Jagtman AMK. Smile line assessment comparing quantitative measurement and visual estimation. Am J Orthod Dentofacial Orthop. 2011;139(2):174-80.

9. Flores-Mir C, Silva E, Barriga MI, Lagravere MO, Major PW. Lay person's perception of smile aesthetics in dental and facial views. J Orthod. 2004;31(3):204-9.

10. Rodrigues CDT, Magnani R, Machado MSC, Oliveira OBO. The perception of smile attractiveness. Angle Orthod. 2009;79(4):634-9.

11. Schabel BJ, Franchi L, Baccetti T, McNamara JA. Subjective versus objetive evaluations of smile esthetics. Am J Orthod Dentofacial Orthop. 2009;135(4):72-9.

12. Sabherwal RS, Gonzalez J, Naini FB. Assessing the influence of skin color and tooth shade value on perceived smile attractiveness. J Am Dent Assoc. 2009;140(6):696-705.

13. Delalíbera HVC, Silva MC, Pascotto RC, Terada HH, Terada RSS. Avaliação estética de pacientes submetidos a tratamento ortodôntico. Acta Scient Health Sci. 2010;32(1):93-100.

14. Reis SAB, Abrão J, Capelozza Filho L, Claro CAA. Análise facial numérica do perfil de brasileiros padrão I. Rev Dental Press Ortod Ortop Facial. 2006;11(6):24-34.

15. Malkinson S, Waldrop TC, Gunsolley JC, Lanning SK, Sabatini R. The effect of esthetic crown lengthening on perceptions of a patient's attractiveness, friendliness, trustworthiness, intelligence, and self-confidence. J Periodontol. 2013;84(8):1126-33.

16. Machado AW, Moon W, Gandini Jr LG. Influence of maxillary incisor edge asymmetries on the perception of smile esthetics among orthodontists and laypersons. Am J Orthod Dentofacial Orthop. 2013;143(5):658-64.

17. Ioi H, Kang S, Shimomura T, Kim SS, Park SB, Son WS, et al. Effects of buccal corridors on smile esthetics in Japanese and Korean orthodontists and orthodontic patients. Am J Orthod Dentofacial Orthop. 2012;142(4):459-65.

Pain, masticatory performance and swallowing threshold in orthodontic patients

Marcos Porto Trein[1], Karina Santos Mundstock[2], Leonardo Maciel[3], Jaqueline Rachor[4], Gustavo Hauber Gameiro[5]

Objective: The aim of this study was to assess pain, masticatory performance and swallowing threshold of patients undergoing orthodontic treatment. **Methods:** Ten patients of both genders (mean age of 17.25 ± 5.21 years), with complete permanent dentition, who underwent orthodontic treatment with fixed appliances were evaluated. The masticatory performance and the swallowing threshold were assessed by patient's individual capacity of fragmenting an artificial test food (Optocal) which was chewed and had the resulting particles processed by a standardized sieving method, presenting the median particle size (MPS) of crushed units. The intensity of pain / discomfort during chewing was evaluated by means of a visual analog scale. All tests were performed at the following times: T_0 – before activating the orthodontic appliance; T_1 – 24 hours after activation, and T_2 – 30 days after activation. **Results:** The results showed a significant increase in pain at T_1 (T_0 – 0.60 ± 0.70 mm; T_1 – 66.2 ± 34.5 mm), returning to baseline values at T_2 (3.20 ± 3.82 mm). Masticatory performance was also reduced in T_1 (MPS 10.15 ± 1.1 mm^2) in comparison to T_0 (MPS 7.01 ± 2.9 mm^2) and T_2 (MPS 6.76 ± 1.3 mm^2). However, particle size was not affected in the swallowing threshold test (T_0 – 5.47 ± 2.37 mm^2; T_1 – 6.19 ± 2.05 mm^2; T_2 – 5.94 ± 2.36 mm^2). **Conclusion:** The orthodontic appliances did not interfere in the size of the particles that would be swallowed, even in the presence of pain.

Keywords: Mastication. Malocclusion. Orthodontics.

[1] Specialist in Orthodontics, Federal University of Rio Grande do Sul (UFRGS).
[2] PhD in Orthodontics, State University of São Paulo (UNESP). Associate professor of Orthodontics, UFRGS.
[3] Undergraduate student of Dentistry, UFRGS.
[4] Undergraduate student of Dentistry, UFRGS.
[5] PhD in Orthodontics, University of Campinas (UNICAMP). Associate professor of Physiology, UFRGS.

» The authors report no commercial, proprietary or financial interest in the products or companies described in this article.

Gustavo Hauber Gameiro
Rua Sarmento Leite 500, 2° andar – Centro
CEP: 90.050-170 – Porto Alegre/RS – Brazil
E-mail: gustavo@gameiro.pro.br

INTRODUCTION

Orthodontic movement pain is caused by the release of different mediators after the application of forces on the periodontal ligament (PDL). These mediators, including substance P, histamine, serotonin, glutamate, prostaglandins, leukotrienes, and cytokines may activate nociceptors within the PDL resulting in orthodontic pain,[1] which usually lasts for 2 or 3 days and gradually reduces by the 5th or 6th day.[2] Studies report that 95% of orthodontic patients experience some pain during treatment and several methods have been used to reduce these symptoms, including low level laser, transcutaneous electric stimulation, vibratory PDL stimulation and use of anti-inflammatory drugs.[1,3,4] Several factors associated with orthodontic pain are still ignored by many clinicians, such as the duration, intensity and functional limitations possibly induced by this symptom.

It has been shown that almost all orthodontic patients report moderate to extreme difficulties in biting and chewing harder foods, and thus tend to choose a less consistent diet.[1] The orthodontic pain is probably the main responsible for the masticatory limitations associated with fixed appliances. The orthodontic pain occurring within 48 hours is so disturbing that approximately 20 per cent of patients report being awakened at night, some of them take medication, and almost all patients report eating difficulties as a result of pain.[5,6] However, an objective analysis of mastication and deglutition in patients during orthodontic therapy was not performed by previous studies. These analyses are necessary considering that patients normally overestimate their masticatory ability when they are evaluated only by subjective methods. For example, many individuals with a compromised dentition and dentures judge their masticatory function as 'good' while an objective test resulted in values much lower than healthy subjects.[7] Therefore, the aims of this study were to evaluate masticatory performance, swallowing threshold and pain after orthodontic fixed appliance activation.

MATERIAL AND METHODS
Sample

Ten patients of both genders, five males and five females (mean age of 17.25 ± 5.21 years) participated in this study. The following inclusion criteria were considered: Approximately equal number of occlusal units with malocclusions requiring orthodontic treatment, the presence of complete permanent dentition (except third molars), uneventful medical history and good oral health. Bonding of at least 10 teeth in the maxillary arch and 0.014 (NiTi), 0.014 or 0.016-in (stainless steel) archwires ligated with elastomeric rings were used during the experimental period. No extractions were performed during this period. Four individuals had Class I malocclusions, four had Class III and two had Class II. The exclusion criteria were: previous orthodontic treatment and symptoms of temporomandibular joint dysfunction. An informed written consent was obtained from all participants or parents prior to their enrolment in the study. The local Institutional Review Board approved the protocol. The study was carried out at the Department of Orthodontics of the Federal University of Rio Grande do Sul (UFRGS), in Brazil. Sample size was determined on the basis of clinically relevant masticatory performance data obtained from the literature,[8,9,10] with a power of 80%, $\alpha = 0.05$, and 10 individuals were deemed adequate for this longitudinal study in which each patient served as their own control.

Timing of evaluations

The subjects were analyzed at three time points: T_0, at their first consultation, before fixed appliances were installed; T_1, 24 hours after installation and engagement of the first archwire; T_2, 30 days after the first activation and before reactivation of the appliance. The data collected included masticatory performance, swallowing threshold and self-reported pain.

Masticatory performance evaluation

Masticatory performance was evaluated by means of the individual capacity of fragmentation of an artificial test-food (Optocal).[11] Subjects were given 17 cubes (3.0 g) and instructed to chew them for 15 cycles, during which they were visually monitored by a trained examiner who also timed them using a digital stopwatch. After 15 chewing cycles, the particles were spat onto a plastic cup and the mouth was rinsed thoroughly until all particles were eliminated into the cup. The collected fragments were then passed through paper filters to eliminate excess water and then placed in an oven at 60 °C for 20 hours. The dried particles were weighed and placed on a series of 10 stacked sieves with progressively smaller mesh sizes, ranging from 5.6 to 0.71 mm. The sieves were submitted to constant vibration for 5 minutes.

The contents of each sieve were then weighed on an analytic scale with a 0.001 g precision. Since the specific mass of the test-food is known, weight was converted into volume using the Rosim-Rammler equation on Statistical Package for the Social Sciences version 18.0 software. The distribution of the particles by weight was described by the cumulative function of median particle size (X50), which represents a virtual sieve mesh where 50% of the particles would pass through. The higher the X50, the worse the masticatory performance.

Swallowing threshold

The individuals were handed another set of 17 Optocal cubes and instructed to chew them until they felt the urge to swallow. A trained examiner counted the number of chewing cycles and registered the total time of the cycles, which was measured with a digital stopwatch. The swallowing threshold particles were submitted to the same fragment size analysis as it was done for the masticatory performance test, described above.

Pain quantification

After the individuals chewed the Optocal cubes they were handed a visual analogic scale (VAS) for registration of the pain experienced on every experimental period. The subjects were instructed to make a mark on the 10 cm line corresponding to the pain experienced during chewing. The left limit of the scale was described as "without discomfort" and the right limit as "worst discomfort possible".

Error of method

The X50 data of 10 subjects with the same age were analyzed with the Dahlberg formula and paired t test after 2 analyses within a 7 day interval. There was no statistical difference between the evaluations (p > 0.05) and the reproducibility error was less than 10% for the X50 (0.5 mm).

Statistical analyses

Shapiro-Wilks test was used to verify data normality. The variables were analyzed by ANOVA for repeated measures, and by Tukey's test when they were normally distributed. The Kruskal-Wallis and Dunn's test were applied when data were not normally distributed. The SPSS software was used and the significance level was set at $p < 0.05$.

RESULTS

The results are presented in Figure 1.

Pain and Masticatory Performance

Figure 1 presents the values of pain level, median particle size chewed for 15 cycles, total chewing time and duration of each cycle.

Pain was significantly higher at T_1 when compared to T_0 and T_2 (Kruskal-Wallis + Dunn, $p < 0.05$). A significant reduction in masticatory performance also occurred in T_1 in comparison to T_0 and T_2 (Kruskal-Wallis and Dunn, $p < 0.05$). However, masticatory performance levels did not show statistical significant difference between T_0 and T_2. Total chewing time and time of each cycle were higher in T_1 than in the other experimental periods (Anova + Tukey, $p < 0.05$).

Swallowing threshold

Figure 2 demonstrates the X50 of the swallowing threshold evaluation, total chewing time, time for each cycle, and number of cycles until deglutition. The median particle size did not show statistical difference between the timepoints. Total chewing time and time for each cycle were increased in T_1 when compared to T_0 but without statistical significance. There was a statistically significant reduction when T_2 was compared to T_1 (Anova + Tukey, $p < 0.05$). Time taken for each cycle was similar in all 3 timepoints and although there was an apparent raise in T_1 it did not reach statistical significance (Kruskal-Wallis, $p = 0.092$).

DISCUSSION

This study evaluated pain, masticatory performance and swallowing threshold in patients undergoing orthodontic treatment with fixed appliances. Although the literature presents some studies on the possible functional impacts of braces,[12,13] no quantitative tool was used for objective evaluation of mastication in these studies.

Objective evaluation of masticatory function is essential in clinical trials, since patients tend to overestimate their chewing ability when evaluated only by subjective methods (e.g. questionnaires). Many patients with compromised dentition or dentures think they have a good chewing ability, even when objective tests show values much lower than in subjects with natural dentition.[7,14]

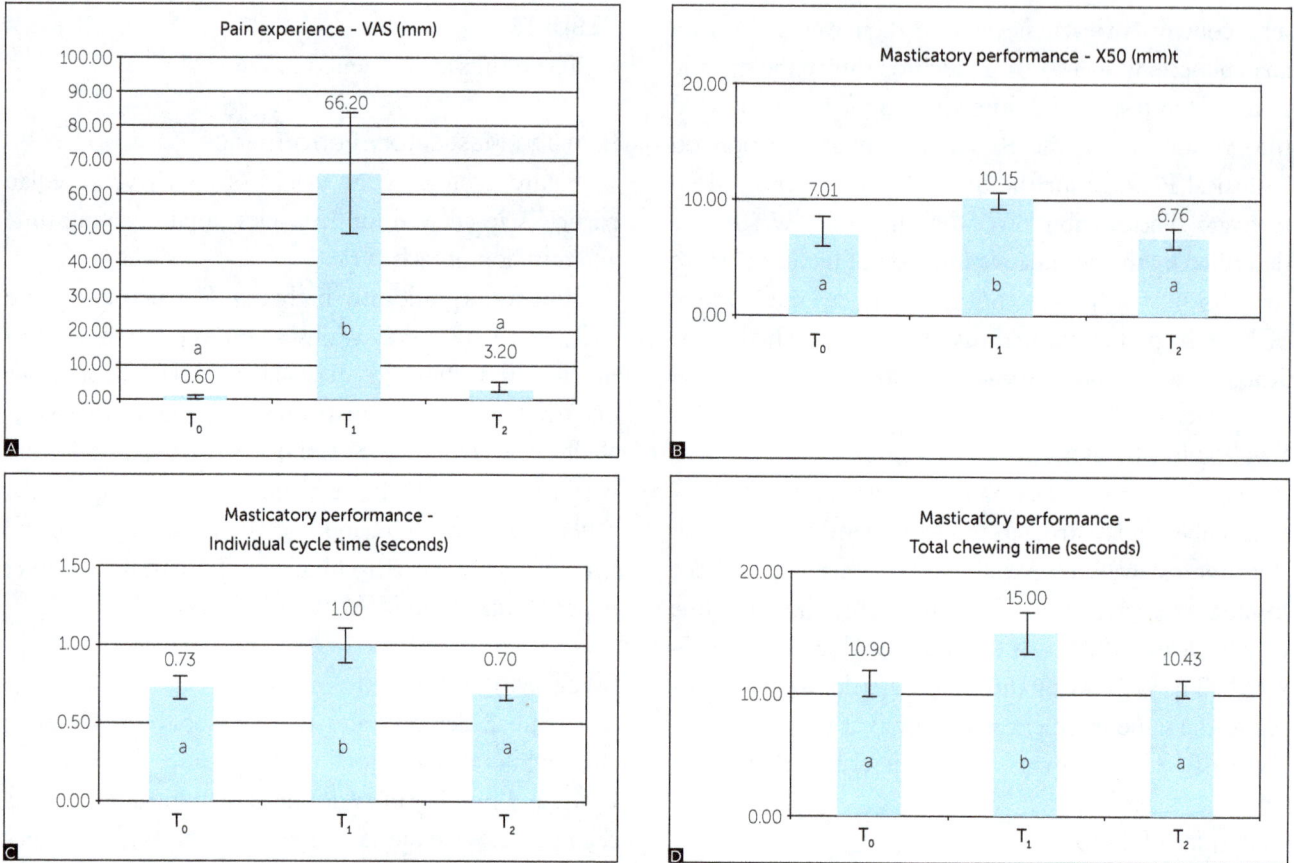

Figure 1 - Masticatory Performance Results. **A**) Pain experience expressed by VAS; **B**) X50 of the particles; **C**) Total chewing time for the 15 cycles; **D**) Individual cycle time. T_0- Before orthodontic appliance activation; T_1- 24 hours after activation; T_2- 30 days after activation. Different letters = statistical significance (Kruskal-Wallis / Dunn or ANOVA / Tukey, p <0.05).

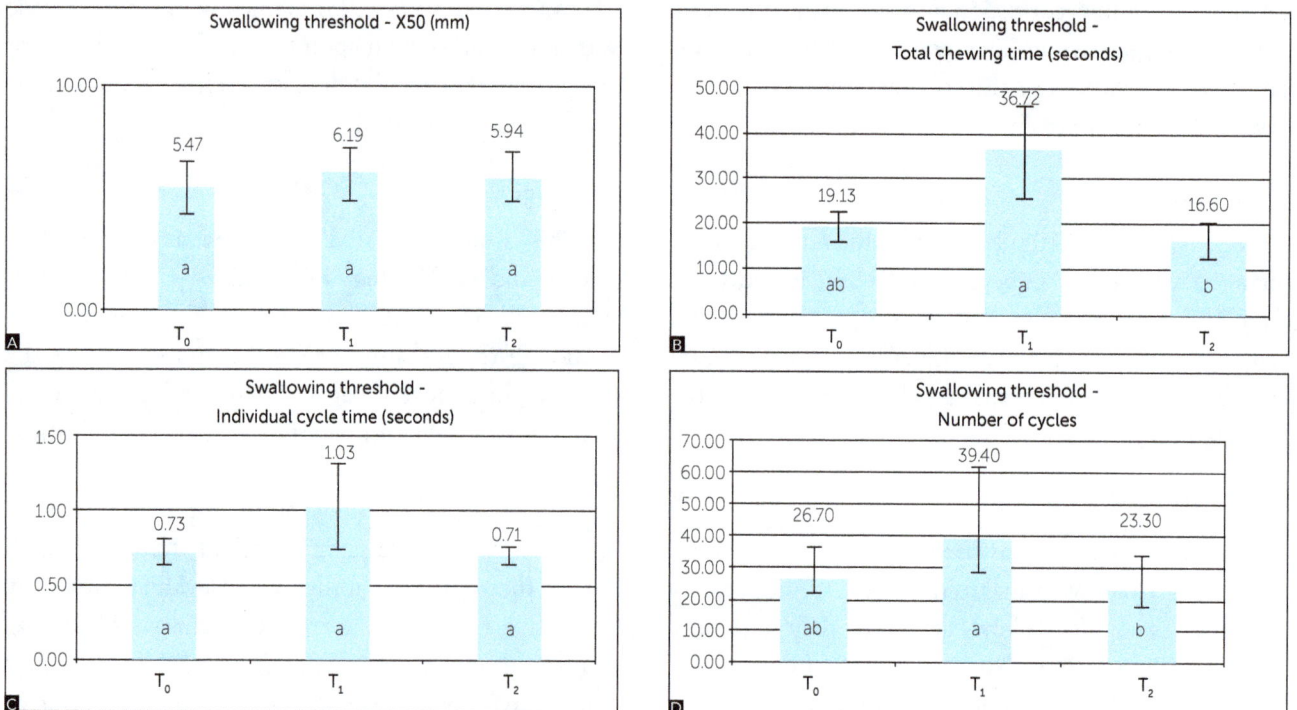

Figure 2 - Swallowing Threshold Results. **A**) X50 of the particles; **B**) Total chewing time until urge of swallowing; **C**) Individual cycle time; **D**) Number of cycles until swallowing. T_0- Before orthodontic appliance activation; T_1- 24 hours after activation; T_2- 30 days after activation. Different letters = statistical significance (Kruskal-Wallis / Dunn or ANOVA / Tukey, p <0.05).

The present study demonstrated that orthodontic patients have low masticatory performance when measured one day after installation and activation of orthodontic appliances. This period represents the peak time of orthodontic pain, which tends to decrease significantly 3 days after insertion of archwires.[2,3,15,16] Erdinç and Dinçer[17] reported the onset of pain as occurring two hours after activation of the device, with a peak within the first 24 hours, in which the recorded average VAS was 48 mm for the group that received a nickel-titanium alloy archwire of 0.016-in section and 49 mm for the group that received a 014-in NiTi alloy archwire. Tortamano et al[18] demonstrated an average registration of 7.25 and 8.25 on a visual scale on the first day after the installation of 0.014-in individualized stainless steel archwires. However, the authors did not use a VAS, but a graduated scale of 1 to 10, in which the subjects had to choose a specific score, which may have resulted in higher average scores. Firestone, Scheurer and Bürgin[19] found an average of 27.5 mm VAS scores for pain caused after the first archwire was installed. It lasted for 7 days with a maximum record of 49.1 mm. In Ong, Ho and Miles study,[16] the peak of reported pain was reached within 24 hours. The work of Fernandes, Ogaard and Skoglund,[20] carried out with subjects from 9 to 16 years old, registered pain experience hourly for the first 11 hours and then on a daily basis for 7 days. The authors found an average of 36 and 37.2 mm VAS scores 24 hours after installation of the first archwire (0.014-in NiTi or 0.014-in Sentalloy). These studies were the basis of our choice of evaluating pain and masticatory performance after 24 hours.

Most studies indicate that there are no gender, age or initial crowding-related differences for pain after orthodontic appliance activation.[2,15,17,21] Firestone, Scheurer and Bürgin[19] did not find gender-related differences for perceived pain. Additionally, Ong, Ho and Miles[16] did not find any relationship between pain and age, gender or initial crowding. The findings of Scott et al[22] demonstrated no correlation between pain and gender or age, either. Therefore, our data was group regardless of gender, age, malocclusion or initial crowding differences. Our results are in agreement with studies that assessed pain associated with braces, and the pain levels reported in the present study (66.2 ± 34.5 mm in T_1) are very similar to those found by Polat, Karaman and Durmus[3] (59.4 ± 31.2 mm), which also recorded the experience of pain by VAS in patients during mastication.

Pain is often underestimated by orthodontists[23] and few studies have assessed the functional impacts of fixed orthodontic appliances.[12,17,24] Pain is often considered the worst aspect of orthodontic treatment, and is also one of the main reasons why patients drop out of treatment.[1,25,26] Some patients report, for example, that the incidence and severity of orthodontic pain is greater than pain caused by tooth extraction.[2] Researchers attribute pain to the hyperalgesia of the periodontal ligament (PDL) caused by induced tooth movement, which is defined as a painful sensation greater than what is expected to a noxious stimulus and felt over a larger area.[27] Orthodontic tooth pressure induces the release of chemical mediators such as histamine, bradykinin, serotonin and prostaglandins, which are capable of activating or sensitizing nociceptors in the PDL.[1,4] In addition to hyperalgesia, orthodontic pain can also be spontaneous or related to non-painful stimuli such as mechanical stimulation of the periodontium during mastication. The pain reported by stimuli that are usually non-painful is called allodynia,[27] and this was clearly observed in our study, since the pain levels were registered right after the masticatory performance and swallowing threshold tests and, after 24 hours, there was significant pain, which is not expected in normal masticatory function. These results are in accordance with those reported by Erdinç and Dinçer,[17] in which approximately 50% of their patients had problems with their daily activities on days 1 and 2 after orthodontic appliance activation and that the discomfort decreased significantly by the third day. In this same study, however, only subjective evaluations were used. In our study, the results of objective evaluation of masticatory function after 24 hours demonstrated that patients presented difficulties in grinding the test food during the masticatory performance test. This can be seen not only by the significant increase in median size of the crushed particles (X50), but also by the increase in the total chewing time and in the time of each cycle during the test.

With regard to the swallowing threshold, there was an increasing trend in time of each cycle and the number of cycles, although not statistically significant. The X50 of the particles right before swallowing was also not increased significantly within 24 hours, indicating that orthodontic patients ingest particles of similar size to that observed prior to the installation of the appliances (T_0). These results suggest that the chewing difficulty presented within 24 hours may have been partially balanced by an upward trend in the number of chewing cycles and time. Other ways to compensate the chewing difficulty during the peak of orthodontic pain may also have been employed, such as changes in the dynamics of jaw movements and bite force, but these variables were not evaluated in this study. Another limitation of our study is that only one test food was evaluated. This test food was chosen because it is less consistent in relation to Optosil® or Cuttersil®,[11] and patients in pain usually avoid harder foods. If we had chosen a harder test-food maybe the results would have pointed towards a more significant difference.

The consequences of inefficient chewing for general health have not been fully elucidated. The particle size ingested, which is determined by the performance of the chewing process, may influence gastric emptying. Some studies suggest that higher masticatory efficiency accelerates gastric emptying,[28,29] although this issue remains controversial. Sierpinska et al[10] found more severe chronic inflammatory changes and infection by Helicobacter pylori in the gastric mucosa in patients with dyspepsia and impaired mastication. If indeed there is a relation of cause and effect between masticatory efficiency and gastric pathologies, orthodontic therapy should not be considered as a potential cause of damage to the patient, since the present results demonstrate that although there is a reduction in masticatory performance within 24 hours, there was no difference in the size of 50X on the verge of swallowing. These findings indicate that orthodontic patients may compensate the functional limitation induced by pain with a more careful mastication until deglutition. To Fontijn-Tekamp et al,[30] individuals with poor masticatory performance tend to swallow larger particles, this observation being similar to that found by English,

Buschang and Throckmorton.[13] In the first article cited,[30] adults with good oral health and varied occlusal conditions were evaluated, while the second[13] evaluated individuals with Class I, II and III malocclusions and normal occlusion, but with no braces installed. Both studies reported that individuals with poor masticatory performance do not compensate this deficiency by increasing the number of cycles until swallowing. However, these results cannot be directly compared to ours, due to the fact that these studies did not evaluate individuals with limitations caused by pain, as in our case, in which the subjects reported significant pain during the evaluation period of 24 hours after orthodontic activation. In the papers mentioned above, the performance was determined only by the dental status of individuals, whereas in our study the experience of pain significantly affected the masticatory performance of patients.

CONCLUSIONS

Patients reported a significant increase in pain during chewing 24 hours after activation of orthodontic appliances, but after 30 days there was no difference compared to baseline values.

By setting a limit of 15 chewing cycles (masticatory performance test), the median size of crushed particles was higher within 24 hours in comparison to initial and final values, which indicates a temporary deterioration in masticatory performance, since this decrease was observed only at the peak of orthodontic pain.

However, when individuals were allowed to perform the number of cycles needed until they felt comfortable to swallow (swallowing threshold test), no statistical difference between the sizes of crushed particles in any of the experimental times was found. These results demonstrate that fixed orthodontic appliances do not interfere in the size of the particles swallowed, even in the presence of orthodontic pain.

REFERENCES

1. Krishnan V. Orthodontic pain: from causes to management-a review. Eur J Orthod. 2007;29(2):170-9.
2. Jones M, Chan C. The pain and discomfort experienced during orthodontic treatment: a randomized controlled clinical trial of two initial aligning arch wires. Am J Orthod Dentofacial Orthop. 1992;102(4):373-81.
3. Polat O, Karaman AI, Durmus E. Effects of preoperative ibuprofen and naproxen sodium on orthodontic pain. Angle Orthod. 2005;75(5):791-6.
4. Gameiro GH, Pereira-Neto JS, Magnani MB, Nouer DF. The influence of drugs and systemic factors on orthodontic tooth movement. J Clin Orthod. 2007;41(2):73-8.
5. Kvam E, Gjerdet N R, Bondevik O. Traumatic ulcers and pain during orthodontic treatment. Community Dent Oral Epidemiol. 1987;15(2):104-7.
6. Scheurer PA, Firestone AR, Bürgin WB. Perception of pain as a result of orthodontic treatment with fixed appliances. Eur J Orthod. 1996;18(4):349-57.
7. van der Bilt A. Assessment of mastication with implications for oral rehabilitation: a review. J Oral Rehabil. 2011;38(10):754-80.
8. Fontijn-Tekamp FA, Slagter AP, van der Bilt A, Van'T Hof MA, Witter DJ, Kalk W, Jansen JA. Biting and chewing in overdentures, full dentures, and natural dentitions. J Dent Res. 2000;79(7):1519-24.

9. van den Braber W, van der Bilt A, van der Glas H, Rosenberg T, Koole R. The influence of mandibular advancement surgery on oral function in retrognathic patients: a 5-year follow-up study. J Oral Maxillofac Surg. 2006;64(8):1237-40.

10. Sierpinska T, Golebiewska M, Dlugosz J, Kemona A, Laszewicz W. Connection between masticatory efficiency and pathomorphologic changes in gastric mucosa. Quintessence Int. 2007;38(1):31-7.

11. Pocztaruk RL, Frasca LC, Rivaldo EG, Fernandes E de L, Gavião MB. Protocol for production of a chewable material for masticatory function tests (Optocal - Brazilian version). Braz Oral Res. 2008;22(4):305-10.

12. Bergius M, Kiliaridis S, Berggren U. Pain in orthodontics. A review and discussion of the literature. J Orofac Orthop. 2000;61(2):125-37.

13. English JD, Buschang PH, Throckmorton GS. Does malocclusion affect masticatory performance? Angle Orthod. 2002;72(1):21-7.

14. Carlsson GE. Masticatory efficiency: the effect of age, the loss of teeth and prosthetic rehabilitation. Int Dent J. 1984;34(2):93-7.

15. Salmassian R, Oesterle LJ, Shellhart WC, Newman SM. Comparison of the efficacy of ibuprofen and acetaminophen in controlling pain after orthodontic tooth movement. Am J Orthod Dentofacial Orthop. 2009;135(4):516-21.

16. Ong E, Ho C, Miles P. Alignment efficiency and discomfort of three orthodontic archwire sequences: a randomized clinical trial. J Orthod. 2011;38(1):32-9.

17. Erdinç AM, Dinçer B. Perception of pain during orthodontic treatment with fixed appliances. Eur J Orthod. 2004;26(1):79-85.

18. Tortamano A, Lenzi DC, Haddad AC, Bottino MC, Dominguez GC, Vigorito JW. Low-level laser therapy for pain caused by placement of the first orthodontic archwire: a randomized clinical trial. Am J Orthod Dentofacial Orthop. 2009;136(5):662-7.

19. Firestone AR, Scheurer PA, Bürgin WB. Patients anticipation of pain and pain-related side effects, and their perception of pain as a result of orthodontic treatment with fixed appliances. Eur J Orthod. 1999;21(4):387-96.

20. Fernandes LM, Ogaard B, Skoglund L. Pain and discomfort experienced after placement of a conventional or a superelastic NiTi aligning archwire. A randomized clinical trial. J Orofac Orthop. 1998;59(6):331-9.

21. Ngan P, Kess B, Wilson S. Perception of discomfort by patients undergoing orthodontic treatment. Am J Orthod Dentofacial Orthop. 1989;96(1):47-53.

22. Scott P, Sherriff M, Dibiase AT, Cobourne MT. Perception of discomfort during initial orthodontic tooth alignment using a self-ligating or conventional bracket system: a randomized clinical trial. Eur J Orthod. 2008;30(3):227-32.

23. Krukemeyer AM, Arruda AO, Inglehart MR. Pain and orthodontic treatment. Angle Orthod. 2009;79(6):1175-81.

24. Brown DF, Moerenhout RG. The pain experience and psychological adjustment to orthodontic treatment of preadolescents, adolescents, and adults. Am J Orthod Dentofacial Orthop. 1991;100(4):349-56.

25. Oliver RG, Knapman YM. Attitudes to orthodontic treatment. Br J Orthod. 1985;12(4):179-88.

26. Kluemper GT, Hiser DG, Rayens MK, Jay MJ. Efficacy of a wax containing benzocaine in the relief of oral mucosal pain caused by orthodontic appliances. Am J Orthod Dentofacial Orthop. 2002;122(4):359-65.

27. Murray GM. Referred pain, allodynia and hyperalgesia. J Am Dent Assoc. 2009;140(9):1122-4.

28. Holt S, Reid J, Taylor TV, Tothill P, Heading RC. Gastric emptying of solids in man. Gut. 1982;23(4):292-6.

29. Pera P, Bucca C, Borro R, Bernocco C, De LA, Carossa S. Influence of mastication on gastric emptying. J Dent Res. 2002;81(3):179-81.

30. Fontijn-Tekamp FA, van der Bilt A, Abbink JH, Bosman F. Swallowing threshold and masticatory performance in dentate adults. Physiol Behav. 2004;83(3):431-6.

17

Occlusal characteristics and orthodontic treatment need in Black adolescents in Salvador/ BA (Brazil): An epidemiologic study using the Dental Aesthetics Index

Arthur Costa Rodrigues Farias[1], Maria Cristina Teixeira Cangussu[2], Rogério Frederico Alves Ferreira[3], Marcelo de Castellucci[4]

Objective: The objective of this article is to evaluate the need of orthodontic treatment, prevalence and severity of the malocclusions in individuals of black ethnicity in a representative sample of schoolchildren of the city of Salvador/Brazil, as well as to verify if the malocclusion was affected by socio-demographic conditions such as age and gender. **Methods:** The reference population was constituted of schoolchildren with age between 12 and 15 years, enrolled in public and private schools. The malocclusion was evaluated in 486 students of black ethnicity, with ages varying from 12 to 15 years, selected in random sample in multiple stages. The adopted significance level was 1% and the power of the test was 90%. A questionnaire registering demographic characteristics was filled out by each individual. The Dental Aesthetics Index (DAI) was used by previously calibrated examiners (kappa 0.89), according to criteria of the World Health Organization. **Results:** It was verified that most of the individuals (76%) had little or any need for orthodontic treatment. About 24% showed a condition of severe malocclusion, culminating in a vital need for orthodontic treatment. The main occlusal characteristics found in the group with high need of orthodontic treatment were dental crowding and accentuated overjet. The age was positively related to the improvement of the maxillary overjet and to the presence of crowding. **Conclusion:** The development of public politics that aim the insertion of orthodontic treatment among the procedures of health programs, with the implementation and development of specialized centers, is fundamental.

Keywords: Malocclusion. Orthodontics. Esthetics. Dental. Dental Health Surveys.

[1] Orthodontist of the Unit of Face Deformities of UFRN.
[2] Associate professor, Department of Social and Pediatric Dentistry, UFBA
[3] Associate professor of Orthodontics, UFBA
[4] Professor, Specialization Course in Orthodontics and Facial Orthopedics, School of Dentistry, UFBA

Arthur Costa Rodrigues Farias
Faculdade de Odontologia da Universidade Federal da Bahia
Av. Araújo Pinho, 62 – Canela – CEP: 40.110-060 – Salvador/BA – Brazil
E-mail: arthurcrfarias@hotmail.com

» The author reports no commercial, proprietary or financial interest in the products or companies described in this article.

INTRODUCTION

Brazil, differently from many other countries, has a population characterized by a large ethnic miscegenation, whose occlusal characteristics have been epidemiologically considered by some studies.[12,26,29] Regarding morphological researches, there seems to be consensus among the orthodontists that some data which indicate normality may vary in the populations from different geographic regions, or in different ethnic groups.

It must also be emphasized the importance of the association of the severity of malocclusions with several factors such as dental caries, early tooth loss and periodontal diseases.

Associated with the ethnic aspects, the socioeconomic factors must also be considered, as according to some authors,[15,18,22] the occlusion must be studied in its social context, giving importance not only to the physical consequences of its bad development, but also to the negative impact it has on the social wellbeing.

In Brazil, the variable "ethnicity" is related to some health problems, including some of oral health, which are often influenced by differences in socioeconomic conditions.[12,25] One of the cities that best fits this situation of ethnic miscellany and socioeconomic disparity is Salvador, in Bahia, where the black ethnicity is the most affected by problems arising from this situation, a fact which can be noticed mainly in the poorest — or in those of social deprivation — areas of the city.

According to Perin's conception,[21] with the evolution of Dentistry, Orthodontics is in a challenging situation, considering that the concern towards the extension of services to the community gradually becomes greater. So, it becomes necessary to know the epidemiological situation of the malocclusions for the planning and rationing of the necessary (human and financial) resources for the efficient provision of orthodontic treatment for the neediest population.

Diagnosis in orthodontics is based primarily on the classification of deviations from normality, and the measure of changes and deviations in relation to it depends on the methods used and the trial of examiners.[23] That is, the traditional orthodontic diagnosis is qualitative, not being suitable for use in public health, since the quantification of problems is the most appropriate solution to get to know the problem in a collective perspective, identify specific factors and subsidize the planning and evaluation of actions as well as the use and distribution of resources. As a result of this, many quantitative methods that are able to classify or evaluate the deviations from normal occlusion have been developed over the past 50 years, allowing a service which is a priority to individuals who show the most severe malocclusions.

The diversity of occlusal indices in the literature is very vast, from those who classify the malocclusions by diagnosis to those who establish the need and complexity of orthodontic treatment, such as: the Treatment Priority Index (TPI), the Summers Occlusal Index, Draker's Handicapping Labio-lingual Deviations Index (HLD), the Handicapping Malocclusion Assessment Record (HMAR), the Index of Orthodontic Treatment Need (IOTN) and the Dental Aesthetic Index (DAI).[6,7,10,13,23,27] All of these indices compile a set of data about malocclusion and expose a final numeric or alphanumeric value that can classify the occlusal situation at a level of severity and of treatment indication.

The Dental Aesthetic Index (DAI) was recommended by the WHO in 1997[30] to assess the severity and need for treatment of malocclusions. The DAI was developed in 1986 at the University of Iowa (USA), based on perceptions of dental esthetics in the United States. It identifies ten occlusal changes, considering dental absence, space and occlusion, resulting mathematically in scores, with weights based on their relative importance according to socially defined esthetic standards. Since it is based on scores of the cases provided by the DAI, in general one may consider it one of the most appropriate criteria to prioritize needs of orthodontic treatment, presenting a clinical approach with an epidemiological character.[8]

In this context, the objective of this study was to identify the main occlusal characteristics of the black ethnicity from a representative sample of the population of schoolchildren in Salvador, in Brazil, and determine the need for orthodontic treatment in this group according to age and gender, in order to provide a solid basis for the estimates of current conditions of oral health of the population and, thus, produce reliable basic data that can be used to develop oral health programs.

MATERIAL AND METHODS

The sample for this survey was drawn from a study conducted by the Institute of Public Health and the Dentistry College of the Federal University of Bahia.

A transversal epidemiological design was used, and the reference population consisted of schoolchildren aged between 12 and 15 years (n = 220300) enrolled in public and private, first and second degree schools in Salvador, Bahia, in 2005. These ages were selected because the World Health Organization (WHO)[18] considers the age of 12 years as a comparison age and international surveillance of oral diseases, and the age of 15 years as the one at which the prevalence of decay is more significant, since permanent teeth are exposed from three to nine years in the oral environment.

This study population consisted of 2100 school born in Bahia (42.5% boys and 57.5% girls), drawn through a multistage probabilistic sample, whose primary sampling units represent the registration of public and private schools of the city, provided by the Ministry of Education. Seventy-two educational establishments (10% of total) were pre-stratified by the Health District and randomly selected, in obedience to the proportionality between public and private schools of basic education and high school. To calculate the sample, data of population of the proportion of malocclusion at 12 years of age with an estimated prevalence of 10% at the highest severity were used. The level of significance was set at 1% and the power of the test was 90%. The number of individuals classified as belonging to a black ethnic group was 486.

The person responsible for each selected student signed the term consent for the study, which was approved by the Committee of Ethics in Research of ISC / UFBA, following the requirements of the Resolution 196/96 of the National Health.

For the categorization of black individuals, the research adopted the classification used by the Brazilian Institute of Geography and Statistics (2004), taking into account the predominant physical features.

The subjects were assessed by means of the Dental Aesthetic Index (DAI) in accordance with the methodology proposed by the World Health Organization.[30]

Periodontal catheters from WHO and disposable wooden spatulas were used for the separation of cheeks and lips.

All data of the malocclusions were collected by six examiners previously calibrated in a pilot study. The overall percentage of agreement was 98.16%, and the kappa 0.89, with the worst agreement between the examiners equal to 85.30%. Both indicators were calculated from the average of the two examiners. An agreement considered satisfactory by WHO[18] for epidemiological surveys on oral health was achieved. Exclusion criteria were:

» Those students who were under orthodontic treatment.
» Students who had already undergone some orthodontic treatment.

Every component registered was multiplied by its corresponding coefficient. The products were summed and added to the constant for the final value of DAI to be obtained (Table 1).

The levels of severity and need for orthodontic treatment can be classified according to the final score of: a) no abnormality or mild malocclusion with little or no need for treatment (≤ 25), b) defined malocclusion in need of elective treatment (26 to 30), c) severe malocclusion with highly desirable indication of treatment (31 to 35) and d) disabling or very severe malocclusion with essential need for treatment (> 36).

Table 1 - Values and data from regression standard equation of DAI. (Source: Cons et al,[8] 1986).

Conditions	Components of DAI	Weight
1	Number of visible missing teeth	6
2	Crowding on incisal segments: 0 = no crowding, 1 = 1 segment with crowding, 2 = 2 segments with crowding	1
3	Spacing on incisal segments: 0 = no spacing, 1 = 1 segment with spacing, 2 = 2 segments with spacing	1
4	Median spacing in mm	3
5	Greater maxillary anterior misalignment in mm	1
6	Greater mandibular anterior misalignment in mm	1
7	Maxillary overjet in mm	2
8	Mandibular overjet in mm	4
9	Anterior open bite in mm	4
10	Molar relationship; greater deviation from normal to mesial or to distal: 0 = normal, 1 = ½ cusp to mesial or to distal, 2 = 1 or more cusps to mesial or to distal	3
11	CONSTANT	13
	Total	Score DAI

Data were entered in the spreadsheet Microsoft Excel® 2003 and subsequently exported and analyzed using SPSS 10.0 for Windows. For purposes of analysis, the severity of malocclusion and need for orthodontic treatment were dichotomized into: mild malocclusion and little need for treatment, and, severe malocclusion and desirable treatment, with set at the score of 30. The level of significance for all tests was $p < 0.05$.

RESULTS

From the 486 black individuals, 236 (48.6%) were male and, 250 (51.4%), female. The average age of subjects examined was 13.5 years (SD = 1.1), with a median of 14. Most individuals (26.5%) were aged 15 years.

It can be statistically measured that male individuals from the age of 15 years have a lower need for orthodontic treatment than the others ($p < 0.05$). The distribution of data according to age, sex and need for treatment is found in Table 2.

With regard to the degree of severity of occlusal condition, two subjects had the more socially acceptable condition, each with a score of 13. Only one individual had the highest severity score (69). The average final value of DAI for the entire sample was 26.28 (SD = 7.87), being 26.01 (SD = 7.78) for males and 26.52 (SD = 7.96) for females. From the total sample, 61% showed a final score equal to or less than average.

It was observed in 76% (n = 369) a low need for orthodontic treatment, with a maximum score of 30, which can be seen in Figure 1. On the other hand, 24% (n = 117) of the group studied had severe malocclusion, with a high need for orthodontic treatment, where the scores were above 31 (Fig 1).

Tables 3 and 4 respectively show the distribution of DAI components according to the classification of the need for treatment and age. The first sub-category within each component characterizes a condition of normal occlusion.[7] Dental crowding is one of the occlusal characteristics that most appear (67.5%) in the group with high need for orthodontic treatment, and their presence increases with age. However, this was the only homogeneous condition in different degrees of severity. In all other components of DAI, like strong maxillary overjet (65%), spacing (43.6%) and open bite (40.2%), we observed an increase in the presence and severity, being these differences statistically significant.

Testing the difference between the values of the various components of DAI between the two age groups (grouped for analysis in 1213 and 1415), the existence of an association between age, the presence of missing teeth and overjet was observed, when the population of younger individuals possessed a greater number of missing teeth and larger overjet. A significant increase in dental crowding with age was also observed.

Table 2 - Number and percentage distribution of individuals according to age, need for treatment and gender. Salvador, BA, 2004.

Gender	Treatment need	Age (years)							
		12		13		14		15	
		n	%	n	%	n	%	n	%
Male	Low	36	70.5	37	64.9	42	71.2	64	92.7
	High	15	29.5	20	35.1	17	28.8	5	7.3
Female	Low	49	80.3	51	72.8	44	74.6	46	76.6
	High	12	19.7	19	27.2	15	25.4	14	23.3

*p > 0.05 (p = 0.001 for the 15 years).

Table 3 - Number and percentage distribution of the variables according to the need for treatment. Salvador, BA, 2004.

Condition		Treatment need				p value
		None/Elective		Highly desirable/ Indispensable		
		n	%	n	%	
Missing teeth	0	362	98.1	100	85.5	0.000
	≥ 1	7	1.9	17	14.5	
Segments with crowding	0	202	54.7	38	32.5	0.785
	1-2	167	45.3	79	67.5	
Segments with spacing	0	240	65	66	56.4	0.000
	1-2	129	35	51	43.6	
Interdental spacing in mm	0	291	78.9	80	68.4	0.000
	> 0	78	21.1	37	31.6	
Anterior maxillary misalignment in mm	0-1	292	79.1	61	52.1	0.000
	> 1	77	20.9	56	47.9	
Anterior mandibular misalignment in mm	0-1	328	88.9	81	69.2	0.000
	> 1	41	11.1	36	30.8	
Maxillary overjet in mm	0-2	210	56.9	41	35	0.000
	> 2	159	43.1	76	65	
Mandibular overjet in mm	0	358	97	104	88.9	0.000
	> 0	11	3	13	11.1	
Open bite in mm	0	351	95.1	70	59.8	0.000
	> 0	18	4.9	47	40.2	
Molar cusps relationship	Normal	236	64	33	28.2	0.018
	Abnormal	133	36	84	71	

Table 4 - Number and percentage of variables according to age. Salvador, BA, 2004.

Condition		Age (years)				p value
		12-13		14-15		
		n	%	n	%	
Missing teeth	0	221	92.5	241	97.6	0.008
	≥ 1	18	7.5	6	2.4	
Segments with crowding	0	124	51.9	116	47	0.160
	1-2	115	48.1	131	53	
Segments with spacing	0	149	62.3	157	63.6	0.427
	1-2	90	37.7	90	36.4	
Interdental spacing in mm	0	180	75.3	191	77.3	0.339
	> 0	59	24.7	56	22.7	
Anterior maxillary misalignment in mm	0-1	172	72	181	73.3	0.412
	> 1	67	28	66	26.7	
Anterior mandibular misalignment in mm	0-1	197	82.4	212	85.8	0.183
	> 1	42	17.6	35	14.2	
Maxillary overjet in mm	0-2	115	48.1	136	55.1	0.075
	≥ 2	124	51.9	111	44.9	
Mandibular overjet in mm	0	225	94.1	237	96	0.232
	> 0	14	5.9	10	4	
Openbite in mm	0	209	87.4	212	85.8	0.348
	> 0	30	12.6	35	14.2	
Molar cusps relationship	Normal	130	54.4	139	56.3	0.372
	Abnormal	109	45.6	108	43.7	

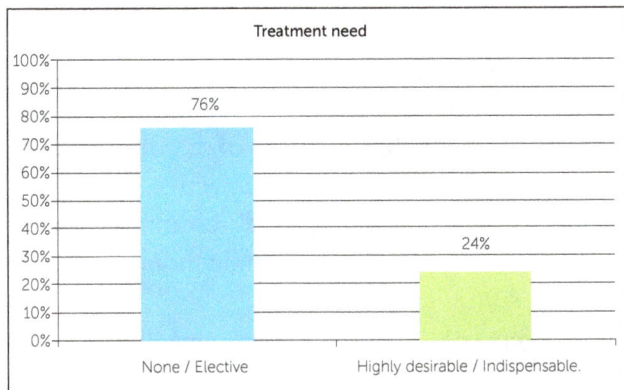

Figure 1 - Numerical and percentual distribution of individuals from Back ethnicity, according to the treatment need. Salvador, BA. 2004.

DISCUSSION

The indices used to assess need for orthodontic treatment ensure that individuals with similar needs have the same priority degree. In addition, the indices work as a communication tool for orthodontists, patients and those responsible for the patients.[2,3,11,23]

However, no index is universally accepted as a means of measuring all aspects of need of orthodontic treatment of individuals or populations. It thus becomes very complicated to elaborate an index that takes into account all circumstances of malocclusions and can also be used consistently by non-specialists in orthodontics. In addition, perceptions of malocclusion may differ between countries and cultures, as well as between age groups, so they may not be valid for different societies.[20,24]

Despite the changes proposed by Cons et al[8] and for the use of DAI in the mixed dentition, it is still the target of much criticism.[20]

Nevertheless, DAI is a product of extensive statistical tests and can be considered a good assessment tool to measure severity and need for orthodontic treatment also in Brazil, according to studies of consistency analysis by Cunha.[9] In other words, it is considered a transcultural index, as it summarizes patterns of dental esthetics which are socially defined in the features it evaluates,[7] besides providing more clinical information than other indices, not underestimating the severity of malocclusion and allowing greater category flexibility to classify the individual.

The present study was conducted in the city of Salvador, in Northeastern Brazil, a city in lack of orthodontic treatment offer in the public sector, where resources are insufficient to meet the population in need of treatment.

The population of the metropolitan region of Salvador is multiethnic, being predominant the African-mestizo segments, i.e., there is a greater number of individuals of black or mixed ethnicity (67.2% of the population).[18] The deprivation that weaves the lives of this population in particular is also unquestionable, with regard to economic and social aspects, which are interconnected with racial issues from the country, where ethnicity contributes to a greater or lesser exposure to different health risks. This generates the hypothesis that individuals belonging to the black race would have a lower dental and medical care and suffer greater physical damage with regard to the presence of malocclusion and therefore present a greater number of individuals with need of essential orthodontic treatment compared to other ethnic groups.

However, according to the findings of this research, 24% of the studied population showed a high need for treatment, not differing from the results of studies without ethnic restriction, such as that by Abdullah and Rock,[1] that found 24.1% of the population requiring orthodontic treatment. Similar results were also found in studies by Jenny et al[16] which analyzed Native Americans, by Estioko, Wright and Morgan[11] which evaluated Australian schoolchildren from 11 to 16 years, despite the final average score of the DAI was slightly larger in this study and by Marques et al,[18] evaluating the schoolchildren aged from 10 to 14 years in Belo Horizonte, in Brazil. Compared to the DAI scores obtained by Cons et al,[8] the proportion of individuals in need of orthodontic treatment was similar in this study.

In another study[14] only with schoolchildren of black ethnicity from Limpopo Province, South Africa, it was observed that 26% of the individuals had severe and defined malocclusion, according to the DAI application.

The occlusal characteristics observed in the group with the highest need of orthodontic treatment were dental crowding, followed by severe maxillary overjet, corroborating the findings of Pires et al,[22] when examining 141 schoolchildren in Salvador / BA, in addition to others.[4,18,26]

Malocclusions characterized by severe crowding and severe maxillary overjet can interfere in social relationships, since facial esthetics is considered significantly determinant in what concerns perception and attribution of society and of individuals about themselves, with dissatisfaction with appearance the main reason for seeking for orthodontic treatment.[18]

In what concerns age, the DAI average fell very little from 12 to 15 years. However, older individuals had a little more acceptable dental appearance than younger individuals. A decrease in the frequency of dental absence and maxillary overjet was observed. This fact probably occurred due to the fact that some younger individuals had clinical absence of some teeth, being in the 2nd transitional period, and in the pubertal growth spurt, harmonizing the horizontal distance of the jaws.[5]

An increase in dental crowding with age was observed. The presence of periodontal diseases, caries and early loss of deciduous elements are facts of frequent occurrence in the poorest populations who live in a situation of lack of basic dental care. Thus, occlusal development is negatively influenced by mesial migration of teeth resulting in dental crowding. As Thilander et al[29] asserts, one must not exclude the hypothesis that the lack of proper oral hygiene explains, at least partially, the high prevalence of dental crowding.

In the facial pattern of black Brazilian individuals, a predominance of maxillary double protrusion is observed, often characterized by earlier dental crowding and consequent double protrusion with labial incompetence. The current trend is the extraction of the four first premolars and maximum retraction of anterior teeth. This treatment tends to retract the lips and reduce the facial convexity.

However, the idea of correcting face convexity of the black is somewhat uncertain from the point of view of many professionals. What are the esthetic goals for these patients? Will the current esthetic values allow a slight facial convexity or that opinion has been modified by society's influence? In essence, what would be the preference of the black ethnic group, a straight or convex profile? Perhaps a middle

ground situation? As society becomes increasingly concerned with the esthetic condition, orthodontists must consider the patient's opinion. The professional must consider the characteristics of the ethnic pattern since the concept of beauty is subjective, an individual matter, where only a general research cannot be applicable to all people of all ethnic groups and from different cultures.

It is impossible not to consider some limitations of the study, mainly based on the indicator used. DAI does not measure certain conditions such as overbite, midline deviation and open and posterior cross bite, clinical findings that could also be present in the analyzed individuals and often significant in severity and complexity of the case.

As the proposed design rigorously followed the requirements for achieving a representative study of schoolchildren from the city of Salvador, when extrapolating these data for the 220,300 students aged between 12 and 15 years, it is estimated that at least 52,872 schoolchildren needed orthodontic treatment. In Salvador, the public health services provided to the population does not offer this treatment. The lack of infrastructure in the political, social and operational aspects regarding the problem is clear.

CONCLUSION

Most individuals (76%) observed in this study had little or no need for orthodontic treatment. About 24% had a condition of severe malocclusion, resulting in a vital need for orthodontic treatment.

The main occlusal characteristics found in the group with higher need for orthodontic treatment were dental crowding and severe overjet;

Age was positively related to improvement of maxillary overjet and to the presence of anterior dental crowding;

There was no statistically significant difference according to gender on the need for treatment.

The development of public policies that aim at the insertion of orthodontic treatment among procedures of health programs, with the implementation and development of specialized centers, thus, becomes essential.

REFERENCES

1. Abdullah MS, Rock WP. Perception of dental appearance using index of treatment need (Aesthetic Component) assessments. Community Dent Health. 2002;19(3):161-5.

2. Baume LJ. A method for measuring occlusal traits. Int Dental J. 1973;23:530-7.

3. Birkeland K, Boe OE, Wisth PJ. Relationship between occlusion and satisfaction with dental appearance in orthodontically treated and untreated groups. A longitudinal study. Eur J Orthod. 2000;22:509-18.

4. Bittencourt LP, Pimentel EC, Modesto A, Bastos E. Frequência dos hábitos orais e a severidade das maloclusões. 17ª Reunião Anual da SBPqO; 2000; Set 2; Águas de Lindoia; 2000.

5. Björk A, Skieller V. Normal and abnormal growth of the mandible. A synthesis of longitudinal cephalometric implant studies over a period of 25 years. Eur J Orthod. 1983;5(1):1-46.

6. Brook PH, Shaw WC. The development of an index of orthodontic treatment priority. Eur J Orthod. 1989;11(3):309-20.

7. Cons NC, Jenny J, Kohout FJ, Songpaisan Y, Jotikastira D. Utility of the dental aesthetic index in industrialized and developing countries. J Public Health Dent. 1989;49(3):163-6.

8. Cons NC, Jenny J, Kohout FJ. DAI: the Dental Aesthetic Index. Iowa: College of Dentistry, University of Iowa; 1986. p. 134.

9. Cunha ACPP. Avaliação da capacidade dos índices DAI e IOTN em estabelecer a necessidade de tratamento ortodôntico [dissertação]. Natal (RN): Universidade Federal do Rio Grande do Norte; 2002.

10. Draker HL. Handicapping labio-lingual deviations: A proposed index for public health purposes. Am J Orthod. 1960;46:295-305.

11. Estioko LJ, Wright FAC, Morgan MV. Orthodontic treatment need of secondary schoolchildren in Heidelberg, Victoria: an epidemiologic study using the Dental Aesthetic Index. Community Dent Health. 1994;11(3):147-51.

12. Frazão P. Epidemiologia da oclusão dentária na infância e os sistemas de saúde [tese]. São Paulo (SP): Universidade de São Paulo; 1999.

13. Grainger RM. Orthodontic treatment priority index. 1000 PHSPN (Public Health Service publication number). ed. 2, n. 25. Washington, DC: Government Priting Office, 1967.

14. Hlongwa P, Plessis JB. Malocclusions among 12-years-old school children in Mankweng, Limpopo Province of South Africa. SADJ. 2005;60(10):455-57.

15. Jenny J. A social perspective on need and demand for orthodontic treatment. Int Dental J. 1975;25:248-56.

16. Jenny J, Cons NC, Kohout FJ, Jakobsen J. Differences in need for orthodontic treatment between Native Americans and the General Population based on DAI scores. J Public Health Dent. 1991;51:234-38.

17. López FU, Cezar GM, Ghisleni GC, Farina JC, Beltrame KP, Ferreira ES. Prevalência de maloclusão na dentição decídua. Rev Fac Odontol Porto Alegre. 2001;43(2):8-11.

18. Marques LS, Barbosa CC, Ramos-Jorge ML, Pordeus IA, Paiva AM. Prevalência da maloclusão e necessidade de tratamento ortodôntico em escolares de 10 a 14 anos de idade em Belo Horizonte, Minas Gerais, Brasil: enfoque psicossocial. Cad Saúde Pública. 2005;21(4):1099-106.

19. Noronha CV, Machado EP, Tapparelli G, Cordeiro TRF, Laranjeira DHP, Santos CAT. Violência, etnia e cor: um estudo dos diferenciais na região metropolitana de Salvador, Bahia, Brasil. Am J Public Health. 1999;5:4-5.

20. Otuyemi D, Ogunyinka A, Dosumu O, et al. Percepções da estética dental nos Estados Unidos e Nigéria. Com Dent Oral Epid. 1998;26:418-20.

21. Perin PCP. Prevalência de má oclusão e necessidade de tratamento ortodôntico, comparando a classificação de Angle e o Índice de Estética Dentária, na cidade de Lins/SP [tese]. Lins (SP): Universidade Estadual Paulista; 2002.

22. Pires DM, Rocha MCBS, Teixeira MCT. Prevalência de oclusopatias na dentadura mista em escolares - Salvador-BA. Rev Bras Odontol. 2001;58(6):414-7.

23. Proffit WR, Fields HW, Moray LJ. Prevalence of malocclusion and orthodontic treatment need in the United States: estimates from the NHANES III survey. Int J Adult Orthodon Orthognath Surg. 1998;13(2):97-106.

24. Saltzmann JA. Handicapping malocclusion assessment to establish treatment priority. Eur J Orthod. 1968;54:749-65.

25. Shaw WC, Lewis HG, Robertson NRE. Perceptions of malocclusion. Br Dent J. 1975;138:211-6.

26. Silva Filho OG, Freitas SF, Cavassan AO. Prevalência de oclusão normal e má oclusão na dentadura mista em escolares da cidade de Bauru (São Paulo). Rev Assoc Paul Cir Dent. 1989;43(6):287-90.

27. Silva CHT, Araújo TM. Prevalência de más oclusões em escolares na Ilha do Governador, Rio de Janeiro. Parte 1: Classes I, II e III e mordida cruzada. Ortodontia. 1983;16(3):10-6.

28. Summers CJ. The Occlusal Index: A system for identifying and scoring occlusal disorders. Am J Orthod. 1971;59(6):552-67.

29. Thilander B, Pena L, Infante C, Parada SS, Mayorga C. Prevalence of malocclusion and orthodontic treatment need in children and adolescents in Bogotá, Colômbia. An epidemiological study related to different stages of dental development. Eur J Orthod. 2001;23:153-67.

30. World Health Organization. Oral health surveys: basic methods. 4th ed. Geneva: ORH/EPID; 1997.

18

Serum insulin-like growth factor-1 levels in females and males in different cervical vertebral maturation stages

Shreya Gupta[1], Anuradha Deoskar[2], Puneet Gupta[3], Sandhya Jain[4]

Objective: The aim of this cross sectional study was to assess serum insulin-like growth factor-1 (IGF-1) levels in female and male subjects at various cervical vertebral maturation (CVM) stages. **Material and methods:** The study sample consisted of 60 subjects, 30 females and 30 males, in the age range of 8-23 years. For all subjects, serum IGF-1 level was estimated from blood samples by means of chemiluminescence immunoassay (CLIA). CVM was assessed on lateral cephalograms using the method described by Baccetti. Serum IGF-1 level and cervical staging data of 30 female subjects were included and taken from records of a previous study. Data were analyzed by Kruska-Wallis and Mann Whitney test. Bonferroni correction was carried out and alpha value was set at 0.003. **Results:** Peak value of serum IGF-1 was observed in cervical stages CS3 in females and CS4 in males. Differences between males and females were observed in mean values of IGF-1 at stages CS3, 4 and 5. The highest mean IGF-1 levels in males was observed in CS4 followed by CS5 and third highest in CS3; whereas in females the highest mean IGF-1 levelswas observed in CS3 followed by CS4 and third highest in CS5. Trends of IGF-1 in relation to the cervical stages also differed between males and females. The greatest mean serum IGF-1 value for both sexes was comparable, for females (397 ng/ml) values were slightly higher than in males (394.8 ng/ml). **Conclusions:** Males and females showed differences in IGF-1 trends and levels at different cervical stages.

Keywords: Female. Male. Cervical vertebrae. Insulin-like growth factor 1.

[1] Senior lecturer, Index Institute of Dental Science, Department of Orthodontics and Dentofacial Orthopedics, Rau, Indore (M.P.), India.
[2] Senior Lecturer, Hitkarini Dental College and Hospital, Department of Orthodontics and Dentofacial Orthopedics, Jabalpur, (M.P.), India.
[3] MDS Public Health Dentistry, Government College of Dentistry, Department of Public Health Dentistry, Indore (M.P.), India.
[4] Professor and Head, Government College of Dentistry, Department of Orthodontics and Dentofacial Orthopedics, Indore (M.P.), India.

» The authors report no commercial, proprietary or financial interest in the products or companies described in this article

Shreya Gupta
E-mail: drshreyagupta@gmail.com

INTRODUCTION

Assessment of growth status plays a vital role in orthodontic treatment planning decisions, including cases involving the use of functional appliances, rapid maxillary expansion, retention appliances, extraoral traction forces, extraction *versus* non-extraction treatment or orthognathic surgery.[1]

Growth modification therapy carried out during the adolescent growth spurt might allow successful outcomes to be achieved within a reduced period of time.[2] An important factor that influences timing of adolescent growth spurt is patient's sex.[3] It is believed that the speed of adolescent spurt is lower in girls and occurs an average of 2 years earlier than boys.[4] This aspect of growth should be taken into account while making clinical decisions. According to Hagg et al,[5] the optimal age of maxillary expansion in girls is 12 to 13 years. However, in boys, maxillary inter-canine dimensions increase is seen until the age of 18. The clinical implication is that, in cases of crowding, any attempt to treat by expansion may not succeed due to the inability to attain a stable increase in inter-canine width. Likewise, pubertal spurt can be easily missed in early maturing girls, while in late maturers the pubertal spurt may not have started at all, but functional treatment would have been completed. Hence, determining the growth trend in each patient becomes crucial for the orthodontic practitioner.

Presently, growth assessment is carried out by means of various skeletal maturity assessing tools, such as hand wrist and cervical vertebrae radiograph.[1] Cervical vertebrae maturation (CVM) assessed on routine lateral cephalograms protects patients from unnecessary radiation exposure by avoiding the need for additional radiograph.[6]

Nevertheless, the use of radiographic methods to predict mandibular growth has been under scrutiny for some time. It has been questioned whether mandible undergoes spurt in growth at the same time as the other skeletal structures or whether it has a late surge. In addition, CVM staging has been documented to involve subjective errors and has a decreased reproducibility.[7] Interobserver and intraobserver disagreement exist with the same radiographs taken at different time intervals.[7] A recent study has proposed that CVM stages cannot accurately identify the onset of the peak in mandibular growth and should be used with other methods of growth assessment.[8] Furthermore, with incorrect neck posture while taking the radiograph, it becomes difficult to visualize the subtle changes in the vertebrae.[9]

There is evidence on accelerated mandibular growth in subjects showing radiographic skeletal maturity termed as residual mandibular growth,[10] and also in certain subjects before the radiographic pubertal growth stage, a phenomenon termed as juvenile acceleration.[11] In such cases, hormonal biomarkers may provide an edge over radiographic skeletal maturity assessment methods.

Puberty is essentially a hormonal phenomenon.[12] Biological changes that occur during puberty include several neurosecretory factors and/or hormones. The entire endocrine system is altered during adolescence, and growth hormone, thyroid and adrenal hormones are all involved in this maturational process. IGF-1 is a hormonal mediator of growth hormone.[13] Studies have documented that serum IGF-1 level has a close association with the growth phenomenon.[13] Hence, in order to gauge the growth status of an individual in the growth trajectory, it would be prudent to assess serum levels of biomarkers such as IGF-1.

Our previous study[14] on serum IGF-1 on female subjects yielded encouraging results, thus, this study aimed at investigating further. The purpose of the present study was to compare the trends and levels of serum IGF-1 in female and male subjects in various CVM stages.

MATERIAL AND METHODS

The study sample consisted of 60 subjects, 30 females and 30 males, in the age range of 8-23 years old. The study sample was randomly selected from the outpatient departments of Orthodontics and Pedodontics, Government College of Dentistry Indore, India, using the simple random sampling technique. Data of 30 female subjects (selected using the same inclusion criteria applied to the male sample) taken from records of our previous study[14] on female subjects, carried out in the same department, were included.

All subjects were included according to the following criteria:

» Normal growth, healthy individuals (height, weight and chronological age of subjects were compared to ideal height, weight and age charts based on ICMR standards 2010 for Indian males and females.[15] Subjects falling in the normal range were included in the study.)

» Absence of systemic disease, serious illnesses, growth abnormality, e.g. craniofacial syndromes, no bone disease or deformities, bleeding disorders or history of any serious trauma or injury to the face, hand and wrist region.

» Absence of signs of acute inflammation or infection at the time of blood sampling. No medication.

» The research protocol was approved by local Institutional Review Board. Parental/patient's informed consent form was taken prior to enrolling each subject in the study.

Lateral cephalograms were obtained and, on the same day, blood samples were collected from the median cubital vein. Time of blood sample collection for all subjects was between 12 noon and 3 pm. Serum was separated from the blood samples and labeled with a patient code (without any mention of patient's details, such as name, age and sex). It was then properly sealed and stored in a thermocol box with ice pack (kept between 2 °C and 8 °C), and sent to the laboratory for chemiluminescence immunoassay for determination of IGF-1 levels by a fully automated, two-site chemiluminescent immunoassay (Siemens Immunolite 2000 immnoassay machine at Metropolis laboratories).

Lateral cephalograms were taken in natural head position. All radiographs were exposed at 80 kVp, 9 mA for 1.25 seconds. The cervical staging technique, as described by Baccetti et al,[16] was used to stage the cervical vertebrae.

CVM staging for all samples was separately performed by two investigators at different times. Both investigators were blinded regarding patient's details, such as name, age, sex and IGF-1 levels. For all samples, the chief investigator assessed CVM stages twice at an interval of 15 days. Intraobserver reliability was 100% (Kappa = 1.0). Another senior investigator assessed the radiographs independently. Interobserver reliability was high (Kappa = 0.918).

Data were checked for assumptions of normality by Shapiro-Wilk test. Since data did not follow normality, non-parametric tests were used.

The IGF-1 levels for male and female subjects between groups were compared by means of Kruskal-Wallis ANOVA (Tables 1 and 2). Individual group differences were tested by means of Mann-Whitney test. Bonferroni correction was used for pair-wise analysis, alpha value was divided by 15 (number of comparisons) and the level of significance was set at $0.05/15 = 0.0033$ (Tables 3 and 4). Data were analyzed using SPSS for Windows (version 18.0).

RESULTS

The IGF-1 level of subjects ranged from 107 to 439 ng/ml (total median IGF-1 = 254 ng/ml and total mean IGF-1 = 281.27 ± 80.26 ng/ml). Tables 1 and 2 give descriptive IGF-1 statistics for different cervical stages in males and females.

In males, highest mean IGF-1 value was observed in CS4 with a mean value of 394.8 ± 50.89 ng/ml at a mean age of 14.08 years. The second highest mean IGF-1 was observed at CS5 followed by CS3. The lowest mean value of IGF-1 was observed at CS1. The IGF-1 values for males with respect to cervical stages in descending order were as follows: CS4 > CS5 > CS3 > CS2 > CS6 > CS1.

In females, the highest mean IGF-1 value was observed in CS3 with a mean value of 397 ± 20.76 ng/ml at a mean age of 12.04 years. The second highest mean IGF-1 was observed at CS4 followed by CS5. The lowest mean value of IGF-1 was observed at CS1. The IGF-1 values for females with respect to cervical stages in descending order were as follows: CS3 > CS4 > CS5 > CS2 > CS6 > CS1.

Kruskal-Wallis ANOVA showed significant differences in IGF-1 levels between different cervical stages in males and female (Tables 1 and 2). Intergroup comparison was performed between different cervical stages within each sex using Mann-Whitney test with alpha at 0.0033 (with Bonferroni correction). Within females, there were statistically significant differences between CS2 and CS3, and CS3 and CS4. Among males, no statistically significant differences were found between the cervical stages at the above mentioned alpha value (Tables 3 and 4).

Figure 1 demonstrates the IGF-1 trends in males and female subjects. In females, IGF-1 levels rose from CS1 towards CS2 with a spike seen from CS2 to peak at CS3, followed by a sudden decline from

CS3 to CS4 continuing to CS6. In males, there was a steady increase in IGF-1 levels from CS1 to CS3 which gradually peaked at CS4, followed by slow decline to CS5 continuing to CS6.

Males and females showed differences in IGF-1 trends in relation to different cervical stages (Tables 1 and 2, Fig 1). The highest mean IGF-1 level in females was observed in CS3 followed by CS4, one cervical stage

Table 1 - IGF-1 levels of female subjects at different cervical stages (n = 30).

Cervical staging	n	Mean age (years)	Mean IGF-1 (ng/ml)	SD	95% confidence interval	Median	IGF-1 Min-Max (ng/ml)
CS1	4	9.36	216 ± 7.53	8.038	208.62 - 223.38	215.5	208 - 225
CS2	6	9.8	244.33 ± 8.41	7.109	237.61 - 251.06	248.5	229 - 250
CS3	8	12.04	397 ± 20.76	9.837	382.61 - 411.39	401.5	364 - 420
CS4	5	16.14	278.8 ± 43.27	18.85	240.87 - 316.73	289	209 - 320
CS5	3	15.97	272 ± 26.15	15.58	242.40 - 301.60	260	254 - 302
CS6	4	19.49	249.25 ± 9.98	8.999	239.47 - 259.03	248	240 - 261

Kruskal-Wallis and ANOVA; significant at $P < 0.000$. Source: Gupta et al,[14] 2012.

Table 2 - IGF-1 levels of male subjects at different cervical stages (n = 30).

Cervical staging	n	Mean age (years)	Mean IGF-1 (ng/ml) ± SD	Standard error	95% confidence interval	Median	IGF-1 Min-Max (ng/ml)
CS1	5	10.04	164.6 ± 36.548	15.705	132.56 - 196.64	164	107 - 200
CS2	4	11.575	214 ± 9.83	8.463	204.37 - 223.63	216	201 - 223
CS3	5	13.4	296.6 ± 55.13	23.36	248.28 - 344.92	292	236 - 369
CS4	5	14.08	394.8 ± 50.889	22.21	350.19 - 439.41	422	330 - 439
CS5	6	15.94	332.83 ± 34.45	14.84	305.26 - 360.4	339	290 - 372
CS6	5	20.28	206 ± 10.9	7.76	196.45 - 215.55	207	194 - 221

Kruskal-Wallis and ANOVA; significant at $P < 0.000$.

Table 3 - Intergroup comparison of various cervical stages in females.

Cervical stage	Compared to stage	P value
CS1	CS2	p = 0.010 (N.S.)
	CS3	p = 0.006 (N.S.)
	CS4	p = 0.086 (N.S.)
	CS5	p = 0.034 (N.S.)
	CS6	p = 0.021 (N.S.)
CS2	CS3	p = 0.002 (Sig.)
	CS4	p = 0.100 (N.S.)
	CS5	p = 0.020 (N.S.)
	CS6	p = 0.453 (N.S.)
CS3	CS4	p = 0.003 (N.S.)
	CS5	p = 0.014 (N.S.)
	CS6	p = 0.006 (N.S.)
CS4	CS5	p = 0.456 (N.S.)
	CS6	p = 0.142 (N.S.)
CS5	CS6	p = 0.212 (N.S.)

Bonferroni's correction for 15 comparisons, alpha value set at 0.05/15=0.0033; (P < 0.0033); Sig = Significant, NS = Non significant. Source: Gupta et al,[14] 2012.

Table 4 - Intergroup comparison of various cervical stages in males.

Cervical stage	Compared to stage	P value
CS1	CS2	p = 0.014 (N.S.)
	CS3	p = 0.009 (N.S.)
	CS4	p = 0.009 (N.S.)
	CS5	p = 0.006 (N.S.)
	CS6	p = 0.028 (N.S.)
CS2	CS3	p = 0.014 (N.S.)
	CS4	p = 0.014 (N.S.)
	CS5	p = 0.011 (N.S.)
	CS6	p = 0.221 (N.S.)
CS3	CS4	p = 0.047 (N.S.)
	CS5	p = 0.234 (N.S.)
	CS6	p = 0.009 (N.S.)
CS4	CS5	p = 1.000 (N.S.)
	CS6	p = 0.009 (N.S.)
CS5	CS6	p = 0.006 (N.S.)

Bonferroni's correction for 15 comparisons, alpha value set at 0.05/15=0.0033; (P < 0.0033); Sig = Significant, NS = Non significant.

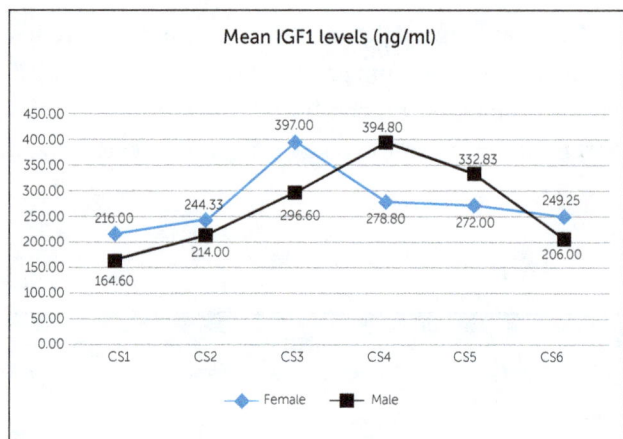

Figure 1 - IGF-1 trends in males and females in relation to the different cervical stages.

earlier than males. Chronologically, it occurred 2 years earlier in females (peak IGF-1 in females observed at a mean age of 12.04 years and at a mean age of 14.08 years in males). The greatest mean serum IGF-1 value for both males and females was compared, for females (397 ng/ml) were slightly higher than in males (394.8 ng/ml).

DISCUSSION

A series of investigations in the field of Medicine, Endocrinology and Dentistry have confirmed that serum IGF-1 estimation is a valid indicator of pubertal growth spurt. IGF-1 is a peptide hormone secreted primarily by the liver in response to growth hormone stimulus. During puberty, IGF-1 levels are regulated by both increased GH and sex steroids.[12]

Serum IGF-1 levels tend to peak whenever there is accelerated growth in the body whether due to the occurrence of pubertal growth spurt,[12] adrenarche,[17] residual mandibular growth,[10] abnormal growth in condylar hyperplasia,[18] acromegaly[19] or tumorous growth occurring in the body.[20] Furthermore, it is established that IGF-1 levels tend to be particularly sensitive with respect to growth occurring in the mandible. Studies have shown that mandibular condyle is more responsive and sensitive to IGF-1 than the femoral head.[21]

In the context of orthodontic diagnosis, treatment planning and treatment, professionals are required to know the mandible growth stage and the amount of mandibular growth that can be anticipated.

A landmark study by Baccetti et al[16] on male and female subjects concluded that the greatest amount of mandibular growth occurred around cervical stage 3 and is the ideal stage to begin functional jaw orthopedics for correction of skeletal Class II malocclusions. It has also been documented that although boys and girls present peak growth speed at different chronological ages, cervical ages showed to be similar.[10]

However, our research data show an irregular pattern. The peak IGF-1 in male and female subjects was recorded at different chronological ages; it was also recorded at different cervical stages. IGF-1 levels increased with each subsequent cervical stages, and maximum mean values were found at CS3 in females (397 ng/ml) and at CS4 (394.8 ng/ml) in males and then decreased in later stages. These findings seem to correlate with a Turkish study[12] in which peak IGF-1 concentrations were recorded a pubertal stage earlier in girls than boys, occurring at Tanner stage III-IV in girls and at stage IV in boys, and started to decline thereafter.

A longitudinal study by Ball et al[8] on male subjects established a pattern of mandibular growth related to CVM stages and found that the greatest amount of mandibular growth in male subjects occurred at CS4. This is in accordance with our data which demonstrate peak IGF-1 at CS4 in male subjects.

Furthermore, our findings also correlate to some extent to the study by Ishaq et al.[22] The study reported peak IGF-1 levels at CS4 in both males and females. Additionally, IGF-1 values in CS3 in females had higher mean values than in males, whereas CS5 in males had higher mean values than females, which corroborates our findings. In addition, the chronological age for peak IGF-1 value in male subjects in their study was found at a mean age of 14.5 years while in our study it was found at 14.08 years.

Nevertheless, in contrast, we found peak mean IGF-1 levels in female subjects at CS3 at a mean age of 12.04 years in comparison to peak value in females found at CS4 at a mean age of 14 years in the study by Ishaq et al.[22] Discordance may be attributed to the difference in ethnic backgrounds, inclusion criteria and methodology. Also, the role of environmental and genetic factors influencing the regulation of sex steroids and IGF-1 system cannot be ruled out.

Though not statistically significant, the greatest mean IGF-1 value in females was slightly higher than males in our study. This is in agreement with the study by Brabent et al[23] in which the authors established reference ranges of serum IGF-1 in male and female subjects separately between age groups of 1 month to 88 years. They reported slightly higher value of mean peak IGF-1 in females (410 ng/ml) as compared to males (382 ng/ml) during adolescence.

On critical assessment of IGF-1 trends, we found that in females IGF-1 levels rose from CS1 towards CS2 with a sudden rise seen from CS2 to peak at CS3, followed by a sudden decline from CS3 to CS4 continuing to CS6; while in males there was a steady increase in IGF-1 levels from CS1 to CS3, which gradually peaked at CS4 followed by a slow decline to CS5 continuing to CS6. Such findings reconfirm previous studies[4] suggesting that females have an earlier and shorter growth spurt denoted by sharp spike and rapid decline in IGF-1 levels. Males, on the other hand, experience a later and longer growth spurt denoted by a relative plateau phase extending from CS3 to CS5 with a gradual increase and decrease in IGF-1 from CS3 to CS4 and from CS4 to CS5, respectively.

On examining the reference values of IGF-1 in both males and females in our study, the mean IGF-1 levels in cervical stages 3, 4 and 5 lie above 250 ng/ml. Considering cervical stages 3, 4 and 5 to be the stages exhibiting significant growth acceleration, as compared to the other cervical stages, it appears that mean IGF-1 level at or above 250 ng/ml indicates a period in which the individual is experiencing growth acceleration. On periodic monitoring, if IGF-1 levels accelerate or decelerate, it may suggest an upward or a downward growth trend, respectively. This hypothesis is supported by the longitudinal study by Masoud et al[24] investigating mandibular growth and IGF-1 levels. The authors found that if IGF-1 levels have an ascending pattern above 250 ng/ml on periodic monitoring, it can be expected an average of 5.5 mm of mandibular growth, whereas if IGF-1 levels have an ascending pattern and average below 250 ng/ml, it can be expected an average of 2 mm of growth. It can be hypothesized that periodic monitoring over quarterly or 6 monthly intervals may guide the clinician regarding ascending and descending growth patterns.

To the present moment, through various studies, it has been established that biomarkers such as growth hormone (GH),[19] IGF-1,[13] PTHrP,[25] sex steroids,[12] osteocalcin,[26] alkaline phosphatase (ALP),[26] etc, play an explicit role in growth phenomenon. However, out of all the suggested biomarkers, IGF-1 has shown to be the most promising marker for growth assessment.

The short half life, pulsatile secretion, diurnal variation and effects of environmental secretion stimuli make growth hormone measurements difficult.[19] According to a recent study,[27] serum PTHrP levels do not correlate with early pubertal stages and hence, its validity to predict peak growth is questionable. Effects of sex steroids[12] on bone growth during adolescence are biphasic, low concentration of sex steroids in early puberty stimulate while higher concentrations inhibit bone formation. Hence, the level may lead to ambiguous assumptions.

Serum osteocalcin and alkaline phosphatase (ALP) levels correlate with pubertal stages in boys, but not in girls.[26] Serum osteocalcin and alkaline phosphatase decrease with advancing sexual development stages (Tanner stages II-IV) in girls; however, it reaches peak levels at Tanner stage IV in boys.

It may be speculated that IGF-1 estimation could have been possible through non invasive sources such as saliva or urine. In a study by Costigan et al,[28] salivary IGF-1 has been shown to be extremely low, less than 1% of serum levels. In addition, gingival fluid or blood can result in inaccurate measurement. Urinary IGF-1 may demand greater patient cooperation, as it would be embarrassing for the patient and contamination of sample can also occur.

In our study, blood samples were taken for IGF-1 estimation in serum. Chemiluminescent immunoassay (CLIA) method was undertaken for IGF-1 estimation which has merits over both enzyme linked immunosorbent assay (ELISA) and radioimmunoassay (RIA). CLIA allows detection of lower analyte concentration and provides a sensitive, high throughput and economical alternative to conventional assays such as ELISA.[29] Additionally, it does not involve hazards of preparing and handling the radioactive antigen as in RIA. CVM staging was also performed using Baccetti et al's[16] technique which has proven to exhibit less intraevaluator and interevaluator errors when compared to other CVM staging methods.[30] However, the drawback of our study design was that it was a cross sectional study with a limited sample size. Further studies on a large sample size is needed to establish more significant evidence even at an alpha value of 0.0033 (i.e. with Bonferroni correction).

The findings of the present study underline the fact that selection of a representative reference population is a delicate task, and that a big sample size collected from different sources reduces the risk of a non desirable impact from a single or a few subpopulations. Longitudinal studies on serum IGF-1

are needed on a larger population for deriving reference intervals, trends, amount of facial growth and the average amount of time span of the accelerated mandibular growth that occurs between males and females and different growth patterns.

CONCLUSIONS

Males and females showed differences in IGF-1 trends and levels at different cervical stages.

IGF-1 values in CS3 in females had higher mean values than in males, whereas CS5 in males had higher mean values than females, thereby indicating earlier onset of pubertal spurt in females and more delayed and longer pubertal spurt in males.

REFERENCES

1. Moore R, Moyer BA, Dubois LM. Skeletal maturation and craniofacial growth. Am J Orthod Dentofacial Orthop. 1990;98(1):33-40.
2. Von Bremen J, Pancherz H. Efficiency of early and late class II division 1 treatment. Am J Orthod Dentofacial Orthop. 2002;121(1):31-7.
3. Tanner JM. Fetus into man. Harvard: Harvard University Press; 1978.
4. Hagg U, Taranger J. Skeletal stages of the hand and wrist as indicators of the pubertal growth spurt. Acta Odontol Scand. 1980;38(3):187-200.
5. Premkumar S. Textbook of craniofacial growth. New Delhi: Jaypee Brothers Medical Publisher; 2011.
6. Soegiharto BM, Moles DR, Cunningham SJ. Discriminatory ability of the skeletal maturation index and the cervical vertebrae maturation index in detecting peak pubertal growth in Indonesian and white subjects with receive operating characteristics analysis. Am J Orthod Dentofacial Orthop. 2008;134(2):227-37.
7. Gabriel DB, Southard KA, Qian F, Marshall SD, Franciscus RG, Southard TE. Cervical vertebrae maturation method: poor reproducibility. Am J Orthod Dentofacial Orthop. 2009;136(4):478.e1-7; discussion 478-80.
8. Ball G, Woodside D, Tompson B, Hunter S. Relationship between cervical vertebral maturation and mandibular growth. Am J Orthod Dentofacial Orthop. 2011;139(5):e455-61.
9. Leite HR, O' Reilly MT, Close JM. Skeletal age assessment using the first, second and third fingers of the hand. Am J Orthod Dentofacial. 1987;92(6):492-8.
10. Masoud M, Masoud I, Kent RL Jr, Gowharji N, Cohen LE. Assessment Skeletal maturity by using blood spot insulin like growth factor I (IGF-I) testing. Am J Orthod Dentofacial Orthop. 2008;134(2):209-16.
11. Proffit WR, Fields HW, Sarver DM. Contemporary Orthodontics. 4th ed. St. Louis: Elsevier; 2007.
12. Kanbur Oksuz N, Derman O, Kynyk E. Corelation of sex steroids with IGF – 1 and IGFBP-3 during different pubertal stages. Turk J Pediatr. 2004;46(4):315-21.
13. Laron Z. Insulin-like growth factors 1 (IGF-1): a growth hormone. Mol Pathol. 2001;54(5):311-6.
14. Gupta S, Jain S, Gupta P, Deoskar A. Determining Skeletal maturation using insulin: like growth factor I (IGF-I) test. Prog Orthod. 2012;13(3):288-95.
15. Nutrient Requirements and Recommended Dietary Allowances for Indians. ICMR 2010. 2010 [Access in 2013 May 15]. Available from: http://www. http://icmr.nic.in/final/RDA-2010.pdf.
16. Baccetti T, Franchi L, McNamara JA. The Cervical Vertebral Maturation (CVM).Method for the assessment of optimal treatment timing in dentofacial orthopedics. Semin Orthod 2005;11(3):119-29.
17. Baquedano MS, Berensztein E, Saraco N, Dorn GV, Davila MT, Rivarola MA, et al. Expression of the IGF system in human adrenal tissues from early infancy to late puberty: implications for the development of adrenarche. Pediatr Res. 2005;58(3):451-8.
18. Meng Q, Long X, Deng M, Cai H, Li J. The expressions of IGF-1, BMP-2 and TGF-b1 in cartilage of condylar hyperplasia. J Oral Rehabil. 2011;38(1)34-40.
19. Insulin-like Growth Factor-1 (IGF-1) - the first-line test for assessing excess growth hormone. Communique. 2006 [Access in 2013 May 15];31(3):1-11. Available from: http://www.mayomedicallaboratories.com/media/articles/communique/mc2831-0306.pdf
20. Daughday WH. The possible autocrine/paracrine and endocrine roles of insulin-like growth factors of human tumors. Endocrinol. 1990;127(1): 1-4.
21. Delatte M, Vonder Hoff J W. Growth stimulation of mandibular condyl and femoral heads of new born rats by IGF-1. Arch Oral Biol. 2004;49(3):165-75.
22. Ishaq RAR, Soliman SAZ, Foda MY, Fayed MMS. Insulin-like growth factor I: a biologic maturation indicator. Am J Orthod Dentofacial Orthop. 2012;142(5):654-61.
23. Brabant G, Muhlen AV, Wuster C. Serum insulin-like growth factor i reference values for an Automated Chemiluminescence Immunoassay System: results from a multicenter study. Horm Res. 2003;60(2):53-60.
24. Masoud MI, Marghalani HY, Masoud IM, Gowharji NF. Prospective longitudinal evaluation of the relationship between changes in mandibular length and blood-spot IGF-1 measurements. Am J Orthod Dentofacial Orthop. 2012;141(6):694-704.
25. Rabie ABM, Tang GH, Xiong H, Hägg U. PTHrP regulates chondrocyte maturation in condylar cartilage. J Dent Res. 2003;82(8):627-31.
26. Kanbur Oksuz N, Derman O, Kynyk E. The relationship between pubertal development, IGF – 1 axis, and bone formation in healthy adolescents. J Bone Miner Metab. 2005;23(1):76-83.
27. Hussain Mohammed Z, Talapaneni Ashok K, Prasad M, Krishnan R. Serum PTHrP level as a biomarker in assessing skeletal maturation during circumpubertal development. Am J Orthod Dentofacial Orthop. 2012;143(4):515-21.
28. Costigan D, Guyda H, Posner B. Free insulin-like growth factor I (IGF-I) and IGF-II in human saliva. J Clin Endocrinol Metab. 1988;66(5):1014-8.
29. Human Growth Hormone Chemiluminescence Immunoassay CAT No: 9020-16. Diagnostic Automation, Inc. Calabasas, CA. 2013 [Access in 2013 May 15]. Available from: http://www.diagnosticautomation.com/inserts06/List_D/PDF/HGH-9020-16.pdf.
30. Jaqueira LMF, Armond MC, Pereira LJ, de Alcântara CEP, Marques LS. Determining skeletal maturation stage using cervical vertebrae: evaluation of three diagnostic methods. Braz Oral Res. 2010;24(4):433-7.

19

Craniofacial skeletal pattern: Is it really correlated with the degree of adenoid obstruction?

Murilo Fernando Neuppmann Feres[1], Tomas Salomão Muniz[2], Saulo Henrique de Andrade[2],
Maurilo de Mello Lemos[3], Shirley Shizue Nagata Pignatari[4]

Objective: The aim of this study was to compare the cephalometric pattern of children with and without adenoid obstruction. **Methods:** The sample comprised 100 children aged between four and 14 years old, both males and females, subjected to cephalometric examination for sagittal and vertical skeletal analysis. The sample also underwent nasofiberendoscopic examination intended to objectively assess the degree of adenoid obstruction. **Results:** The individuals presented tendencies towards vertical craniofacial growth, convex profile and mandibular retrusion. However, there were no differences between obstructive and non-obstructive patients concerning all cephalometric variables. Correlations between skeletal parameters and the percentage of adenoid obstruction were either low or not significant. **Conclusions:** Results suggest that specific craniofacial patterns, such as Class II and hyperdivergency, might not be associated with adenoid hypertrophy.

Keywords: Mouth breathing. Diagnosis. Angle Class II malocclusion.

[1] Associate professor, Universidade São Francisco, Department of Orthodontics, Bragança Paulista, São Paulo, Brazil.
[2] Private practice, Bragança Paulista, São Paulo, Brazil.
[3] Full professor, Universidade Guarulhos, Department of Orthodontics, Guarulhos, São Paulo, Brazil.
[4] Adjunct professor of Otolaryngology, Universidade Federal de São Paulo, Department of Otolaryngology, Head and Neck Surgery, São Paulo, São Paulo, Brazil.

» The authors report no commercial, proprietary or financial interest in the products or companies described in this article.

Murilo Fernando Neuppmann Feres
Av. São Francisco de Assis, 218, Jardim São José, Bragança Paulista/SP – Brazil
CEP: 12916-900 – E-mail: murilo.feres@usf.edu.br

INTRODUCTION

Studies on the relationship between respiratory pattern and the development of craniofacial characteristics have been published for a considerable period of time.[1-8] The persistence of the interest in this topic might be partially explained by the high prevalence of mouth breathing,[9] even among orthodontic patients.[10]

The presence of this habit is correlated with a number of muscular[11] and dento-craniofacial alterations, including maxillary constriction, posterior crossbite, retrusion and clockwise rotation of the mandible, Class II skeletal pattern and excessive vertical growth.[1-8]

One of the main causes of mouth breathing is adenoid hypertrophy.[12] In addition, several studies have demonstrated a significant correlation between long face morphology and anatomical reduction in the nasopharyngeal airway.[1,7,8,13,14,16-19] Class II malocclusion or mandibular retrognathia have also been frequently related to smaller dimensions of the nasopharynx.[13,20-23] Therefore, some of these studies[7,14,16,18,24] suggest that dimensional reduction of the nasopharynx, due to hyperdivergent craniofacial pattern or mandibular retrusion, might predispose patients to an obstructive breathing status derived from adenoid hypertrophy. However, such inferences might be considered mere assumptions rather than scientific evidence, since most of these studies have relied upon inaccurate methods, such as rhinomanometry[1,13,21] or lateral cephalometric radiographs,[7,8,14,16,17,18,19,20,22] to assess patients' respiratory pattern. On the other hand, nasofiberendoscopic examination has been considered as the gold standard method for adenoid evaluation.[23]

The primary objective of this study was to describe the craniofacial morphology of patients with complaints of nasopharyngeal obstruction. In addition, comparative analysis of cephalometric skeletal features was conducted on patients with and without adenoid hypertrophy, as assessed by nasofiberendoscopic examination. Finally, this study also aimed to investigate the correlations established between skeletal characteristics and the percentage of adenoid obstruction.

MATERIAL AND METHODS

This research was a descriptive-analytical, cross-sectional study approved by Universidade Federal de São Paulo Institutional Review Board (protocol #0181/08).

Between February 2009 and June 2010, 170 children who attended or were referred to a public pediatric otolaryngology outpatient clinic, were invited to take part in the study, from which 43 refused to participate. The convenience sample thus consisted of 127 individuals, both males and females, aged between four to 14 years old. In order to be eligible to the study, the children should have presented complaints of nasopharyngeal obstruction and/or mouth breathing. At this point, no objective information regarding the degree of adenoid hypertrophy was available.

Children with syndromes or craniofacial malformation, as well as those which had been previously subjected to orthodontic treatment, were not included in the sample.

All eligible participants, along with their parents or legal guardians, were properly informed about the study objectives and procedures, as well as the examinations that would be performed. Those who agreed to participate formalized their intent by signing an informed consent form previously prepared according to Universidade Federal de São Paulo Institutional Review Board.

Initially, the children selected underwent lateral cephalometric radiographic examination performed by a radiology specialist who used the same device for all of them (Instrumentarium Ortopantomographic OP100; General Electric Healthcare, Tuusula, Finland). The focus-film distance was 140 cm, while X-ray exposure settings were 70 kV and 12 mA for 0.40 to 0.64 s. During record taking, patients were instructed to breathe exclusively through the nose, keep their mouth closed and their teeth in occlusion. We used 20 x 25 cm films (Kodak, Rochester, NY) and processed them according to a standardized protocol. Radiographs were identified by codes, so as to prevent patient identification.

Lateral cephalometric radiographs were manually traced by two independent blind examiners, and subsequent measurements (Table 1, Figs 1, 2, and 3) were performed on Ultraphan acetate sheets, with the aid of a light box, a protractor and a digital caliper (model 799A-8/200; Starrett , Itu, Brazil), with 0.01 mm precision.

Subsequently, patients underwent flexible nasofiberendoscopic examination (model ENFP4, 3.4 mm; Olympus, Melville, NY) through both nostrils. The examination was conducted by experienced otolaryngologists and performed after topical anesthesia application (2% lidocaine). All examinations were recorded by a DVD recorder (model DVD-R150/XAZ; Samsung, Manaus, Brazil), and a digital file derived from the

Craniofacial skeletal pattern: Is it really correlated with the degree of adenoid...

133

Table 1 - Cephalometric variables evaluated.

Cephalometric variables	
SNA	Anteroposterior position of the maxilla
SNB	Anteroposterior position of the mandible
ANB	Relative anteroposterior position of the maxilla and mandible
NAPg	Facial convexity
NSGn	Direction of facial growth
SNGoGn	Mandibular plane angle
SNPP	Inclination of the palatal plane (ANS/PNS)
BaNPtGn	Facial axis
AFHi	Anterior facial height index (ANS-Me/N-Me)
FHi	Total facial height index (S-Go/N-Me)

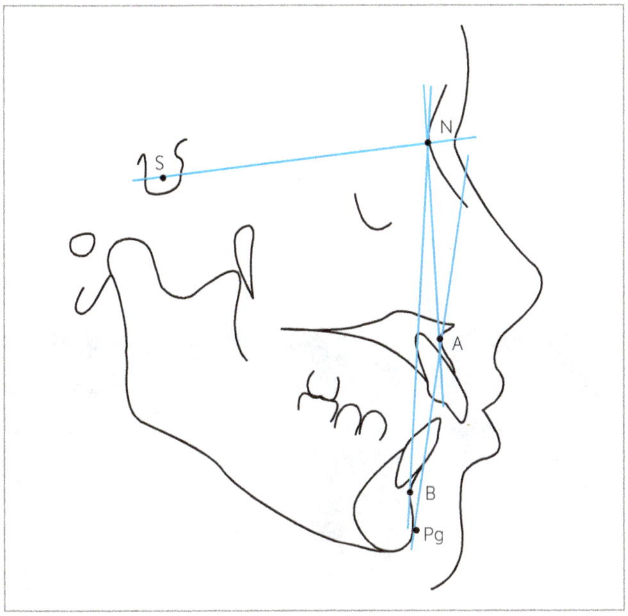

Figure 1 - Horizontal cephalometric variables (SNA, SNB, ANB, NAPg).

primary video was edited to prevent patient identification. Edited video clips were then forwarded to another experienced and independent otolaryngologist who had not been involved with subjects' enrollment, videonasopharyngoscopic examination performance, record taking or editing.

In order to evaluate the edited video clips, the examiner used an assessment method originally designed to quantify the degree of obstruction caused by the adenoid tissue: measured choanal obstruction (MCO) which has previously proven to be satisfactorily reproducible.[25] The evaluator was instructed to choose the frame that provided the best view of the

adenoid in relation to the choana, obtained from the most distal portion of the inferior turbinate. In these frames, the patient had to be breathing exclusively through the nose, with no evidence of soft palate elevation. The selected frame was then converted into a JPEG file and the MCO was calculated by means of Image J,[26] an image processing software. MCO represented the percentage of the choanal area occupied by adenoid tissue (Fig 4). When images from both nostrils were available, the mean between right and left side evaluations was calculated to minimize potential variations, as proposed by Feres et al.[25]

Statistical analysis

At first, radiographic parameters reliability was determined after intra and inter-reproducibility analysis calculated by intraclass correlation coefficient (ICC).

Then, radiographic variables were described (means, standard deviations, minimum and maximum values) for all subjects. Subsequently, the sample was divided into two groups, according to the degree of obstruction caused by adenoid hypertrophy. According to previous parameters,[27] patients with MCO ≥ 66.7% were considered to have pathological adenoid hypertrophy, herein denominated the "positive" group; while patients with MCO < 66.7% were not considered to present pathological adenoid hypertrophy ("negative" group). Both groups were compared regarding all cephalometric variables, according to Mann-Withney test.

Finally, Pearson correlation analysis between cephalometric measurements and MCO was determined for the whole sample. The "strength" of the correlation was characterized according to Vieira[28] as: "irrelevant" ($0.00 < r \leq 0.25$), "weak" ($0.25 < r \leq 0.50$), "moderate" ($0.50 < r \leq 0.75$), or "strong" ($0.75 < r \leq 1.00$).

Significance level for statistical tests was set at 5% ($\alpha \leq 0.05$). All analyzes were performed using SPSS 10.0 for Windows.

RESULTS

From the initial sample comprising 127 patients who met the eligibility criteria and agreed to participate in the study, seven were excluded due to inadequate exams and 20 presented inconsistent repeated radiographic measurements. For the 100 remaining patients, all of them had radiographic parameters with satisfactory reproducibility (Table 2).

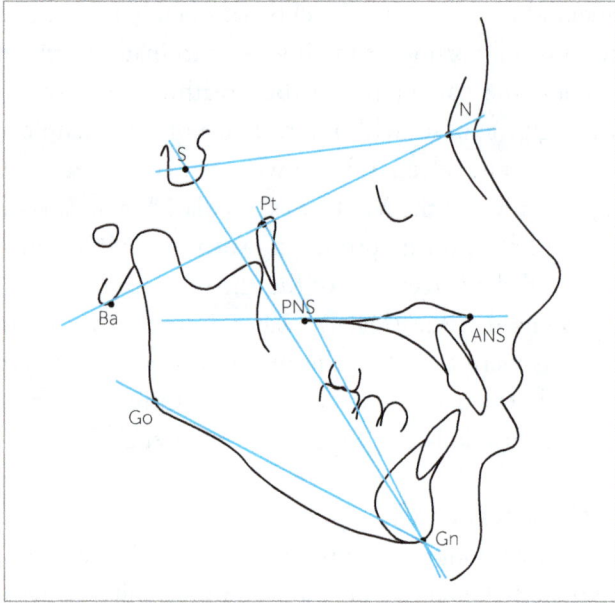

Figure 2 - Vertical cephalometric variables (NSGn, SNGoGn, SNPP, BaNPtGn).

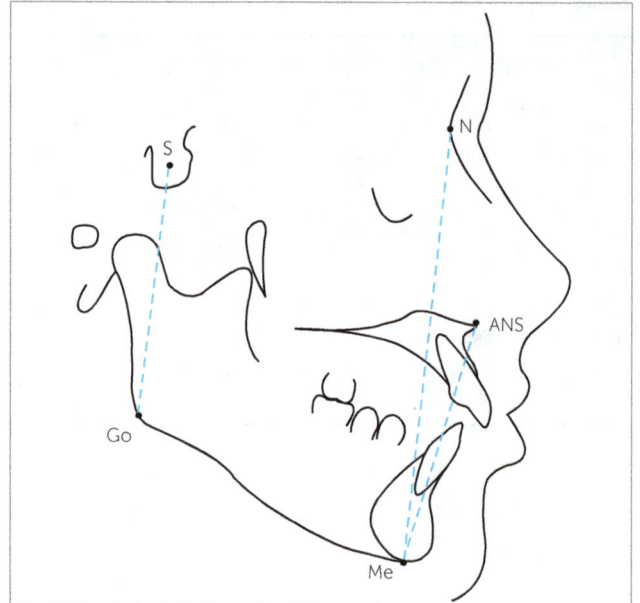

Figure 3 - Cephalometric variables related to the facial indices AFHi and FHi.

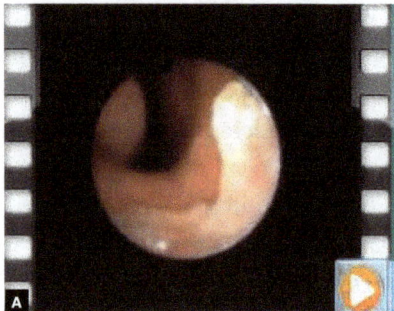

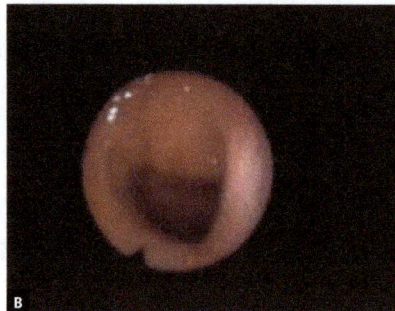

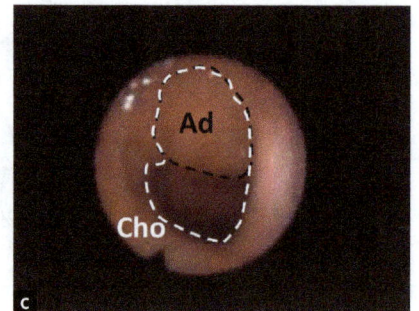

Figure 4 - Final frame selection (**B**) derived from the video clip (**A**), and MCO calculation (**C**): MCO = (Ad/Cho) x 100.

The final sample comprised 48 female children (48.0%) and 52 male children (52.0%), with a mean age of 9.0 years old (standard deviation = 2.4). The descriptive analysis of all cephalometric variables is presented in Table 3. According to universally accepted parameters, the sample of this study showed skeletal patterns with a slight tendency towards excessive vertical growth, a convex profile and mandibular retrusion. However, comparison between the cephalometric variables of the positive (n = 58, 58.0%) and negative groups (n = 42, 42.0%) showed no statistically significant differences (Table 4).

Furthermore, amongst all radiographic variables evaluated herein, SNA, SNB, NSGn, SNGoGn and BaNPtGn were significantly correlated with MCO. Although statistically significant, the magnitude of these correlations was considered either irrelevant (SNA, SNB, SNGoGn, BaNPtGn) or weak (NSGn) (Table 4).

Craniofacial skeletal pattern: Is it really correlated with the degree of adenoid...

135

Table 2 - Interclass correlation coefficient (ICC) of skeletal parameters (intra and inter-examiner analysis).

Variables	Intraexaminer	p value	Inter-examiner	p value
SNA (degrees)	0.942	< 0.001	0.950	< 0.001
SNB (degrees)	0.966	< 0.001	0.970	< 0.001
ANB (degrees)	0.928	< 0.001	0.913	< 0.001
NAPog (degrees)	0.940	< 0.001	0.926	< 0.001
NSGn (degrees)	0.961	< 0.001	0.945	< 0.001
SnGoGN (degrees)	0.911	< 0.001	0.908	< 0.001
SNPP (degrees)	0.923	< 0.001	0.910	< 0.001
BaNPtGn (degrees)	0.988	< 0.001	0.975	< 0.001
AFHi	0.890	< 0.001	0.877	< 0.001
FHi	0.869	< 0.001	0.868	< 0.001

Table 3 - Descriptive analysis of radiographic variables.

Variables	Mean	Standard deviation	Minimum	Maximum
SNA (degrees)	82.910	4.3376	70.0	97.5
SNB (degrees)	78.195	3.7281	70.0	93.0
ANB (degrees)	4.715	2.6412	-6.0	11.5
NAPog (degrees)	10.050	5.4802	-8.0	24.0
NSGn (degrees)	69.300	3.9222	56.0	79.0
SnGoGN (degrees)	37.679	5.2047	19.0	48.0
SNPP (degrees)	6.975	3.7902	-4.0	16.0
BaNPtGn (degrees)	87.470	4.1261	78.0	101.0
AFHi	0.588	0.026	0.528	0.705
FHi	0.612	0.041	0.517	0.784

Table 4 - Comparative analysis between positive (MCO ≥ 66.7%) and negative groups (MCO < 66.7%) in relation to the radiographic variables.

Variables	Groups	Mean	Standard deviation	Mann-Withney (p value)
SNA (degrees)	Positive	82.129	4.0410	0.058
	Negative	83.988	4.5472	
SNB (degrees)	Positive	77.612	3.1247	0.290
	Negative	79.000	4.3407	
ANB (degrees)	Positive	4.517	2.9289	0.296
	Negative	4.988	2.1878	
NAPog (degrees)	Positive	9.276	5.8115	0.150
	Negative	11.119	4.8525	
NSGn (degrees)	Positive	69.957	3.8824	0.105
	Negative	68.393	3.8390	
SnGoGN (degrees)	Positive	38.257	4.5389	0.419
	Negative	36.881	5.9703	
SNPP (degrees)	Positive	6.724	3.6685	0.241
	Negative	7.321	3.9707	
BaNPtGn (degrees)	Positive	86.905	4.0819	0.324
	Negative	88.250	4.1072	
AFHi	Positive	0.591	0.027	0.157
	Negative	0.582	0.023	
FHi	Positive	0.611	0.030	0.772
	Negative	0.613	0.054	

Table 5 - Correlation coefficient (r) between radiographic variables and MCO.

Variables	r	Spearman (p value)
SNA	-0.250	0.012
SNB	-0.202	0.044
ANB	-0.052	0.605
NAPog	-0.078	0.443
NSGn	0.304	0.002
SNGoGn	0.233	0.020
SNPP	-0.014	0.888
BaNPtGn	-0.242	0.015
AFHi	0.183	0.069
FHi	-0.105	0.298

DISCUSSION

The association between specific skeletal patterns and the presence of obstructive adenoid is a topic which has been debated for years,[1,7,8,13-19] although controversy still remains. One of the reasons that might contribute for this debate to persist is related to the varied sorts of assessment methods used to evaluate the level of adenoid obstruction.

This study has demonstrated that children with respiratory complaints might present skeletal features associated with hyperdivergency and retrognathia. However, despite currently accepted hypotheses according to which dolichofacial or Class II patients are more anatomically susceptible to present adenoid obstruction, evidence presented herein suggests that children are likely to experience it regardless of their skeletal characteristics.

According to most studies, the size of the nasopharyngeal airway is significantly correlated with excessively vertical cephalometric features. Researchers have suggested that this dimensional reduction of the nasopharynx might be attributed to skeletal characteristics which are inherent to hyperdivergent patients, such as maxillomandibular retrusion.[7,14,16,18,23] Nevertheless, Santos-Pinto et al[16] refuted this hypothesis when they demonstrated that individuals with varying nasopharyngeal dimensions did not significantly differ in relation to the anteroposterior position of the maxilla and the mandible. The data obtained in our study support their findings,[16] since the anteroposterior position of the maxilla and the

mandible showed no relevant correlation with the degree of adenoid obstruction, as determined by flexible nasofiberendoscopic examination. Moreover, according to our results, the subjects who were considered to be positive presented similar maxillomandibular sagittal position as those considered to be negative for adenoid obstruction.

That finding might explain why no significant differences were found in relation to ANB when positive and negative groups were compared. In addition, ANB revealed no relevant correlation with the degree of adenoid obstruction. These findings corroborate the results of Freitas et al,[17] according to which sagittal malocclusions are not correlated with nasopharyngeal airway depth.

Further evidence provided by this study contradicts what other studies[7,20,23,25] claim. Some of these researches,[7,23] after lateral cephalometric analysis, reported that Class II patients had significantly smaller airway areas. In their latest study on tomographic measurements, Claudino et al[28] were unable to detect a significant association between nasopharyngeal dimensions and the sagittal skeletal pattern in adolescents. The authors demonstrated that more obvious influence of the skeletal pattern could be observed in relatively lower portions of the pharynx, such as the oropharynx, rather than at the nasopharyngeal level.[28]

Similarly to Claudino et al,[29] this study found no significant differences between participants with distinct grades of adenoid obstruction, whether vertical or sagittal skeletal parameters. Likewise, no relevant

Craniofacial skeletal pattern: Is it really correlated with the degree of adenoid...

137

correlations were observed between the percentage of adenoid obstruction and any of the skeletal variables investigated. It is our opinion that most of the studies that have been carried out to date[7,8,13,14,16-22,24] have actually failed to infer that patients with specific skeletal patterns (dolichofacial and/or Class II) significantly present higher frequencies of pathological adenoid obstruction. Considering the data obtained herein, it no longer seems reasonable to assume that a reduction in the nasopharyngeal airway is directly related to an actual clinical obstruction. Thüer et al[13] have already reported that there is no significant correlation between nasal airflow parameters, derived from rhinomanometry, and the nasopharyngeal space observed in lateral cephalometric radiograph. The absence of a significant correlation between respiratory capacity and anatomical traits of dolichocephaly has been also reported by Solow et al[21] who sought to correlate skeletal morphological patterns with data obtained from rhinomanometry examination.

In addition, although imaging techniques may indeed indicate nasopharyngeal anatomical reduction, these might not be able to promote significant influence on patient's clinical respiratory conditions, nor necessarily predispose one to effectively develop obstruction. Unlike many other researches, in this study, a direct and visual nasopharyngeal evaluation method was used, which, according to relevant literature,[23] is considered to be the gold standard for adenoid evaluation.

However, this study presents significant limitations, with the most important one being associated with single cross-sectional evaluation of adenoid hypertrophy. As previously reported,[31] the adenoid lymphoid tissue might be susceptible to sudden dimensional changes as a consequence of allergic sensitization. Therefore, the authors suggest that future studies should address this limitation by performing serial adenoid evaluations, so as to minimize potential variations. In addition, new research is still required to investigate the influence of other morphological parameters, such as those related to the cranial base,[30] on the dimensional reduction of the nasopharynx and the potential establishment of an obstructive respiratory process, since this study was limited to assess only maxillary or mandibular parameters.

CONCLUSION

The sample studied herein showed skeletal patterns with a discrete tendency towards excessive vertical growth, a convex profile and mandibular retrusion. However, no statistically significant differences were found between patients with or without adenoid hypertrophy. The correlations established between the characteristics of craniofacial morphology and the percentage of choanal obstruction were weak or not significant.

Acknowledgements

This research was financially supported by Fundação de Amparo à Pesquisa do Estado de São Paulo (FAPESP) under the protocol #08/53538-0.

Author contributions

Conceived and designed the study: MFNF, SSNP. Data collection: TSM, SHA. Data analysis: MML, MFNF. Wrote the article: TSM, SHA, MML, SSNP, MFNF. Critical revision of the article: MFNF, MML, SSNP. Final approval of the article: TSM, SHA, MML, SSNP, MFNF.

REFERENCES

1. Their effect on mode of breathing and nasal airflow and their relationship to characteristics of the facial skeleton and the dentition. A biometric, rhino-manometric and cephalometro-radiographic study on children with and without adenoids. Acta Otolaryngol Suppl. 1970;265:1-132.

2. Melsen B, Attina L, Santuari M, Attina A. Relationships between swallowing pattern, mode of respiration, and development of malocclusion. Angle Orthod. 1987;57(2):113-20.

3. Löfstrand-Tideström B, Thilander B, Ahlqvist-Rastad J, Jakobsson O, Hultcrantz E. Breathing obstruction in relation to craniofacial and dental arch morphology in 4-year-old children. Eur J Orthod. 1999;21(4):323-32.

4. Sabatoski CV, Maruo H, Camargo ES, Oliveira JHG. Estudo comparativo de dimensões craniofaciais verticais e horizontais entre crianças respiradoras bucais e nasais. J Bras Ortodon Ortop Facial. 2002;7(39):246-57.

5. Lopatiene K, Babarskas A. Malocclusion and upper airway obstruction. Medicina (Kaunas). 2002;38(3):277-83.

6. Lessa FC, Enoki C, Feres MF, Valera FC, Lima WT, Matsumoto MA, Breathing mode influence in craniofacial development. Braz J Otorhinolaryngol. 2005;71:156-60.

7. Wysocki J, Krasny M, Skarzyński PH. Patency of nasopharynx and a cephalometric image in the children with orthodontic problems. Int J Pediatr Otorhinolaryngol. 2009;73:1803-9.

8. Ucar FI, Uysal T Orofacial airway dimensions in subjects with Class I malocclusion and different growth patterns. Angle Orthod. 2011;81(3):460-8.

9. de Menezes VA, Leal RB, Pessoa RS, Pontes RM. Prevalence and factors related to mouth breathing in school children at the Santo Amaro project-Recife, 2005. Braz J Otorhinolaryngol. 2006;72(3):394-9.

10. di Francesco RC, Bregola EGP, Pereira LS, Lima RS. A obstrução nasal e o diagnóstico ortodôntico. Rev Dent Press Ortod Ortop Facial. 2006;11(1):107-13.

11. Valera FC, Travitzki LV, Mattar SE, Matsumoto MA, Elias AM, Anselmo-Lima WT. Muscular, functional and orthodontic changes in pre school children with enlarged adenoids and tonsils. Int J Pediatr Otorhinolaryngol. 2003;67(7):761-70.

12. Farid M, Metwalli N. Computed tomographic evaluation of mouth breathers among paediatric patients. Dentomaxillofac Radiol. 2010;39(1):1-10.

13. Thüer U, Kuster R, Ingervall B. A comparison between anamnestic, rhinomanometric and radiological methods of diagnosing mouth-breathing. Eur J Orthod. 1989;11:161-8.

14. Joseph AA, Elbaum J, Cisneros GJ, Eisig SB. A cephalometric comparative study of the soft tissue airway dimensions in persons with hyperdivergent and normodivergent facial patterns. J Oral Maxillofac Surg. 1998;56(2):135-9;

15. Akcam MO, Toygar TU, Wada T. Longitudinal investigation of soft palate and nasopharyngeal airway relations in different rotation types. Angle Orthod. 2002;72(6):521-6.

16. Santos-Pinto A, Paulin RF, Melo ACM, Martins LP. A influência da redução do espaço nasofaringeano na morfologia facial de pré-adolescentes. Rev Dental Press Ortod Ortop Facial. 2004;9(3):19-26.

17. Freitas MR, Alcazar NM, Janson G, Freitas KM, Henriques JF. Upper and lower pharyngeal airways in subjects with Class I and Class II malocclusions and different growth patterns. Am J Orthod Dentofacial Orthop. 2006;130(6):742-5.

18. Feres MFN, Enoki C, Anselmo-Lima WT, Matsumoto MAN. Dimensões nasofaringeanas e faciais em diferentes padrões morfológicos. Dental Press J Orthod. 2010;15(3):52-61.

19. Macari AT, Bitar MA, Ghafari JG. New insights on age-related association between nasopharyngeal airway clearance and facial morphology. Orthod Orthod Craniofac Res. 2012;15(3):188-97.

20. Mergen DC, Jacobs RM. The size of nasopharynx associated with normal occlusion and Class II malocclusion. Angle Orthod. 1970;40(4):342-6.

21. Solow B, Siersbaek-Nielsen S, Greve E. Airway adequacy, head posture, and craniofacial morphology. Am J Orthod. 1984;86(3):214-23.

22. Krasny M, Wysocki J, Zadurska M, Skarżyński PH. Relative nasopharyngeal patency index as possible objective indication for adenoidectomy in children with orthodontic problems. Int J Pediatr Otorhinolaryngol. 2011;75(2):250-5.

23. Mlynarek A, Tewfik MA, Hagr A, Manoukian JJ, Schloss MD, Tewfik TL, et al. Lateral neck radiography versus direct video rhinoscopy in assessing adenoid size. J Otolaryngol. 2004;33(6):360-5.

24. Alves M Jr, Franzotti ES, Baratieri C, Nunes LK, Nojima LI, Ruellas AC. Evaluation of pharyngeal airway space amongst different skeletal patterns. Int J Oral Maxillofac Surg. 2012;41(7):814-9.

25. Feres MF, Hermann JS, Sallum AC, Pignatari SS. Endoscopic evaluation of adenoids: reproducibility analysis of current methods. Clin Exp Otorhinolaryngol. 2013;6(1):36-40.

26. ImageJ. US National Institutes of Health. 1997 [Access in: 2014 Jan 09]. Available from: http://imagej.nih.gov/ij.

27. Chien CY, Chen AM, Hwang CF, Su CY. The clinical significance of adenoid-choanae area ratio in children with adenoid hypertrophy. Int J Pediatr Otorhinolaryngol. 2005;69(2):235-9.

28. Vieira S. Introdução à Bioestatística. Rio de Janeiro: Elsevier; 2008.

29. Claudino LV, Mattos CT, Ruellas AC, Sant' Anna EF. Pharyngeal airway characterization in adolescents related to facial skeletal pattern: a preliminary study. Am J Orthod Dentofacial Orthop. 2013;143(6):799-809.

30. Martin O, Muelas L, Viñas MJ. Comparative study of nasopharyngeal soft-tissue characteristics in patients with Class III malocclusion. Am J Orthod Dentofacial Orthop. 2011;139(2):242-51.

31. Modrzynski M, Zawisza E. The influence of birch pollination on the adenoid size in children with intermittent allergic rhinitis. Int J Pediatr Otorhinolaryngol. 2007;71(7):1017-23.

20

Evaluation of metallic brackets adhesion after the use of bleaching gels with and without amorphous calcium phosphate (ACP): *In vitro* study

Sissy Maria Mendes Machado[1], Diego Bruno Pinho do Nascimento[2], Robson Costa Silva[2],
Sandro Cordeiro Loretto[3], David Normando[4]

Objective: To evaluate *in vitro* the effects of tooth whitening using gel with Amorphous Calcium Phosphate (ACP) on the bond strength of metal brackets. **Methods:** Thirty-six bovine incisors were sectioned at the crown-root interface, and the crowns were then placed in PVC cylinders. The specimens were divided into 3 groups (n = 12) according to whitening treatment and type of gel used, as follows: G1 (control) = no whitening; G2 = whitening with gel not containing ACP (Whiteness Perfect - FGM), G3 = whitening with gel containing ACP (Nite White ACP - Discus Dental). Groups G2 and G3 were subjected to 14 cycles of whitening followed by an interval of 15 days before the bonding of metal brackets. Shear bond strength testing was performed on a Kratos universal test machine at a speed of 0.5 mm/min. After the mechanical test, the specimens were assessed to determine the adhesive remnant index (ARI). The results were subjected to ANOVA, Tukey's test and Kruskal-Wallis test (5%). **Results:** Significant differences were noted between the groups. Control group (G1 = 11.10 MPa) showed a statistically higher shear bond strength than the groups that underwent whitening (G2 = 5.40 Mpa, G3 = 3.73 MPa), which did not differ from each other. There were no significant differences between the groups in terms of ARI. **Conclusion:** Tooth whitening reduces the bond strength of metal brackets, whereas the presence of ACP in the whitening gel has no bearing on the results.
Keywords: Tooth whitening. Dental bonding. Shear bond strength. Orthodontics. Tooth enamel.

[1] Professor, Specialization Course of Orthodontics, Brazilian Dental Association - Pará (ABO-PA).

[2] Student of the Specialization Course of Orthodontics, ABO-PA.

[3] Associate Professor of Dentistry. Professor of the MSc Program of the School of Dentistry, Federal University of Pará (UFPa).

[4] Associate Professor, Division of Orthodontics, School of Dentistry, Federal University of Pará (UFPa), Professor of the Specialization Program of Orthodontics, ABO-PA.

» The authors report no commercial, proprietary or financial interest in the products or companies described in this article.

Sissy Maria Mendes Machado
Specialite Saúde Oral – Rua Diogo Móia, 295
CEP: 66.055-170 – Umarizal – Belém/Pará – Brazil
E-mail: dra.sissy@specialite-saudeoral.com.br

INTRODUCTION

Human beings' motivation towards body esthetics and beauty has been increasingly extended to the smile.[29] Dental esthetics is now a primary factor in seeking dental treatment, thus rendering teeth whitening a very sought procedure. Therefore, today this procedure is usually performed prior to different treatments in dentistry, such as tooth alignment with orthodontic appliances.

To be successful, orthodontic treatment with fixed appliances depends, among other factors, on proper bonding of brackets and a lasting retention of these attachments to the teeth. The need to rebond orthodontic attachments can severely hinder treatment progress, thereby increasing biological and financial costs.[22] These attachments are placed on the tooth enamel and are subject to a wide range of intraoral forces, which is often entirely delivered to the bonding adhesive layer and the adhesive/enamel interface.[6] Thus, any treatment of the tooth surface using chemicals – such as whitening agents – could potentially affect bond strength.[22]

Nowadays, teeth whitening is a widespread cosmetic procedure in society, with a number of whitening products available in the market. Among the existing techniques, at-home whitening, which involves low concentrations, has evolved into a very popular technique given its effectiveness and convenience.[7] However, even with the use of low concentrations, several studies report changes in tooth structure in the whitened areas.[18,31] There are differences in the degree of adverse effects caused by whitening vital teeth.[30]

Although it has been found that whitening teeth with carbamide peroxide at 10% does not interfere with bond strength to the enamel when performed prior to the bonding of brackets,[2] there have been reports[18] of interferences with the mechanical bonding of orthodontic appliances to enamel previously subjected to the whitening procedure. Remnants from the whitening material possibly interfere with the composite by changing or preventing the formation of tags, thus impairing mechanical bond strength.

Some of the noteworthy changes occur in the mineral content of the whitened teeth, which can generate: Increased porosity and permeability of the enamel, which reduces its microhardness, undermines

bond strength after whitening, and an increase in dentin hypersensitivity during and after treatment.[5] In an attempt to avoid or minimize the undesirable effects that may occur in the whitened tooth structure dental products have been launched on the market with some changes in their composition.

Recently, whitening gels and amorphous calcium phosphate (ACP), or just calcium, have been added to the composition. Manufacturers claim that these substances can supply minerals to the whitened tooth structure and thereby prevent the emergence of porosities and erosions. Additionally, they contribute to reducing trans- and postoperative sensitivity by decreasing enamel permeability, inhibiting neural activation and/or obliterating exposed and open dentinal tubules.[11] However, few studies have been published on the behavior of these whitening gels as well as how their use can influence the bond strength of orthodontic appliances. The present study therefore aimed to use these new products as a means to investigate the potential effects of employing them prior to bracket bonding.

OBJECTIVE

To evaluate, *in vitro,* the bond strength of orthodontic brackets after tooth whitening with and without ACP through mechanical shear bond tests. The adhesive remnant index (ARI) of orthodontic brackets after the use of different dental whitening agents was also examined.

MATERIAL AND METHODS

This study was approved by the Ethics Committee for Animal Research (CEPAN) of the Pará State University (UEPA) under file nº 067-2009.

The study included 36 recently extracted bovine teeth, all permanent mandibular incisors, supplied by a slaughterhouse in the city of Belem, Pará State (PA). The selection criteria required that each tooth enamel be intact, with no cracks and no prior use of chemical agents. Teeth with anatomical irregularities in their labial surfaces were also excluded from the study. The specimens were stored in aqueous solution, and the water was changed every 5 days at room temperature.

After the extractions, followed by removal of periodontal tissues and rinsing, the teeth were stored in distilled water. Thereafter, the root portion was removed with a stainless steel disc (Starret - Germany) at low speed, the pulp was removed with endodontic curettes (Ice - SP). Subsequently the crowns were attached to 25 x 20 mm PVC cylinders with self-curing acrylic resin (JET, São Paulo, SP), so that the most prominent portion and central labial surface of the teeth was exposed perpendicularly to the cylinder. This position was obtained with the aid of a square by determining a 90° angle between the labial surface of the crown and the cylinder base.

Prophylaxis was performed on the labial surface of the teeth with a rubber cup and pumice (fine-grained and without fluoride - JET-São Paulo/SP) for 10s and then each specimen was rinsed with water/air sprays for an equal time length.

Groups

The specimens were randomly divided into three groups (n = 12) according to whether or not they had been whitened, and the type of whitening gel (Table 1). The gels were applied as recommended by the manufacturers on the labial surface of the enamel in a layer about 0.5 mm thick, which corresponded to one cycle. Upon completion of each gel application cycle the specimens were washed with air/water jets for 30 seconds, and thereafter immersed in distilled water renewed weekly and stored at 34° C room temperature on average. Fourteen cycles were carried out spanning a 15-day time interval since the end of the whitening treatment. Only then were the brackets bonded to the teeth.

Standard Edgewise metal brackets with slots 0.022 x 0.028-in (Abzil, 3M/Unitek, São José do Rio Preto/SP, Brazil) were bonded to the maxillary central incisors. The size of the bracket base, as informed by the manufacturer, was 14.35 mm.^{2} The base featured

metal mesh type mechanical retention. Transbond XT adhesive system (3M Unitek, Monrovia, CA, USA) was used for bonding the brackets. The brackets were bonded to the tooth surface with the slot parallel to the base of the cylinder, following the manufacturer's protocol.

To perform the shear bond strength test of the specimens a Kratos TRCV59DUSB universal mechanical testing machine (Jundiaí, SP, Brazil) was utilized at a speed of 0.5 mm/min (ISO 11405:2003)[14] with a chisel tip. Shear bond strength results were obtained in kgf, converted to N, and divided by the bracket base area (14.35 mm^2), yielding the results in MPa.

After conducting the test, the labial surface of each specimen was evaluated by stereomicroscopy (Opton, Germany) with 8x magnification to measure Adhesive Remnant Index (ARI), as recommended by Årtun and Bergland,[1] where 0 = no composite remnant adhered to the enamel, 1 = less than half of composite adhered to the enamel, 2 = more than half of composite adhered to enamel, 3 = all composite adhered to the enamel.

Statistical analysis

All data were analyzed for normality by the Shapiro-Wilk test was used for normality analysis of all data. Data were considered normal after excluding an outlier (Group 2). If this specimen had been included the data would have been considered abnormal.

Shear bond strength test results were subjected to analysis of variance (ANOVA) at 5% significance level, and subsequently Tukey's test to compare the control group with the other treatments, and also between the experimental groups (G2 and G3). Kruskal-Wallis test at 5% was used in evaluating ARI scores.

Table 1 - Experimental groups, product/manufacturer and basic composition of whitening gels.

EXPERIMENTAL GROUPS	PRODUCT/MANUFACTURER	BASIC COMPOSITION
GROUP 1		
G1 (n = 12): Standardized bracket bonding, and shear bond test without prior whitening - control group.	_____	_____
GROUP 2		
G2 (n = 12): 14 cycles of at-home whitening without ACP – 15-day time interval immersed in distilled water. Bracket bonding and shear bond test.	Whiteness Perfect / FGM Lot 181209	Carbamide peroxide at 16% + Potassium Nitrate + Fluoride
GROUP 3		
G3 (n = 12): 14 cycles of at-home whitening with ACP – 15-day interval immersed in distilled water. Bracket bonding and shear bond test.	NiteWhite ACP / Discus Dental Lot 08315151	Carbamide peroxide 16% + Potassium nitrate + Calcium + Phosphate

RESULTS

ANOVA analysis of variance results with p values are depicted in Table 2.

Differences in bond strength between groups are displayed in Figure 1, which shows a significant difference between Group 1 – control (not whitened), and the groups after whitening (Group 2 – conventional whitening product, and Group 3 – whitening product containing ACP). No significant differences were found between the whitened groups.

The value of the Kruskal-Wallis statistical test for ARI was p = 0.0509, indicating a statistically insignificant difference. Figure 2 shows ARI in both groups.

DISCUSSION

A number of studies have evaluated the bond strength of orthodontic brackets bonded to different surfaces.[3,20,27] In this context, preference has been given to central incisor brackets as they feature a flatter base surface, which adapts more easily to the surfaces being tested. These surfaces are normally flat since specimens are seldom fabricated with crown contours, which explains the brackets used in this experiment.

Nevertheless, it is noteworthy that *in vitro* tests exhibit numerous differences compared with *in vivo* tests. The key difference lies in the fact that the forces which occur during mastication are compressive in nature and pose a greater risk of damage to enamel than forces applied to the bracket/adhesive during shear bond tests.[13] These peculiarities of laboratory tests should be emphasized as they improve variable control. Conversely, clinical studies do not allow these variables to be controlled, which warrants further studies on this topic.

In actuality there is no such thing as a pure shear force *in vivo*, given that the different components combine to influence the bond. Moreover, *in vitro* results undergo significant effects, as shown by Swift Jr., Perdigão;[29] Bishara and Sulieman.[4] Despite the above, this investigation followed the methodology adopted by the ISO/TS11405 standard.

As regards the type of substrate used, bovine teeth have long been considered a good alternative since not only are they more readily available but their enamel structure is similar to that of human teeth. Assessments made by comparative studies involving different substrates show that the bond strength of bovine enamel is quite acceptable, although their bond strength may be lower compared to human teeth.[9,21]

Another noteworthy aspect concerns the storage medium adopted in the present study (distilled water). In bond strength tests of whitened substrates the storage medium used for the specimens plays a role as relevant as it is controversial. Artificial saliva, which

Table 2 - P values of the statistical test between experimental groups.

Groups	p value
Groups 1 and 2	< 0.05
Groups 1 and 3	< 0.01
Groups 2 and 3	n.s.

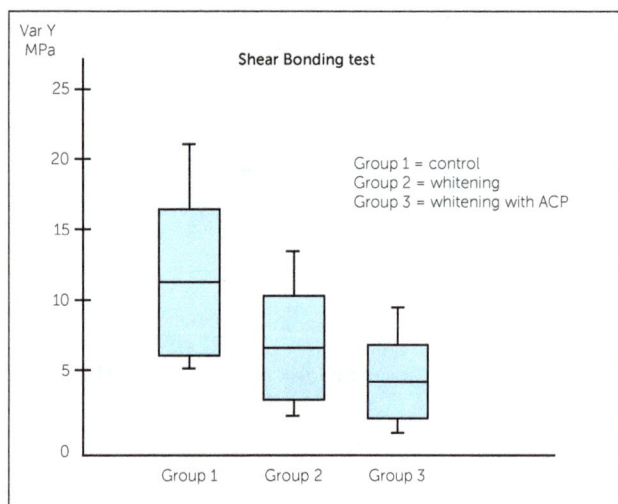

Figure 1 - Shear bond strength values, means and standard deviations of groups 1, 2 and 3.

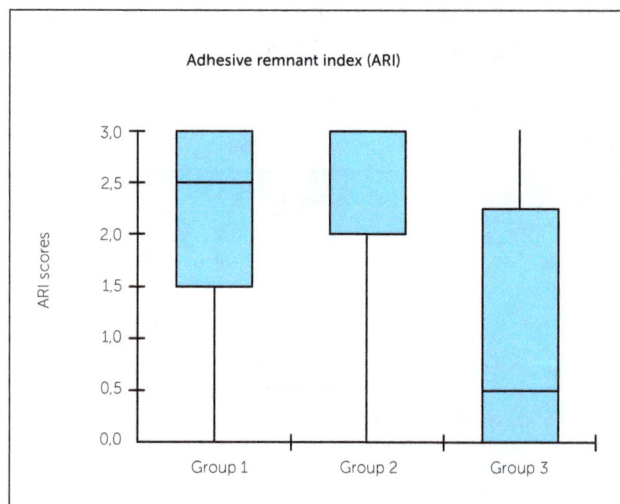

Figure 2 - Adhesive remnant index (ARI), median and quartile in groups 1, 2 and 3.

has been employed in different studies,[8,10,16,17,28] is primarily aimed at making laboratory tests resemble as closely as possible the clinical conditions actually experienced in routine practice.

As to the mechanical test, it is a known fact that orthodontic brackets require a bond strength capable of withstanding masticatory forces and activation of the mechanics utilized.[21] The minimum acceptable bond strength for routine orthodontic procedures ranges from 6 to 8 Mpa.[21] The results showed unacceptable mean bond strength values for whitened teeth.

Thus, artificial saliva has often been blamed for the lack of differences in bond strength after whitening, according to published studies.[15,19] This finding could be attributed to the remineralizing effect of saliva cited by Souza,[28] who argued that enamel samples treated with 10% carbamide peroxide and stored in artificial saliva display smaller spaces in between the hydroxyapatite crystals. However, other studies[29,30] claim that this potential remineralizing effect of saliva has not yet been properly explained.

Therefore, in order to avert a possible potentiating (remineralizing), or deleterious effect by artificial saliva, which could interfere with the analysis of the results, a storage medium. i.e., distilled water, was chosen as it exerts little or no effect on bond strength.

Residues derived from the degradation of peroxide or oxygen leads to a lower amount of shorter resinous tags compared to teeth not subjected to whitening,[7,18] resulting in lower bond strength as hydrogen peroxide negatively affects the curing of adhesive systems.[12,14,16,23,30]

Therefore, teeth whitening can change the mineral structure of tooth enamel and, hence, affect the bond between this substrate and adhesive systems.[24,25] It is thus necessary to wait for a post-whitening period long enough for the enamel's mineral structure to be restored, and for the residual oxygen of the whitening agent to be completely removed. Although the literature shows significant variation in the length of the post-whitening period recommended before bonding brackets (24h to 4 weeks), Cavalli[8] showed that a minimum of two weeks would be required for the structure to recover its adhesive properties. The results led the authors to believe that 15 days were not sufficient to restore the enamel, suggesting therefore

that a longer time interval should be allowed to elapse prior to bonding any orthodontic appliances.

Furthermore, removal of the remaining resin from the tooth surface does not pose a challenge since removal of adhesive remnants from tooth surfaces after removal of the fixed orthodontic appliance is a routine procedure. Thus, the choice of bonding materials depends on a careful assessment of their clinical properties. This finding concerning the adhesive remnant index (ARI) is of great interest to the orthodontist, who can thus choose materials that respond clinically by presenting a greater amount of adhesive remnants on the tooth surface after removal of the brackets. This should ensure greater safety, preventing enamel fractures and preserving tooth integrity.

Although the use of hydrogen peroxide at 35% significantly reduces the amount of resin on the tooth surface after debonding,[31] this study did not reveal any differences in terms of ARI in both whitened and non-whitened teeth, with and without ACP.

Proper orthodontic treatment requires scientific knowledge and special technical skills. It is also paramount that orthodontists be instructed about the wide array of materials of different types and manufacturers currently available for clinical use. There are various products of different origins, both domestic and imported, manufactured specifically for direct bonding of orthodontic attachments to enamel. It is therefore extremely important that these results be applied in clinical practice in order to optimize professional orthodontic treatment, thus avoiding frequent bond failures due to poor bond strength between brackets and tooth enamel.

CONCLUSION

Significant differences were found in the bond strength of metal brackets between whitened and non-whitened teeth. There was a considerable reduction in bond strength in the groups that were subjected to tooth surface whitening. Both whitened groups (2 and 3) failed to achieve a clinically efficient bond strength, especially group 3 (whitened with ACP), underscoring the need to restore the tooth surface and remove all chemical whitening agents prior to bonding the brackets. As regards ARI, there was no statistically significant difference between the 3 groups tested.

REFERENCES

1. Artun J, Bergland S. Clinical trials with crystal growth conditioning as an alternative to acid-etch enamel pretreatment. Am J Orthod. 1984;85(4):333-40.

2. Bishara SE, Ostby AW. Bonding and debonding from metal to ceramic: research and its clinical application. Semin Orthod. 2010;16(1):24-36.

3. Bishara SE, VonWald L, Laffoon JF, Warren JJ. Effect of a self-etch primer/adhesive on the shear bond strength of orthodontic brackets. Am J Orthod Dentofacial Orthop. 2001;119(6):621-4.

4. Bishara SE, Sulieman AH, Olson M. Effect of enamel bleaching on the bonding strength of orthodontic brackets. Am J Orthod Dentofacial Orthop. 1993;104(5):444-7.

5. Bitter NC. Bleaching agents. J Am Dent Assoc. 1999;130:26.

6. Buonocore MG. Simple method of increasing the adhesion of acrylic filling materials to enamel surface. J Dent Res. 1955;34(6):849-53.

7. Cal Neto JOAP, Miguel JAM. Uma análise dos testes in vitro de força de adesão em Ortodontia. Rev Dental Press Ortod Ortop Facial. 2004;9(4):44-51.

8. Cavalli V, Reis AF, Giannini M, Ambrosano GM. The effect of elapsed time following bleaching on enamel bond strength of resin composite. Oper Dent. 2001;26(6):597-602.

9. Cavalli V, Arrais CA, Giannini M, Ambrosano GM. High concentrated carbamide peroxide bleaching agent effect on enamel surface. J Oral Rehabil. 2004;31(2):155-9.

10. Cavalli V, Carvalho RM, Giannini M. Influence of carbamide peroxide-based bleaching agents on the bond strength of resin-enamel/dentin interfaces. Braz Oral Res. 2005;19(1):23-9.

11. Dishman MV, Covey DA, Baughan LW. The effects of peroxide bleaching on composite to enamel bond strength. Dent Mater. 1994;10(1):33-6.

12. Dunn WJ. Shear bond strength of an amorphous calcium-phosphate-containing orthodontic resin cement. Am J Orthod Dentofacial Orthop. 2007;131(2):243-7.

13. Eliades T, Brantley WA. Orthodontics materials, scientific and clinical aspects. 1st ed. Stuttgart: Thieme; 2001.

14. International Organization for Standardization. Dental materials. [Access 2011 may 17]. Available from: http://www.iso.org.

15. Josey AL, Meyers IA, Romaniuk K, Symons AL. The effect of vital bleaching technique on enamel surface morphology and the bonding of composite resin to enamel. J Oral Rehabil. 1996;23(4):244-50.

16. Loretto SC, Braz R, Lyra AMVC, Lopes LM. Influence of photopolymerization light source on enamel shear bond strength after bleaching. Braz Dent J. 2004;15(2):133-7. Epub 2005 Mar 11.

17. Kalili T, Caputo AA, Mito R, Sperbeck G, Matyas J. In vitro toothbrush abrasion and bond strength of bleached enamel. Pract Periodontics Aesthet Dent. 1991;3(5):22-4.

18. Miles PG, Pontier JP, Bahiraei D, Close J. The effect of carbamide peroxide bleach on the tensile bond strength of ceramic brackets: an in vitro study. Am J Orthod Dentofacial Orthop. 1994;106(4):371-5.

19. Murchison DF, Charlton DG, Moore BK. Carbamide peroxide bleaching: effects on enamel surface hardness and bonding. Oper Dent. 1992;17(5):181-5.

20. Newman GV. Epoxy adhesives for orthodontic attachments: progress report. Am J Orthod. 1965;51(12):901-12.

21. Perdigão J, Francci C, Swift EJ, Ambrose WW, Lopes M. Ultra-morphological study of the interaction of dental adhesives with carbamide peroxide-bleached enamel. Am J Dent. 1998;11(6):291-301.

22. Oesterle LJ, Shellhart WC, Belanger GK. The use of bovine enamel in bonding studies. Am J Orthod Dentofacial Orthop. 1998;114(5):514-9.

23. Øgaard B, Fjeld M. The enamel surface and bonding in Orthodontics. Semin Orthod. 2010;16:37-48.

24. Oshiro M, Yamaguchi K, Takamizawa T, Inage H, Watanabe T, Irokawa A, et al. Effect of CPP-ACP paste on tooth mineralization: an FE-SEM study. J Oral Sci. 2007;49(2):115-20.

25. Perdigão J, Francci C, Swift EJ Jr, Ambrose WW, Lopes M. Ultra-morphological study of the interaction of dental adhesives with carbamide peroxide-bleached enamel. Am J Dent. 1998;11(6):291-301.

26. Reynolds IR. A review of direct orthodontic bonding. Br J Orthod. 1975;2(3):171-8.

27. Spyrides GM, Perdigão J, Pagani C, Araújo MA, Spyrides SM. Effect of whitening agents on dentin bonding. J Esthet Dent. 2000;12(5):264-70.

28. Souza MAL. Clareamento caseiro de dentes: ação do peróxido de carbamida sobre dentes e mucosa bucal [tese]. Porto Alegre (RS): Pontifícia Universidade Católica; 1993.

29. Swift EJ Jr, Perdigão J. Effects of bleaching on teeth and restorations. Compend Contin Educ Dent. 1998;19(8):815-20; quiz 822.

30. Türkün M, Kaya AD. Effect of 10% sodium ascorbate on the shear bond strength of composite resin to bleached bovine enamel. J Oral Rehabil. 2004;31(12):1184-91.

31. Uysal T, Basciftci FA, Uşümez S, Sari Z, Buyukerkmen A. Can previously bleached teeh bonded safely? Am J Orthod Dentofacial Orthop. 2003;123(6):628-32.

21

Brazilian primary school teachers' knowledge about immediate management of dental trauma

Matheus Melo Pithon[1], Rogério Lacerda dos Santos[2], Pedro Henrique Bomfim Magalhães[3], Raildo da Silva Coqueiro[4]

Objective: To assess the level of knowledge of primary school teachers in the public school network of Northeastern Brazil with respect to management of dental trauma and its relationship with prognosis. **Methods:** A questionnaire was applied to 195 school teachers of public schools in Northeastern Brazil. The questionnaire comprised 12 objective questions about dental trauma and methods for its prevention and management. Data were submitted to chi-square test and Poisson regression test ($P > 0.05$). **Results:** Out of the 141 teachers who responded the questionnaires, the majority were women (70.2%) and most of them had experienced previous dental accidents involving a child (53.2%). The majority (84.4%) had incomplete college education and few were given some training on how to deal with emergency situations during their undergraduate course (13.5%) or after it (38.3%). Their level of knowledge about dental trauma and emergency protocols showed that unsatisfactory knowledge level was associated with the male sex: 46% higher for men in comparison to women ($P = 0.025$). **Conclusions:** Approximately half of teachers evaluated had unsatisfactory knowledge about dental trauma and emergency protocols, with female teachers showing more knowledge than men.

Keywords: Knowledge. Teaching. Dental care.

[1] Professor, Department of Orthodontics, State University of Southwestern Bahia (UESB).
[2] Professor, Department of Orthodontics, Federal University of Campina Grande (UFCG).
[3] DDS, State University of Southwestern Bahia (UESB).
[4] Professor, Department of Epidemiology, State University of Southwestern Bahia (UESB).

» The authors report no commercial, proprietary or financial interest in the products or companies described in this article.

Matheus Melo Pithon
Av. Otávio Santos, 395, sala 705,
Centro Odontomédico Dr. Altamirando da Costa Lima, Bairro Recreio,
Cep: 45020-750 – Vitória da Conquista / BA —Brazil
E-mail: matheuspithon@gmail.com

INTRODUCTION

Dentoalveolar trauma is frequent among children and adolescents.[1,2,3] It may affect teeth, soft tissues and supporting structures, and may lead to psychological, social, masticatory, phonological and esthetic changes.[4] At present, this is considered a public health problem due to the growing rates of violence, automobile accidents, contact sports and injuries in the school environment.[3,5] Some studies assert that the number of cases with dental trauma will exceed cases with dental caries or periodontal problems,[6,7] and may result in high costs to Public Health Services.[8]

Accidents are the main cause of dental trauma[1,9,10] and frequently occur when the child reaches school age. Dental lesions may range from slight to extensive maxillofacial damage.[1]

Parents and teachers who deal with children must be familiarized with dental emergency maneuvers.[1,2] However, studies[1,3,4,9-12] have shown lack of teacher's knowledge regarding emergency management of dental trauma.[1] Lack of knowledge on these questions lead to implementation, frequently inadequate, of health policies that do not achieve ideal results.[1,2,9,10]

Bearing in mind the importance of this issue and the lack of information in Northeastern Brazil, the aim of this study was to investigate the knowledge of school teachers working in the public school network of the municipality of Jéquie / BA about dental injuries caused by trauma, and the procedures to be carried out when they occur.

MATERIAL AND METHODS

A field research was conducted. Data was collected by means of a questionnaire answered by 195 full-time teachers working in the public school network of the city of Jequié / BA in 2012. Data on the total number of teachers was provided by the Municipal Secretary of Education in the city of Jequié and by the Regional Board of Education (DIREC-13). The questionnaire comprised 12 objective questions and was self-applied in the presence of the main researcher. The first part of the questionnaire consisted in collecting general information about teachers' personal and professional profiles, including age, sex, career time-span, and whether or not they had received any training about dental trauma. The second part consisted of questions with reference to knowledge about dental trauma and dental emergency protocols,

hypothesizing situations that could occur in the school environment. To assess teachers' level of knowledge, those who correctly answered 4 to 6 questions were classified as having satisfactory level of knowledge, and those who correctly answered 0 to 3 questions, as having an unsatisfactory level of knowledge. The research project was approved by the Institutional Review Board of UESB, Protocol N°.089/011.

The frequency of responses given by the teachers was compared by means of chi-square test (P > 0.05). Associations between the dependent variable (level of knowledge) and explanatory variables (sex, age group, educational level, career time-span, first-aid, dental trauma and first aid training during academic education and having witnessed an accident) were tested by means of Poisson regression technique. Simple robust models were calculated to estimate the prevalence ratios (PR) with their respective confidence interval of 95% (CI: 95%). Significance level was set at 5% (α = 0.05). Data were tabulated and analyzed in Statistical Package for Social Sciences for Windows (SPSS. 15.0, 2006, SPSS, Inc, Chicago, IL, USA) software.

RESULTS

Teachers' response rate was 72.3% (n = 141). A total of 54 teachers (n = 27.7) decided not to participate in the research. Career time-span ranged from 1 to 33 years, with a mean of 13.5 ± 9.5 years. The majority of teachers (64.5%) aged between 31 and 50 years and had a level of incomplete professional college education (84.4%). They had not had first aid training during their academic education (86.5%) or after it (61.7%), but the majority had witnessed accidents (53.2%) (Table 1).

Associations between knowledge (Table 2) and the variables presented in Table 1 were tested. Chi-square test highlighted a single association: Knowledge about the type of tooth (Question 1) vs. witnessed an accident. Results showed that teachers who had witnessed some type of accident had a higher frequency of correct answers in comparison to those who had never witnessed one (P = 0.048) (Fig 1). For the other questions, no statistical differences were observed. (P > 0.05).

In the six questions asked, the mean score for right answers was 3.5 ± 1.2 questions. Results revealed that nearly half of teachers had unsatisfactory knowledge with respect to dental trauma and emergency protocols (Fig 2).

Table 1 - Characteristics of study participants.

Characteristics	n	%
Sex		
Male	42	29.8
Female	99	70.2
Age group		
≤ 30 years	34	24.1
31 to 40 years	46	32.6
41 to 50 years	45	31.9
> 50 years	16	11.3
Educational level		
Incomplete college education	119	84.4
Complete college education	22	15.6
Career time-span*		
≤ 6 years	49	34.8
7 to 19 years	47	33.3
> 19 years	45	31.9
First aid training		
Yes	54	38.3
No	87	61.7
Dental trauma and first aid information during academic education		
Yes	19	13.5
No	122	86.5
Witnessed accident		
Yes	75	53.2
No	66	46.8

* For categorization of career time-span, distribution into terciles was taken into consideration: 1st tercile = 6 years and 2nd tercile = 19 years.

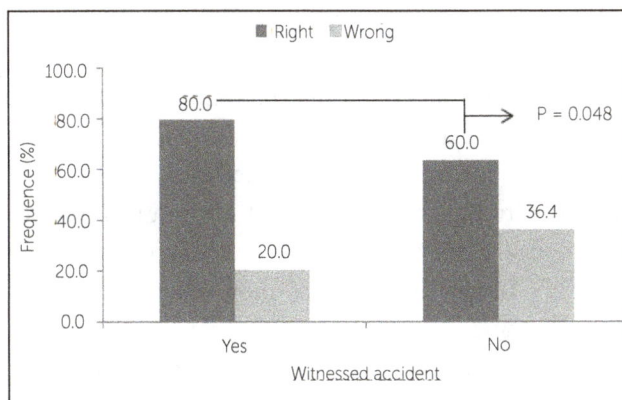

Figure 1 - Teachers distribution according to knowledge about the type of tooth fractured and whether or not they witnessed an accident.

Table 2 - Teachers distribution with regard to knowledge of dental trauma and emergency protocol.

Question	Correct	Incorrect
1. A 9-year-old child is hit on the face by a ball and fractures two anterior teeth. Are the affected teeth:		
( ) Permanent teeth.	102	39
( ) Milk teeth.	(72.3%)	(27.7%)
2. Which of the following actions do you consider most adequate?		
( ) You will look for the parts of broken tooth and after class, would contact his parents to explain what had happened.		
( ) You will look for the parts of broken tooth and then give him a warm drink and would contact her parents.	83 (58.9%)	58 (41.1%)
( ) You will look for the parts of broken tooth and would contact his parents and then send him immediately to the dentist.		
3. At school, a 12-year-old child falls down the stairs and hits his/her mouth on the floor. One of his/her top front teeth was knocked out of the mouth. What would be the first thing you do?		
( ) You would look for the tooth and wash it with tap water.		
( ) You would ask the child to bite on a tissue paper to control bleeding.		
( ) You would ask the child to hold the tooth carefully in his mouth and take her immediately to the nearest dentist.	70 (49.6%)	71 (50.4%)
( ) You would look for the tooth and put it back into the socket.		
4. If you decide to reimplant the tooth back in its place, but it had fallen on the floor, what would you do?		
( ) You would scrub the tooth gently with a toothbrush.		
( ) You would rinse the tooth under tap water.	108 (76.6%)	33 (23.4%)
( ) You would put the tooth straight back into the socket without any pretreatment.		
5. If you chose to wash the tooth, which solution would you use to wash it?		
( ) Tap water.		
( ) Saline solution.		
( ) Alcohol.	103 (73.0%)	38 (27.0%)
( ) Filtered water.		
( ) Antiseptic solution.		
6. If you do not reimplant the tooth, how would you transport it to the dentist?		
( ) Tap water.		
( ) Milk.		
( ) Child's mouth.	24 (17.0%)	117 (83.0%)
( ) Paper tissue.		
( ) Filtered water.		

The results of regression for the level of knowledge about dental trauma and emergency protocols as regards the explanatory variables of the study (Table 3), demonstrated that unsatisfactory level of knowledge was associated with the male sex: 46% higher for men in comparison to women (P = 0.025). The other variables were not associated with teachers' level of knowledge (P > 0.05).

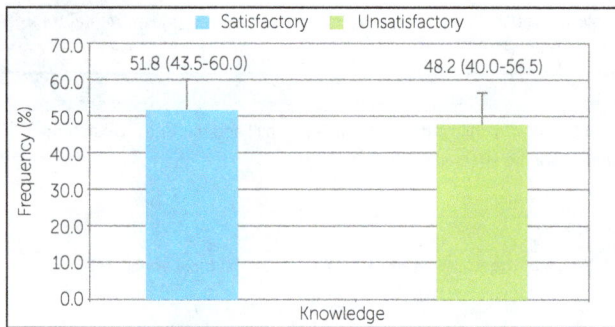

Figure 2 - Teachers distribution [prevalence (CI 95%)] according to level of knowledge about dental trauma and emergency protocols.

Table 3 - Association between the level of unsatisfactory knowledge about dental trauma/emergency protocols and characteristics of the studied sample.

Variables	%	PR (CI 95%)	P value
Sex			
Male	61.9	1.46 (1.05 – 2.03)	
Female	42.4	1	0.025
Age group			
≤ 30 years	50.0	1.00 (0.55 – 1.81)	
31 to 40 years	41.3	0.83 (0.45 – 1.50)	
41 to 50 years	53.3	1.07 (0.61 – 1.87)	0.721
> 50 years	50.0	1	
Educational level			
Incomplete college education	54.5	1.16 (0.56 – 1.32)	
Complete college education	47.1	1	0.497
Career time-span			
≤ 6 years	49.0	1.05 (0.69 – 1.60)	
7 a 19 years	48.9	1.05 (0.68 – 1.61)	0.969
> 19 years	46.7	1	
First aid training			
Yes	46.3	1	
No	49.4	1.07 (0.75 – 1.53)	0.720
Learning about dental trauma and first aid in academic education			
Yes	47.4	1	
No	48.4	1.02 (0.61 – 1.70)	0.936
Witnessed an accident			
Yes	46.7	1	
No	50.0	1.07 (0.76 – 1.51)	0.692

PR, prevalence ratio; CI 95%, confidence interval at 95%.

DISCUSSION

At least half of schoolchildren face the possibility of suffering dentoalveolar trauma during school time.[3,13] Dental trauma is relevant in children and adolescents, since their permanent teeth are erupting at this phase.[14] Additionally, at school, during sporting and recreational activities, children and adolescents are the main groups with an increased likelihood of dental trauma,[3,5,15] thereby rendering investigation of school teachers knowledge with regard to dental injuries and treatment approaches.[1,2,11,12,15-21]

In the present study, approximately half teachers surveyed (48.2%) had unsatisfactory knowledge (correctly answered up to three questions) about dental trauma and emergency protocols. Their mean career time-span was 13.5 years. Only 38.3% of teachers had received first aid training on dental trauma, which was higher than the percentage found by Al-Obaida[1] who showed only 1.5%. A total of 53.2% teachers who had received training experienced some type of accident involving a child in the school environment, a higher percentage than the 20% found by Arikan.[2]

As for the most adequate solution for washing an avulsed tooth,[22] 73% of the teachers answered the question correctly by stating filtered water or saline solution; however, only 17% correctly stated milk, the oral cavity, or filtered water as being adequate for sending the avulsed tooth to the dentist.[22] These findings are similar to those observed in studies conducted in other countries[1,2,11,12,16-21] and are important for defining educational strategies, because storing a tooth in an inappropriate environment, in addition to rapidly transporting the child and the tooth to a dentist is crucial for favorable prognosis.[2,15,23]

Variables such as age, educational level, career timespan, having undergone a first aid training course, having received training on how to deal with emergency situations during their undergraduate course, and having witnessed an accident did not result in greater knowledge about dental trauma and emergency protocols.[2,11,15] Female teachers had more knowledge about dental trauma and emergency protocols in comparison to male teachers. This may be related to the fact that women have more contact with children in outdoor environments, in addition to the fact that the majority of them were mothers.

Freitas et al[24] showed evidence of great lack of knowledge about dentoalveolar trauma in Physical Education professionals, and indicated that they should be better informed on the subject, as they will have to deal with risk situations related to dentoalveolar trauma on a daily basis.[7,8,13,22]

Children spend great part of their time at school where sporting activities become predisposing factors for dental trauma.[15] Thus, including emergency procedures in the curriculum of these professionals and implementing educational preventive programs is necessary,[2,15] as favorable prognosis will depend on how these injuries are managed.[9] Therefore, multidisciplinary interaction between dentists and teachers in the public school network is necessary for positive interference in health promotion and prevention of more severe complications.[9,25] This includes the dissemination of posters, leaflets, and information through lectures,[2,19] television, magazines, radio and newspapers,[10] or the Internet (http://www.iadt-dentaltrauma.org.).[2]

An educational program[1,15] that discusses the importance of preventing dental trauma and the benefits of immediate treatment, conservation of fractures or avulsed teeth would significantly reduce dentoalveolar trauma and sequelae.[26]

Another relevant factor is knowledge about primary and permanent dentitions, and their period of transition.[27] In the present study, nearly 28% of teachers were unable to differentiate a permanent to a primary anterior tooth in a 9 year-old-child. A large portion of the population is not aware of the period of primary dentition in a child's development. Early loss of a primary tooth due to trauma may affect the physiological sequence of permanent teeth, and may be etiological factors for malocclusions,[14] thus stimulating incorrect exercise of perioral musculature and/or cause phonological changes related to teeth.[5,11,14]

Studies[20,28] have shown that teachers with a rudimentary level of learning about dental trauma expressed the desire to receive more information about the subject, totaling 95% of respondents. On the other hand, many primary schools in Japan have nurse teachers with knowledge of emergency care, which is considered a good approach when dealing with children and adolescents.[29]

Knowledge about teachers' ability in dealing with traumatized patients in Northeastern Brazil will make it possible to conduct adequate programs for guidance, prevention[3] and management of dental trauma, thereby improving prognosis in cases of dental trauma.[2,4,9,10,14]

CONCLUSION

Based on the results of this study it is reasonable to conclude that:

» Approximately half of teachers has unsatisfactory knowledge about dental trauma and emergency protocols.

» Female teachers had more knowledge about dental trauma and emergency protocols than male teachers.

» Being older, having a better educational level, longer career time-span, having undergone first aid training related to dental trauma during academic education, and having witnessed an accident did not provide more knowledge of dental trauma and emergency protocols.

REFERENCES

1. Al-Obaida M. Knowledge and management of traumatic dental injuries in a group of Saudi primary schools teachers. Dent Traumatol. 2010;26(4):338-41.

2. Arikan V, Sonmez H. Knowledge level of primary school teachers regarding traumatic dental injuries and their emergency management before and after receiving an informative leaflet. Dent Traumatol. 2012;28(2):101-7.

3. Faus-Damiá M, Alegre-Domingo T, Faus-Matoses I, Faus-Matoses V, Faus-Llácer VJ. Traumatic dental injuries among schoolchildren in Valencia, Spain. Med Oral Patol Oral Cir Bucal. 2011;16(2):e292-5.

4. Bittencourt AM, Pessoa OF, Silva JL. Evaluation of the knowledge of teachers in relation to the management of tooth avulsion in children. J Dent UNESP. 2008;37:15-9.

5. Marcenes W, Zabot NE, Traebert J. Socio-economic correlates of traumatic injuries to the permanent incisors in schoolchildren aged 12 years in Blumenau, Brazil. Dent Traumatol. 2001;17:222-6.

6. Marchiori EC, Santos SE, Asprino L, Moraes M, Moreira RW. Occurrence of dental avulsion and associated injuries in patients with facial trauma over a 9-year period. Oral Maxillofac Surg. 2013;17(2):119-26.

7. Al-Khateeb S, Al-Nimri K, Alhaija EA. Factors affecting coronal fracture of anterior teeth in North Jordanian children. Dent Traumatol. 2005;21(1):26-8.

8. Bonini GAVC, Marcenes W, Oliveira LB, Sheiham A, Bonecker M. Trends in the prevalence of traumatic dental injuries in Brazilian preschool children. Dent Traumatol. 2009;25(6):594-8.

9. Caglar E, Ferreira LP, Kargul B. Dental trauma management knowledge among a group of teachers in two south European cities. Dent Traumatol. 2005;21(5):258-62.

10. Young C, Wong KY, Cheung LK. Emergency management of dental trauma: knowledge of Hong Kong primary and secondary school teachers. Hong Kong Med J. 2012;18(5):362-70.

11. Tzigkounakis V, Merglova V. Attitude of Pilsen primary school teachers in dental trauma. Dent Traumatol. 2008;24(5):528-31.

12. Vergotine RJ, Govoni R. Public school educator's knowledge of initial management of dental trauma. Dent Traumatol. 2010;26(2):133-6

13. Glendor U. Aetiology and risk factors related to traumatic dental injuries: a review of the literature. Dent Traumatol. 2009;25(1):19-31.

14. Campos MICC, Henriques KAM, Campos CS. Level of Information about the conduct of emergency trauma dental front. Pesq Bras Odontoped Clin Integr. 2006;6:155-9.

15. Trope M, Chivian N, Sigurdsson A, Vann WF. Traumatic injuries. In: Cohen S, Burns RC, editors. Pathways of the pulp. 8th ed. St Louis: Mosby; 2002. p. 603-49.

16. Feldens EG, Feldens CA, Kramer PF, Silva KG, Munari CC, Brei VA. Understanding school teacher's knowledge regarding dental trauma: a basis for future interventions. Dent Traumatol. 2010;26(2):158-63.

17. Haragushiku GA, Faria MI, Silva SR, Gonzaga CC, Baratto-Filho F. Knowledge and attitudes toward dental avulsion of public and private elementary schoolteachers. J Dent Child (Chic). 2010;77(1):49-53.

18. Skeie MS, Audestad E, Bardsen A. Traumatic dental injuries: knowledge and awareness among present and prospective teachers in selected urban and rural areas of Norway. Dent Traumatol. 2010;26:243-7.

19. Lieger O, Graf C, El-Maaytah M, Von Arx T. Impact of educational posters on the lay knowledge of school teachers regarding emergency management of dental injuries. Dent Traumatol. 2009;25:406-12.

20. Sae-Lim V, Lim LP. Dental trauma management awareness of Singapore pre-school teachers. Dent Traumatol. 2001;17(2):71-6.

21. Mesgarzadeh AH, Shahamfar M, Hefzollesan A. Evaluating knowledge and attitudes of elementary school teachers on emergency management of traumatic dental injuries: a study in an Iranian urban area. Oral Health Prev Dent. 2009;7:297-308.

22. Andersson L, Andreasen JO, Day P, Heithersay G, Trope M, Diangelis AJ, et al. International Association of Dental Traumatology guidelines for the management of traumatic dental injuries: 2. Avulsion of permanent teeth. Dent Traumatol. 2012;28:88-96.

23. Donaldson M, Kinirons MJ. Factors affecting the time of onset of resorption in avulsed and replanted incisor teeth in children. Dent Traumatol. 2001;17(5):205-9.

24. Freitas DA, Freitas VA, Antunes SLNO, Crispim RR. Assessment of knowledge of Physical Education academics about avulsion / tooth replantation and the importance of using mouthguard during physical activities. Rev Bras Cir Cabeça Pescoço. 2008;37:215-8.

25. Panzarini SR, Pedrini D, Brandini DA, Poi WR, Santos MF, Correa JP, et al. Physical education undergraduates and dental trauma knowledge. Dent Traumatol. 2005;21:324-8.

26. Walker A, Brenchley J. It's a knockout: survey of the management of avulsed teeth. Accid Emerg Nurs. 2000;8(2):66-70.

27. Silva MB, Costa AMM, Almeida MEC, Maia SA, Carvalhal CIO, Resende GB. Evaluation of the knowledge of the approach of dental trauma by daycare professional. ConScientiae Saúde. 2009;8:65-73.

28. Blakytny C, Surbuts C, Thomas A, Hunter ML. Avulsed permanent incisors: knowledge and attitudes of primary school teachers with regard to emergency management. Int J Paediatr Dent. 2001;11:327-32.

29. Kinoshita S, Kojima R, Taguchi Y, Noda T. Tooth replantation after traumatic avulsion: a report of ten cases. Dent Traumatol. 2002;18(3):153-6.

22

Assessment of motivation, expectations and satisfaction of adult patients submitted to orthodontic treatment

Patrícia Gomide de Souza Andrade Oliveira[1], Rubens Rodrigues Tavares[2], Jairo Curado de Freitas[3]

Objective: The purpose of this study was to analyze the psychological aspects of adult patients who sought and underwent orthodontic treatment, evaluating their expectations and discomfort during treatment, as well as their satisfaction after completion of dental movement. **Results and Conclusions:** Data obtained from previous published papers, and also from questionnaires answered by 54 patients, showed that adult patients stood out for their attention to details and high interest in the esthetic improvements provided by treatment, and also for a greater perception of their initial malocclusion. On the other hand, the same data showed that adult patients, once informed about the limitations of their treatment and having confidence on the orthodontist, presented a high level of satisfaction with treatment results, revealing themselves as good patients for indication and execution of orthodontic procedures.

Keywords: Orthodontics. Psychology. Behavior. Adults.

» The author reports no commercial, proprietary or financial interest in the products or companies described in this article.

[1] Specialist in Orthodontics.
[2] Professor of the Orthodontics Specialization Program at the Brazilian Dental Association - Goiás Section (ABO-GO).
[3] Head of the Orthodontics Specialization Program, ABO-GO.

Patrícia Gomide de Souza Andrade Oliveira
Rua 1028 nº. 131, ap. 503, setor Pedro Ludovico
CEP: 74.823-130 – Goiânia / GO, Brazil
E-mail: drapatriciagomide@yahoo.com.br

INTRODUCTION

Many authors confirm what orthodontists have been noticing on a daily basis in their private practices: The increasing number of adult patients seeking orthodontic treatment.[3,4,6]

When planning orthodontic treatment for patients in that scope, we should bear in mind that, generally, adults present a different experience in relation to buccal pathologies, and psychological limitations when compared to teenagers and children.

Focusing in the psychological aspects concerning adult patients, many studies prove that these patients have a greater awareness of their malocclusion, which may generate very optimistic expectations about the final results of their treatment.[4,10,11] In search for delivering a more efficient treatment to such patients, it is mandatory that orthodontists investigate and understand the expectations, difficulties, and motivations of this increasing group, in order to offer assistance that matches their concerns.

The offer of orthodontic treatment to adult patients, albeit becoming more common in the last decades, is not a product of our time. The first reference to it was made by Pierre Fauchard, author of the first scientific Dentistry book known to us as Le Chirurgien Dentiste from 1723.[6]

Epidemiologic data that has been gathered since the 80's confirms the increase of the demand of patients in that age group (18 +) who want and need orthodontic treatment. In the United States, in 1988, it became clear that in large urban business centers, this demand represented between 60 to 70% of all the patients looking for treatment. In Europe, studies from the beginning of the 80's also show an increase in adult patients seeking orthodontic care.[6,11]

Recent studies show that the frequency of malocclusion in adults is similar, if not higher to that observed in children and teenagers. According to official data released by the North American government in the NHANES III (Third National Health and Nutrition Survey), in the 90's, only 41.1% of all American adults had an optimal overjet, 49% presented deep bite, 3.3% open bite, and there was also a significant occurrence of misalignment in upper and lower incisors, respectively 56% and 62.9%.[3,12] In a similar way, the prevalence of malocclusion in Eastern Europe adults, according to studies conducted within populations from Germany and Sweden, reached between 40 and 76% of the total adult population from these regions.[3]

In 2003, a study made with 200 adult patients, evaluated the reasons which led them to initially reject the suggestion to undergo orthodontic treatment. The researchers found out the reasons to be, from the highest to the lowest prevalence: Long treatment time, the discomfort of wearing orthodontic appliances, rejection to the anti-esthetic appearance of brackets, concerns about pain, and fear of disappointment with the final treatment result.[7]

Within the large demand of adult patients who seek and need orthodontic assistance, literature has shown that most of these patients are females,[6,10] and that the indication for them to seek for an orthodontist comes from the family dentist.[6]

Just like every health related treatment, orthodontic treatment in adults has its indications and contraindications, which must be carefully assessed before any action takes place.

Highlighted among the indications are: The possibility of improving teeth implantation in the periodontal tissues, determining a more stable and harmonious occlusive pattern, distribution of edentulous spaces so that they can be restored later, improvement of the occlusal condition and protection of the stomatognathic system (especially the temporomandibular joint - TMJ) and satisfaction of the patients esthetical demands.

The cases where orthodontic treatment would be contraindicated in adult patients are: Existence of severe skeletal discrepancies (in these cases surgical treatment would be preferable), patients with systemic or advanced local diseases, cases of severe alveolar bone loss, when the results might not fulfill the expectations of both the patient and the professional in charge of the treatment, questionable prognostic stability, and lack of patient interest or motivation.[13]

The main reason that leads adult individuals to search for orthodontic care is their dissatisfaction with their dental and/or facial appearance; and many studies confirm that adult patients have greater perception of their dental esthetics thus presenting higher demands concerning the results achieved after orthodontic therapy.[4,5,6,9] Another frequent reason is the need for isolated dental movements so that other procedures aiming the control of periodontal disease prosthetic rehabilitation (implants or prosthesis), or cosmetic (dental reconstructions) can be executed within a multidisciplinary planning.[6]

Previous studies that proposed to evaluate the psychological profile of adult patients seeking orthodontic treatment showed that many of these patients presented a neurotic or unstable psychological profile along with problems of self-esteem. These same studies alert orthodontists that this kind of patient tends to nurture great expectations, some of them even being unreal, regarding treatment results, and suggesting that the tangible results should be made as clear as possible to them in order to avoid future disappointments.[4,10,11]

In 2005, researchers gave a satisfaction questionnaire to be answered by 100 patients treated in the Academic Center of Dentistry in Amsterdam three years after they completed their orthodontic treatment. In that study it was observed that the most important issue in determining patient satisfaction was the good orthodontist/patient relationship during treatment and that female patients revealed lower satisfaction levels with the dentofacial improvements achieved by treatment when compared to male patients.

The objective of the present study was to analyze, through questionnaires the psychological profile of adult patients, most of them living in the city of Goiânia/GO, Brazil, who underwent orthodontic treatment, assessing their expectations, discomfort during treatment, and final satisfaction after completion of the dental movements, in order to serve as a guideline for orthodontists during planning and executing their clinical treatment focusing on the satisfaction of their patients, minimizing their discomfort, and establishing special procedure protocols for such patients.

MATERIAL AND METHODS

The material used in the present study was a set of 54 questionnaires given to adult patients, most of them residents in the city of Goiânia/GO (Brazil), who had received orthodontic treatment from dentists specialized in orthodontics living in that same city. Among the selected patients, 12 had completed their treatment at the Orthodontics Specialization Program Clinic at the ABO-GO and 42 had been treated in private practices of orthodontists registered in the Regional Dental Council (CRO) as specialists.

The patients were selected according to the following inclusion criteria: 1 – completion of orthodontic treatment; 2 – Submitted to only one corrective orthodontic treatment; 3 – Treatment initiated after reaching the age of 20 years; 4 – Orthodontic treatment did not involve orthognathic surgical procedures; 5 – Absence of any health problem that could influence in the orthodontic treatment.

Once selected, the patients were contacted by phone and were motivated to come either to the Orthodontics Specialization Program Clinic at the ABO-GO (patients who had been treated at that institution) or to the private practice of their respective orthodontists.

Concerning gender, 40 female patients and 14 male patients were evaluated (Fig 1).

The age which the patients started treatment ranged from 20 up to 61 years old, being that 29 of them started treatment in their second decade of life, 12 in their third decade of life, 07 in their fourth, and 06 after being 50 years old (Fig 2).

At the moment each patient arrived to the practice, they were given the Informed Consent and after signing it, they all answered a questionnaire with 9 objective questions concerning the topic that was being investigating. The questions were tailored so that they could answer them fast and objectively, and some blank space was given so that they could include personal considerations.

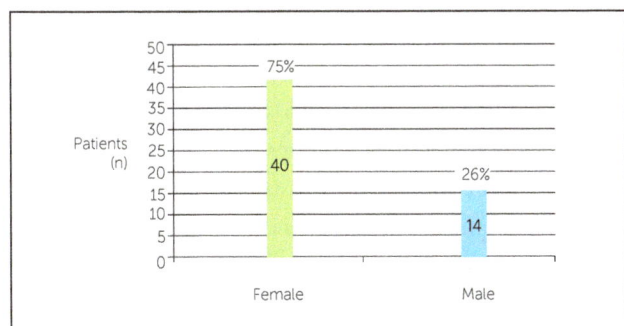

Figure 1 - Distribution of the sample by gender.

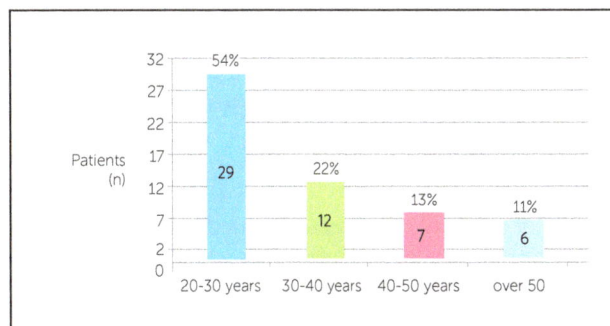

Figure 2 - Distribution of the sample according to the age at the beginning of the performed orthodontic treatment.

The data contained in the questionnaires were classified and transformed into tables and descriptive statistics were made.

RESULTS
Assessment of the answers to the questionnaire.

When the patients were asked about the reason for them to seek treatment only when adults, the answers were: 31% for a previous lack of financial means; 30% were not previously bothered with the position of their teeth; 14% looked for treatment after being told (insistently) by their general dentists; 9% said they didn't know orthodontics could solve their dental problems; 2% believed orthodontic treatment was only suitable for teenagers and children, and 14% mentioned other reasons, and among these we found: The wish and the need of a better facial look, the need of preparation for dental implants, speech therapist recommendation, and TMJ discomfort (Fig 3).

Trying to assess the perception of malocclusion, before the beginning of orthodontic treatment, the patients informed that the aspects that were most annoying them were: The poor appearance of the smile, 36 patients (61%); 09 patients pointed to problems with chewing (15.2%); 08 patients pointed to the empty spaces due to tooth loss (13.5%); 04 pointed to periodontal problems (inflammation, tooth mobility) corresponding to 6.7% of the answers; and 02 pointed to difficulty in speaking (3.3%), being that 05 out of the 54 patients marked 2 answers to this question (Table 1).

When answering about the reasons for rejecting the initial indication to undergo orthodontic care, the answers were: 55.3% felt concerned with the perspective of the long duration of treatment; 17.8% had doubts about the true efficiency of orthodontic intervention; 12.5% were afraid of feeling pain during treatment; 10.7% rejected the unpleasant appearance of braces; and 3.5% said they had never rejected the idea of undergoing an orthodontic treatment (Table 2).

In relation to the reasons which led the patients to make the choice for receiving orthodontic treatment it was found that: 35.5% said about the suggestion of a general dentist; 27.1% already wanted to undergo treatment; 22% made up their minds after talking to an orthodontist; 11.8% told they were influenced by the opinion of their relatives and friends; and 3.3% mentioned different reasons, such as the opportunity to

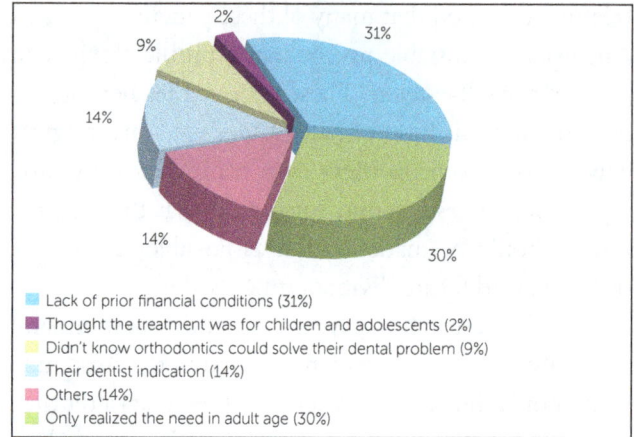

Figure 3 - Reasons that led patients to seek orthodontic treatment only in adult age.

avoid a possible orthognathic surgery and the wish to receive dental implants afterwards. The data referring to the previous question are available on Table 3, and each patient could check more than one answer.

Regarding the discomforts experienced throughout treatment, 22 patients complained of pain after activation appointments (40%); 13 complained about the long time of active treatment (23.6%); 09 patients (16.3% from the total) claimed they hadn't felt any discomfort during orthodontic treatment; 06 pointed to difficulties in dental hygiene and flossing, associated with wounds on their inner cheeks, as the main reason for discomfort (10.9%); 03 people were concerned about the unpleasant look of their braces (5.4%); 01 patient complained about periodontal inflammations linked to the treatment (1.8%); 1 complaint about recurrent aphthous lesions during treatment, and none felt embarrassed about being among much younger patients at the orthodontic practice environment (Table 4).

The most important positive change observed by patients after treatment conclusion was: The improvement of facial appearance for 39 patients (72.2%); 13 noticed changes in their chewing and/or speaking pattern (24%); 07 reported improvements in their periodontal conditions along with a better implantation of their teeth (12.9%); 01 patient checked all the answers above and 08 checked two answers (Table 5).

When comparing the actual results obtained with the pre-treatment expectations: 50% considered the obtained results to be better than what they had expected; for 46.2% the results were similar to what they had expected; 3.7% considered that their expectations

Table 1 - Patients perception of their smile, prior to orthodontic treatment.

Before the treatment, what was your chief complaint about your teeth?	
Bad esthetics	36
Mastication problems	09
Edentulous space (closed during treatment)	08
Gingival problems (inflammations, tooth mobility)	04
Speaking problems	02
Number of patients that checked two answers	05

Table 2 - Reasons most mentioned for initial rejection of the treatment suggested.

What was bothering the most in the orthodontic treatment idea?	
Long duration	31
Doubts on the treatment efficiency	10
Fear of feeling pain	07
Unaesthetic aspect of the appliance	06
Nothing	02
Number of patients that checked two answers	05

Table 3 - Determining factor in deciding for starting the treatment.

What made you start the orthodontic treatment?	
Dentist orientation	21
You wanted already to receive the treatment	16
Chat with the orthodontist	13
Opinion and support from family, spouse and friends	07
Others (avoid orthognathic surgery, implants need)	02

Table 4 - Main discomfort brought by the treatment.

During treatment, what most displeased you?	
Pain during and after activation sessions	22
Found the treatment too long	13
Nothing	09
Difficulty in cleaning and wounds in the mucosa.	07
Felt embarrassed with the appearance with appliance	03
Gingiva inflammation	01
Recurrent ulcer	01
Embarrassment in contact with children and adolescents	00

Table 5 - Subjective perception of patients front orthodontic treatment results.

After treatment, which motivation did you noticed more?	
More beautiful smile (facial esthetic improvement)	39
Speech and mastication pattern improvement	13
Gingival and tooth implantation condition improvement	07
Others	04

Note: A patient marked all the answers and eight others marked two answers.

before treatment were fairly achieved; and none of them considered the treatment results to be inferior to their initial expectations.

In a question aiming to know if they would undergo orthodontic treatment again, it was concluded that 100% of patients did not regret undergoing it, and all of them said they would, based on their personal experience, encourage other adults to go through orthodontic treatment if necessary

DISCUSSION

This study consisted in the subjective evaluation of 54 adult patients in the fixed retention stage. The predominance of female patients (74%) is consistent with data found in previous studies that suggested that women have a greater motivation to undergo orthodontic treatment when compared to men.

As seen in the results, when questioned about the reasons that led them to look for orthodontic assistance for the first time when in a more advanced age, the most common answers were the following in order of importance: 31.5% showed a previous lack of financial means; 29.8% reported that the awareness of the need for orthodontic treatment only raised at adult age. The high relevance of treatment costs seen in this local sample shows that this specific population has serious financial constraints, which sometimes may prevent them from gaining access to better health and well-being conditions.

When assessing the chief concern of adult patients who sought late orthodontic treatment, it is clear that most of the patients had esthetic reasons (61%). This data corroborates with previous studies that show that the great majority of patients seek treatment to improve their smile esthetics and their facial esthetics.[2,8]

A previous study also evaluated the reasons that led some adult patients to initially reject the indication for orthodontic treatment and found the following reasons, in relevance order: Long duration of the proposed treatment; discomfort caused by the braces, rejection to the anti-esthetic look of brackets, fear of pain, and the fear of disappointment with the final results.[7] When comparing the results achieved in this research with those of the one mentioned above, it is possible to observe in general, that patients showed similar doubts and concerns.

Among the factors indicated as determinant for the beginning of treatment were: A previous will to undergo it (27.1% of the patients), which shows a good acceptance of adults when confronted with the indication for orthodontic treatment; 22% decided only after consulting with an orthodontist, which also highlights the importance of a good professional/patient relationship, and 11.8% made the decision influenced by spouses, friends and relatives.

In relation to the main discomforts experienced throughout the active treatment, the majority of patients complained about pain during treatment and immediately after the activation sessions (40%); some complained about the long period of treatment (23.6%); and 16.3% said they did not feel any discomfort or constraint. In previous studies, patients highlighted discomfort as the worst aspect of orthodontic treatment, although classifying this discomfort as mild and short lasting (with a duration average of 2 days after clinical activation of the appliances). In these same studies, orientation on the controlled use of painkillers and restriction in the ingestion of hard foods on the days following the activations were enough to significantly minimize the aforementioned discomfort.[2,3]

In a research made in 1981, all adult patients assessed, who were undergoing orthodontic care, considered the treatment advantageous despite the discomfort related to treatment; they did not regret having started it, and would suggest it to others who were in doubt about the cost-benefit ratio of orthodontic treatment.[13] Other authors also found high level of satisfaction in patients when faced with the results achieved through the orthodontic treatment performed.[3] These informations were also confirmed by the present study.

When evaluating the level of satisfaction of patients after treatment, it should be kept in mind that the analysis made by patients are based on subjective aspects and not technical ones, thus being under influence of different agents, such as, the kind of professional/patient relationship and variables such as gender. Another research in 2005 concluded that the most important aspect to affect the level of satisfaction of patients is not the final quality of the treatment done, but a good relationship between the patient and his orthodontist. According to that same research, women were more critical regarding treatment results, although in previous studies mentioned by these authors, men had shown to be more demanding and critical about the results of orthodontic treatment.

CONCLUSION

When assessing the characteristics of adult individuals that underwent orthodontic treatment, it was found that this group is mainly constituted by women, between 20 and 30 years old (53%) who were not satisfied, mainly, with their smile esthetics (61%).

When patients were asked about the reason for not seeking orthodontic treatment earlier, the great majority answered that they did not have financial conditions, or did not feel inconvenienced by the malocclusion they had. Unfortunately, the lack of economical conditions proved, at least in this set of Brazilian patients, to be a major restraint for them, having prevented their previous access to the facial and smile esthetics improvements they were longing for.

Individual clinical planning and clarity in procedures, previously discussed with patients, can minimize the main reasons for initial rejection from patients when faced with orthodontic treatment, which were: Aversion to the long duration of treatment (55.3%), doubts about the efficiency of treatment (17.8%), fear of pain (12.5%), and discomfort with the esthetical aspect of fixed braces (10.7%). A good relationship between the orthodontist, the general practitioner and other professionals involved with the patient, along with a clear and careful initial appointment can be considered decisive in making adult patients fell safe to effectively start orthodontic treatment.

Once the treatment is initiated, the information gathered suggests that orthodontists should be aware about reducing the discomfort felt during and after appliance activation appointments, which was a reason of complaint in 40% of the people interviewed; also to instruct their patients on dental hygiene techniques, and to elaborate a simplified treatment plan to reduce, according to the possibilities, the total treatment time (regarded as uncomfortably long for 23.6% of patients).

At last, when assessing patients already in retention, a high level of satisfaction was found for patients interviewed with regard to the final treatment results. This only shows that once patients are aware and clarified about the peculiar limitations of each clinical case, and when a trusting relationship between the patient and their orthodontist is established, adults are excellent candidates for orthodontic treatment.

Assessment of motivation, expectations and satisfaction of adult patients submitted to orthodontic...

157

REFERENCES

1. Bos A, Vosselman N, Hoogstraten J, Prahl-Andersen B. Patient compliance: a determinant of patient satisfaction? Angle Orthod. 2005;75(4):526-31.

2. Breece GL, Nieberg LG. Motivation for adult orthodontic treatment. J Clin Orthod. 1986;20(3):166-71.

3. Buttke TM, Proffit WR. Referring adult patients for orthodontic treatment. J Am Dent Assoc. 1999 Jan;130(1):73-9.

4. Capelloza Filho L, Braga SA, Cavassan AO, Ozawa TO. Tratamento ortodôntico em adultos: uma abordagem direcionada. Rev Dental Press Ortod Ortop Facial. 2001;6(5):63-80.

5. Carvalho KV, Miguel JAM, Carlini MG. Satisfação dos pacientes submetidos a tratamento ortocirúrgico. Ortod Gaúch. 2001;5(1):49-56.

6. Khan RS, Horrocks EN. A study of adult orthodontic patients and their treatment. Br J Orthod. 1990;18(3):183-94.

7. Langlade M. Terapêutica ortodôntica. 3ª ed. São Paulo: Ed. Santos; 2003. 844 p.

8. McKiernan EX, McKiernan F, Jones ML. Psychological profiles and motives of adults seeking orthodontic treatment. Int J Adult Orthodon Orthognath Surg. 1992;7(3):187-98.

9. Moyers RE. Ortodontia. 4ª ed. Rio de Janeiro: Guanabara Koogan; 1999. 482 p.

10. Nattrass C, Sandy JR. Adult orthodontics: a review. Br J Orthod. 1995;22(4):331-7.

11. Proffit WR, Fields WH. Ortodontia contemporânea. 2ª ed. Rio de Janeiro: Guanabara Koogan; 1995.

12. Proffit WR, Fields HW Jr, Moray LJ. Prevalence of malocclusion and orthodontic treatment need in the United States. Estimates from the NHANES III survey. Int J Adult Orthodon Orthognath Surg. 1998;13(2):97-106.

13. Tayer BH, Burek MJ. A survey of adult's attitudes toward orthodontic therapy. Am J Orthod. 1981;79(3):305-15.

14. Varela M, García-Camba JE. Impact of orthodontics on the psychologic profile of adult patients: a prospective study. Am J Orthod Dentofacial Orthop. 1995;108(2):142-8.

23

Flexural strength of mini-implants developed for Herbst appliance skeletal anchorage: A study in Minipigs br1 cadavers

Klaus Barretto Lopes[1], Gladys Cristina Dominguez[2], Caio Biasi[3], Jesualdo Luiz Rossi[4]

Objective: The present study was designed to verify if mini-implant prototypes (MIP) developed for Herbst appliance anchorage are capable of withstanding orthopedic forces, and to determine whether the flexural strength of these MIP varies depending on the site of insertion (maxilla and mandible). **Methods:** Thirteen MIP were inserted in three minipig cadavers (six in the maxilla and seven in the mandible). The specimens were prepared and submitted to mechanical testing. The mean and standard deviation were calculated for each region. A two-way Student's t test was used to compare the strength between the sites. A one-way Student's t test was performed to test the hypothesis. Orthopedic forces above 1.0 kgf were considered. **Results:** The MIP supported flexural strength higher than 1.0 kgf (13.8 ± 2.3 Kg, in the posterior region of the maxilla and 20.5 ± 5.2 Kg in the anterior region of the mandible) with a significantly lower flexural strength in the anterior region of the mandible (P < 0.05). **Conclusion:** The MIP are capable of withstanding orthopedic forces, and are more resistant in the anterior region of the mandible than in the posterior region of the maxilla in Minipigs br1 cadavers.

Keywords: Functional appliances. Dental implants. Orthodontic appliances. Orthodontic anchorage procedures. Angle Class II malocclusion.

[1] Postdoc in Orthodontics, State University of Rio de Janeiro (UERJ).
[2] Full professor, Department of Orthodontics, College of Dentistry, University of São Paulo (USP).
[3] PhD Resident, Veterinary Medicine, University of São Paulo (USP).
[4] Postdoc in Materials Science and Engineering, University of Surrey.

» The author Klaus Barretto Lopes asserts to be the developer and patent holder of the mini-implant prototypes used in this study.

Klaus Barretto Lopes
Rua Visconde de Pirajá, 550/1407 – Ipanema
Rio de Janeiro/RJ — Brazil — CEP: 22.410-002
E-mail: klausbarretto@uol.com.br

INTRODUCTION

Implants and mini-implants have been used as orthodontic anchorages for different purposes in different locations.[1,2,3] Some researchers have suggested the use of mini-implants as orthopedic anchors in animals[4,5] and in the treatment of Class III malocclusions with retrusive maxillae in humans.[6] However, there is little information about the use of mini-implants as orthopedic anchorage in the treatment of Class II malocclusions.

The Herbst appliance has often been used in the treatment of Class II malocclusions, because of its efficiency[7] and also because of positive effects in orthodontic and orthopedic correction.[8] Nevertheless, some investigators have stated that the correction of Class II malocclusion is a result of anchorage loss, and could be responsible for negative effects, such as protrusion and gingival recession,[9] on lower incisors.

Many attempts have been made to reduce the negative effects caused by the Herbst appliance on lower incisors, such as increasing the number of teeth in the mandibular anchorage, using soft-tissue anchorage, splints, and cast splints anchorage.[10,11] However, these attempts were unsuccessful.

With the intention of solving these problems, a mini-implant prototype was developed for Herbst appliance anchorage, and its flexural resistance was measured in an *in vitro* study.[12]. However, a question arose with respect to the resistance strength of this mini-implant prototype when inserted into the bone. The present study was designed to evaluate if the mini-implant prototype developed for Herbst appliance anchorage is capable of withstanding orthopedic forces in Minipigs br1, and to compare the prototype resistance between the sites of insertion.

MATERIAL AND METHODS

Thirteen mini-implants (Neodent, Curitiba, Brazil), 2 mm in diameter and 10 mm in length, with attachment to Herbst appliance telescopic tubes, were inserted in three Minipigs br1[13,14] (15-month old) after they had been euthanized.

A calculation of the sample size[15] was carried out by means of two pilot studies, one for the posterior region of the maxilla and another for the anterior region of the mandible of one minipig.

Based on the performance of the specimens on the graph, the sample size was calculated with the values ob-

tained with a dislocation of 1.2 mm, because after this point the strength values increased abruptly, indicating the resistance of the metal block.

Afterwards, the following statistical formula was used:

$$n= \frac{(Z \times Cv)^2}{Er^2}$$

Where n = number of specimens, Z = Standard deviation from normal distribution, Cv = Coefficient of variation, and Er = Relative error.

After sample size calculation, the number of specimens needed for the final study was 6 in the maxilla and 7 in the mandible.

In order to test sample normality, the Kolmogorov-Smirnov test was carried out. To test the hypothesis, a one-way Student's t test was performed with Minitab 15 (State College, PA, USA). Orthopedic forces above 1 Kgf were considered.[16,17]

Thereafter, the hypotheses of withstanding orthopedic forces were defined (H0: $\mu = 1.0$ and H1: $\mu > 1.0$).

The criterion to reject the null hypothesis was:

tcal > tα, n - 1,

where α =0.05 or calculated:

t > t from t table.

To compare the flexural strength between the posterior region of the maxilla and the anterior region of the mandible, a two-way Student's t test was calculated using Minitab 15.

Experiment

The animals were euthanized before the experiment and frozen at a temperature of - 20°C.

Two minipigs received four mini-implants (two in each maxilla and two in each mandible), and one minipig received five mini-implants (two in the maxilla and three in the mandible).

Six specimens with the new mini-implant were obtained from the posterior region of the maxilla, and seven specimens were obtained from the anterior region of the mandible, which were the possible places where the mini-implants could be used to anchor the Herbst appliance.

After that, the straight telescopic tube was placed in the head of the mini-implant with a suitable screw (Fig 1).

To create a guide for the mini-implant, a drill with torque control with a 1.3 mm diameter bur (Neodent, Curitiba, Brazil) was used. The insertion sites were in the posterior region of the maxilla, between the roots of the upper first molar and the anterior region of the mandible, between the roots of the second premolar and the roots of the third premolar.

To insert the mini-implant, a torque key with a torque meter calibrated at a measure not greater than 30 Kgf.cm was used. When the insertion was completed, new radiographs were taken to check the final positioning of the mini-implants.

To prepare the specimens, the maxilla and the mandible were sectioned into small pieces, using an electric cutting machine. Metal blocks were used to protect the specimens during the experiment. Afterwards, an acrylic resin was used to fix the bone fragments with the mini-implants (Fig 2).

The specimens were placed in an Instron 4400R test machine (Instron, Norwood, MO, USA), with the metal block in the lower part and the telescopic tube in the upper part (Fig 3).

The specimens were submitted to a single cantilever flexure test. Traction was applied at 0.5 mm per minute until 1.5 mm of dislocation was obtained. This value was based on a pilot study carried out by Brettin et al.[18] The values were recorded, and a graph of strength x dislocation was constructed.

RESULTS

Single cantilever flexure tests were successfully carried out on 13 specimens. The graphs illustrate the performance of the specimens during the tests in the maxilla and the mandible (Figs 4 and 5). The mini-implant prototypes showed a flexural strength of 13.86 ± 2.30 Kgf for the posterior region of the maxilla, and 20.5 ± 5.20 Kgf for the anterior region of the mandible.

The normality of the two samples was confirmed with the Kolmogorov-Smirnov test.

For the hypothesis test, the calculated t was 13.71 (P< 0.001) for the posterior region of the maxilla. The critical t obtained from the table was 2.015. The criterion used to reject the null hypothesis revealed that:

tcal > tα, *n-1*, where α = 0.05 → 13.71 > 2.015

Therefore, the value calculated for t for the posterior region of the maxilla is outside the region of H_0 acceptance. The null hypothesis was rejected, and the hypothesis that mini-implants cannot withstand orthopedic forces could not be confirmed for the posterior region of the maxilla.

Using the same criterion for the anterior region of the mandible, the calculated t was 9.94 (P < 0.001). The critical t obtained from the table was 1.943.

The criterion used to reject the null hypothesis revealed that:

tcal > tα, *n-1*, where α = 0.05 → 9.94 > 1.943

Similarly to the maxilla, the value calculated for t is outside the region of H_0 acceptance. The null hypothesis was rejected, and the hypothesis that mini-implants cannot withstand orthopedic forces could not be confirmed for the anterior region of the mandible.

A statistically significant difference was found in the flexural strength between the posterior region of the maxilla and the anterior region of the mandible (P = 0.015): the anterior region of the mandible was significantly more resistant.

DISCUSSION

One of the purposes of this study was to quantify the flexural resistance of the mini-implant prototypes when inserted in the posterior region of the

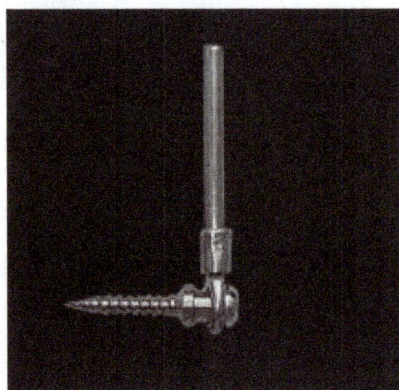

Figure 1 - Straight telescopic tube placed in the head of the mini-implant with a suitable screw.

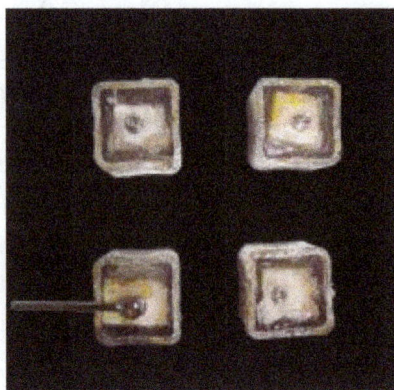

Figure 2 - Bone fragments with mini-implants inserted which were included in the metal block.

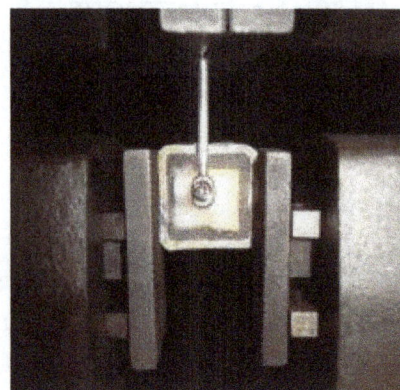

Figure 3 - Specimen ready for flexure test.

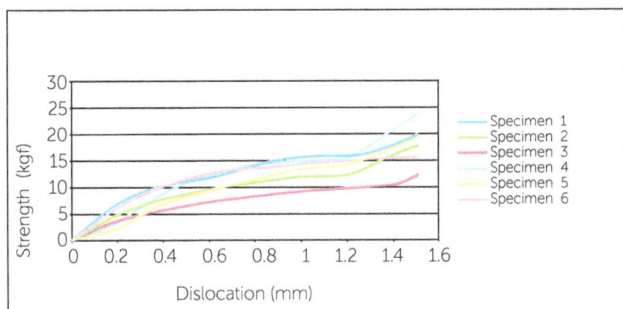

Figure 4 - Graph of strength x dislocation of six specimens tested in the posterior region of the maxilla.

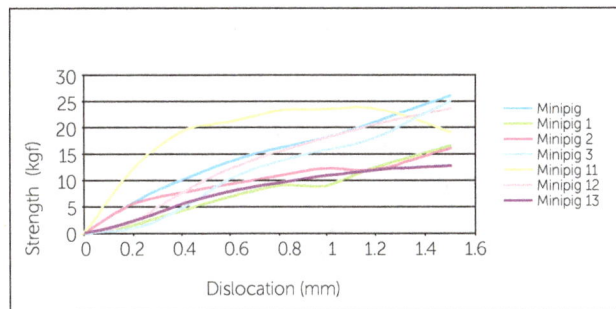

Figure 5 - Graph of strength x dislocation of the seven specimens tested in the anterior region of the mandible.

maxilla and the anterior region of the mandible. Although studies involving extrapolations from animals to humans should be viewed with caution, the authors' intention was to assess the strength that the mini-implant prototypes could withstand in specific regions in a Minipig br1. The mini-implant prototype showed a flexural strength of 13.86 ± 23.0 Kgf for the posterior region of the maxilla, and 20.55 ± 5.20 Kgf for the anterior region of the mandible. Another purpose of this study was to test the hypothesis that mini-implant prototypes are not capable of withstanding orthopedic forces. The hypothesis was rejected.

Miyawaki et al[3] reported that the success rate of mini-implants with a 1.0-mm diameter was significantly lower than that of other mini-implants with 1.5-mm or 2.3-mm diameters. This author suggested the use of mini-implants with a 1.5-mm diameter for patients with average-to-low mandibular plane angle, and a 2.3-mm diameter for patients with a high mandibular plane angle (i.e., with a thin cortical bone). Miyawaki et al[3] did not find a significant association between the success rate and the mini-implant length. However, Brettin et al[18] concluded that bicortical mini-implants provide superior anchorage resistance, reduced cortical bone stress, and superior stability when compared with monocortical mini-implants. Also, according to Barros et al[19] increases in mini-implant diameters significantly influenced the increases in placement torque and fracture torque on quantities that progressively reduced the fracture risk. Therefore, in order to increase the resistance of the mini-implant prototype, the diameter was increased to 2.0 mm and the length to 10 mm, so as to achieve bicortical anchorage.

It could be argued that the 2.0-mm diameter mini-implant is too large for the inter-radicular space. However, Poggio et al.[20] showed that, in humans, this size is compatible with the inter-radicular distance between the upper first molars and second premolars and between the lower cuspids and the first premolars (3 mm when the distance from the alveolar crest is 8 mm). This is the location suggested for the insertion of the mini-implant prototypes for the Herbst appliance anchorage.

Two pilot studies were performed before the experiment to test the researchers' abilities and to calculate the sample size.[15] The number of specimens was calculated in order to obtain scientific validation with the fewest possible specimens and animals.

In the present study, the mini-implant prototypes were inserted after the animals had been euthanized. Huja et al[21] explained that no healing period or adaptive response could occur, and resistance strength was an indication of primary stability. Therefore, the values found in the present study are similar to the experiments of immediate loading after placement. Some studies have evaluated bone contact according to the healing period, recommending immediate loading after placement.[1,22,23]

Storage conditions of the specimens used in the study have been associated with differences in pull-out strengths during mechanical traction testing. Simonian et al[24] found lower pull-out strengths in frozen specimens. However, Roe et al[25] reported no significant difference when the test was performed no later than one week after storage at - 20° C. Therefore, to avoid any influence of storage conditions on the results, the specimens used in this study were prepared on the same day or on the day after insertion of mini-implants, frozen at - 20° C and tested between one and seven days after mini-implant insertion.

A single cantilever flexure test was performed instead of a shear force test and traction test, because there was a distance of 4 mm between the block base and the point of force application. In a shear force test, the point of force application should be parallel to the block base. A traction test would not reproduce the perpendicular strength received by the mini-implant when used as an anchorage for the Herbst appliance.

Brettin et al[18] also performed a cantilever flexure tests, but in human cadavers. They found lower values than those of the present study (20.55 kgf for bicortical mandibular mini-implants and 13.86 kgf for monocortical maxillary mini-implants in Minipigs, against 11.0 kgf for bicortical mandibular mini-implants and 9.0 kgf for bicortical maxillary mini-implants, 5.0 kgf for monocortical maxillary mini-implants and 7.0 kgf for monocortical mandibular mini-implants in human cadavers). This difference may be related to the larger diameter of the mini-implants used in the Minipigs (2.0 mm in the Minipigs against 1.6 mm in the human cadavers) or increased cortical bone thickness in the Minipigs.

The cantilever test is a static test. Probably, if dynamic forces had been applied to the mini-implants, different results would have been obtained. Future *in vivo* studies using the Herbst appliance anchored in bone will answer this question.

According to Huja et al[21] some possible problems were related to cantilever tests, namely: standardization, reproducibility, bone flexure and collision of the mini-implants with adjacent root of the tooth. These problems could negatively influence accuracy of results regarding the flexural strength of the mini-implants. In this research, these possible problems were avoided, because the flexural strength of the mini-implants was obtained following the experiment performed by Brettin et al[18] in which the mini-implants were tested with dislocation of 1.5 mm. Those authors performed a pilot study in cadavers in which they concluded that the mini-implants could present mobility with dislocation above 1.5 mm.

To test the hypothesis, orthopedic forces above 1.0 kgf were considered. This value is very common in Orthodontics, in clinical work and research,

because of the headgear which functions with 500 g per side.[16,17] Other studies showed the use of orthopedic forces (from 500 to 800 g) on implants[4,5,6] and a few focused on the use of orthopedic forces in mini-implants, such as the study by Büchter et al[26] who found that mini-implants resisted up to 900 g without mobility.

The flexural strength differed significantly between the posterior region of the maxilla and the anterior region of the mandible. However, this result may have been influenced by the fact that the mini-implants fixed in the mandible had bicortical anchorage while those fixed in the maxilla apparently did not have this anchorage. Probably, the distance between the cortical bones in the maxilla in the posterior region was greater than 6 mm or the cortical-lingual was not accessible due to the palate being too low. Because the mini-implant was 10 mm long, the active part was only 6 mm. This suggests that in future studies the mini-implants should be constructed according to the distance between the cortical bone, as Brettin et al[18] did with human cadavers.

Other forces that could affect the resistance of the mini-implant prototypes could be those originating from muscles and soft tissues of the face, due to mandibular advancement caused by functional appliances. However, earlier studies[27,28] showed that the forces delivered to the teeth by functional appliances were of low intensity (80 and 160 gf).

The question that arises is whether to use mastication forces as a parameter rather than the orthopedic forces. According to Pancherz and Anehus-Pancherz[29], there is no contact in the posterior teeth after the installation of the Herbst appliance. The contact occurs only in the anterior teeth. This is responsible for the decrease in mastication efficiency as well as in temporal and masseter muscle activity in the first three months of treatment. After that, the authors observed an increase in the mastication forces during six months of treatment.

The forces transmitted to the teeth when using the Herbst appliance are probably the best parameter. However, it was not possible to locate studies with the data that is necessary to carry out a statistical analysis, and the force transmitted to the mini-implants in the skeletal anchorage of the Herbst appliance remains unknown.

Thus, *in vivo* and clinical studies are necessary to assess the possibility of using the Herbst appliance skeletal anchorage in humans.

CONCLUSION

The mini-implant prototypes developed for Herbst appliance skeletal anchorage are capable of withstanding orthopedic forces in Minipigs br1 cadavers. The prototypes are more resistant in the anterior region of the mandible than in the posterior region of the maxilla.

REFERENCES

1. Deguchi T, Takano-Yamamoto T, Kanomi R, Hartsfield JK, Roberts WE, Garetto LP. The use of small titanium screws for orthodontic anchorage. J Dent Res. 2003;82(5):377-81.

2. Kanomi R. Mini-implant for orthodontic anchorage. J Clin Orthod. 1997;(31):763-7.

3. Miyawaki S, Koyama I, Inoue M, Mishima K, Sugahara T, Takano-Yamamoto T. Factors associated with the stability of titanium screws placed in the posterior region for orthodontic anchorage. Am J Orthod Dentofacial Orthop. 2003;124(4):373-8.

4. De Pauw GA, Dermaut L, De Bruyn H, Johansson C. Stability of implants as anchorage for orthopedic traction. Angle Orthod. 1999;69(5):401-7.

5. Smalley WM, Shapiro PA, Hohl TH, Kokich VG, Bränemark PI. Osseointegrated titanium implants for maxillofacial protraction in monkeys. Am J Orthod Dentofacial Orthop. 1988;94(4):285-95.

6. Enacar A, Giray B, Pehlivanoglu, M, Iplikcioglu H. Facemask therapy with rigid anchorage in a patient with maxillary hypoplasia and severe oligodontia. Am J Orthod Dentofacial Orthop. 2003;123(5):571-7.

7. Bremen JV, Pancherz H. Efficiency of Class II division 1 and Class II division 2 treatment in relation to different treatment approaches. Semin Orthod. 2003;(9):87-92.

8. Franchi L, Baccetti T, McNamara J. Treatment and posttreatment effects of acrylic splint Herbst appliance therapy. Am J Orthod Dentofacial Orthop. 1999;115(4):429-38.

9. Yared KF, Senobio EG, Pacheco W. Periodontal status of mandibular central incisors after orthodontic proclination in adults. Am J Orthod Dentofacial Orthop. 2006;130(1):6.e1-8.

10. El-Fateh T, Ruf S. Herbst treatment with mandibular cast splints-revisited. Am J Orthod Dentofacial Orthop. 2011;81(5):820-7.

11. Weschler D, Pancherz H. Efficiency of three mandibular anchorage forms in Herbst treatment: a cephalometric investigation. Angle Orthod. 2005;75(1):23-7.

12. Barretto-Lopes K, Dominguez G, Tortamano A, Rossi JL, Vigorito JW. Avaliação in vitro da resistência à flexão de um protótipo de mini-implante desenvolvido para ancoragem do aparelho de Herbst. Dental Press J Orthod. 2010;15(4):38e1-6. Disponível em: http://www.scielo.br/pdf/dpjo/v15n4/06.pdf.

13. Mariano M. Minisuíno (minipig) na pesquisa biomédica experimental. O Minipig br1. Acta Cir Bras. 2003;18(5):387-91.

14. Oltramari PVP, Navarro RL, Henriques JFC, Capelozza ALA, Granjeiro JM. Dental and skeletal characterization of the BR-1 minipig. Vet J. 2007;173(2):399-407.

15. Aguilar-Nascimento JE. Fundamental steps in experimental design for animal studies. Acta Cir Bras. 2005;20(1):2-8.

16. Tanne K, Matsubara S. Association between the direction of orthopedic headgear force and sutural responses in the nasomaxillary complex. Angle Orthod. 1996;66(2):125-30.

17. Almeida-Pedrin RR, Henriques JFC, Almeida RR, Almeida MR, McNamara JA. Effects of the pendulum appliance, cervical headgear, and 2 premolar extractions followed by fixed appliances in patients with Class II malocclusion. Am J Orthod Dentofacial Orthop. 2009;136(6):833-42.

18. Brettin BT, Grosland NM, Qian F, Southard KA, Stuntz TD, Morgan TA, et al. Bicortical vs monocortical orthodontic skeletal anchorage. Am J Orthod Dentofacial Orthop. 2008;134(5):625-35.

19. Barros SE, Janson G, Chiqueto K, Garib DG, Janson M. Effect of mini-implant diameter on fracture risk and self-drilling efficacy. Am J Orthod Dentofacial Orthop. 2011;140(4):e181-92.

20. Poggio PM, Incorvati C, Velo S, Carano A. "Safe zones": A guide for miniscrew positioning in the maxillary and mandibular arch. Angle Orthod. 2006;76(2):191-7.

21. Huja SS, Litsky AS, Beck FM, Johnson KA, Larsen PE. Pull-out strength of monocortical screws placed in the maxillae and mandibles of dogs. Am J Orthod Dentofacial Orthop. 2005;127(3):307-13.

22. Huja SS, Rao J, Struckhoff JA, Beck FM, Litsky AS. Biomechanical and histomorphometric analyses of monocortical screws at placement and 6 weeks postinsertion. J Oral Implantol. 2006:32(3):110-6.

23. Salmória KK, Tanaka OM, Guariza-Filho O, Camargo ES, Souza LT, Maruo H. Insertional torque and axial pull-out strength of mini-implants in mandibles of dogs. Am J Orthod Dentofacial Orthop. 2008;133(6):790.e15-22.

24. Simonian PT, Conrad EU, Chapman JR, Harrington RM, Chansky HA. Effect of sterilization and storage treatments on screw pullout strength in human allgraft bone. Clin Orthop Relat Res. 1994:302:290-6.

25. Roe SC, Pijanowski GJ, Johnson AL. Biomechanical properties of canine cortical bone allografts: effects of preparation and storage. Am J Vet Res. 1988:49:6:873-7.

26. Büchter A, Wiechmann D, Gaertner C, Hendrik M, Vogeler M, Wiesmann HP, et al. Load-related bone modelling at the interface of orthodontic micro-implants. Clin Oral Implants Res. 2006;17(6):714-22.

27. Noro T, Tanne K, Sakuda M. Orthodontic forces exerted by activators with varying construction bite heights. Am J Orthod Dentofacial Orthop. 1994;105(2):169-79.

28. Katsavrias EG, Halazonetis DJ. Intermaxillary forces during activator treatment. Am J Orthod Dentofacial Orthop. 1999;115(2):133-7.

29. Pancherz H, Anehus-Pancherz M. The effect of continuous bite jumping with the Herbst appliance on the masticatory system: a functional analysis of treated Class II malocclusions. Eur J Orthod. 1982;4(1):37-44.

24

Comparison of arch forms between Turkish and North American

Ahmet A. Celebi[1], Hakan Keklik[2], Enes Tan[3], Faruk I. Ucar[4]

Objective: The aim of this study was to clarify the morphological differences in the mandibular arches of Turkish and North American white subjects. **Methods:** The sample included 132 Turkish (34 Class I, 58 Class II, and 40 Class III) and 160 North American (60 Class I, 50 Class II, and 50 Class III) subjects. The most facial portion of 13 proximal contact areas was digitized from photocopied images of patients' mandibular dental arches. Clinical bracket points were calculated for each tooth based on mandibular tooth thickness data. Four linear and two proportional measurements were taken. The subjects were grouped according to arch form types (tapered, ovoid and square) in order to have frequency distribution compared between ethnic groups in each Angle classification. **Results:** The Turkish group showed significantly lower molar depth and more significant molar width-depth (W/D) ratio in all three Angle classifications. On the other hand, the Turkish group also showed a significantly larger intercanine width in Class III malocclusion and intermolar width in Class II malocclusion. The most frequent arch forms seen were the ovoid arch form in the Turkish group and the tapered form in the white group. **Conclusions:** Our results demonstrate that when treating Turkish patients, one should expect to use preformed ovoid arch form orthodontic wires in a significant percentage of patients.

Keywords: Dental arch. Dental model. Ethnic groups. Malocclusion.

[1] Assistant professor, Zirve University, Department of Orthodontics, School of Dentistry, Gaziantep, Turkey.

[2] Postgraduate student, Kirikkale University, Department of Orthodontics, School of Dentistry, Kirikkale, Turkey.

[3] Assistant professor, Kirikkale University, Department of Orthodontics, School of Dentistry, Kirikkale, Turkey.

[4] Assistant professor, Selcuk University, Department of Orthodontics, School of Dentistry, Konya, Turkey.

» The authors report no commercial, proprietary or financial interest in the products or companies described in this article.

Enes Tan
E-mail: dentistan@yahoo.com

INTRODUCTION

The dental arch, fundamental principle in orthodontic planning and therapy, is an important element in Orthodontics.[1] Therefore, correct identification of a patient's arch form is a crucial parameter in achieving a stable, functional and esthetic orthodontic treatment result, since failure to preserve the arch form might increase the probability of relapse.[2,3]

Over the years, human dental arch form has been recognized to be variable in shape and size. It is described by many authors in geometric forms (ellipse, parabolic curve and hyperbolic) and mathematical functions.[4] A number of studies have used normal, untreated samples to determine arch form mathematically[5,6] or to characterize arch form through various measurements, with incisal edges and cusp tips as landmarks.[7,8,9]

Classic studies have described that well-aligned dental arches are roughly categorized as square, ovoid, and tapered.[10] These arch forms can also be expressed as narrow, normal and wide.[11] Especially when determining the arch wire forms to be used at the initial phase of treatment, Chuck[12] advocated that making a choice between these three forms would be better than using a single arch form. Due to this cause, the most convenient arch form type, according to patient's ethnical origin and malocclusion, should be chosen for preformed superelastic arch wires in leveling and arrangement phases.[13,14]

The dolichocephalic head form is the most common among North American whites. The Turkish population, however, originates from heterogeneous ethnic backgrounds: Asiatic Turks, Kurds, the Balkans, Caucasus, Middle East, Iran as well as from ancient Romans, Byzantines, and Arabs; also, Turkey, is an Eurasian country located in Western Asia (mostly in the Anatolian peninsula) and in Southeastern Europe (East Thracian).[15] Therefore, head form of the Turkish might well differ from the white population.

Studies on the arch forms of the Turkish and comparisons with other ethnic groups have not been performed previously. The aim of this study was to determine the morphological differences between Turkish and North American white clinical mandibular arches in Class I, Class II, and Class III malocclusions by measuring patients' arch dimensions. The subjects were grouped according to arch form (tapered, ovoid and square) in order to have the frequency distribution of the three arch forms clarified for comparison between the ethnic groups in each Angle classification.

MATERIAL AND METHODS

This study was based on two sample groups of Turkish and North American white subjects. The Turkish group consisted of pretreatment mandibular dental models from 34 Class I, 58 Class II, and 40 Class III patients obtained from the Kirikkale University Department of Orthodontics, Turkey. The North American white group consisted of models from 60 Class I, 50 Class II, and 50 Class III patients from the University of Southern California, Department of Orthodontics, Los Angeles, and a private practice in San Diego, California, USA (Table 1).

The samples were selected to match the following criteria: (1) Angle dental Class I, II, and III malocclusions; (2) permanent dentition with normal tooth size and shape; (3) no supernumerary teeth; (4) arch-length discrepancy of 3 mm or less; (5) absence of restorations extending to contact areas, cusp tips, or incisal edges; and (6) no previous orthodontic treatment.

The occlusal surfaces of the mandibular models were photocopied, with a ruler included for magnification correction. The photocopied images were placed on a digitizer, and the most facial portions of 13 proximal contact areas around the arch were digitized (Fig 1). These points are used to estimate corresponding bracket slot locations (clinical bracket point) for each tooth. The proximal contact between the two central incisors was used as the origin of the x-y coordinate.

The original x-y coordinate on the digitizer was corrected for magnification and adjusted to establish a new x-y coordinate, so that the mean inclination of straight lines connecting the right and left contact points between the first and second premolars as well as those between the second premolars and first molar became parallel to the original x-axis.

The perpendicular to a line connecting mesial and distal contact points of each tooth on the coordinate was drawn from the midpoint of the mesiodistal line for incisors, canines, and premolars and from the mesial third of the line for molars. The perpendicular was extended labially or buccally to locate a clinical bracket point for each tooth, according to mandibular teeth thickness data of Andrews.[16]

The following four linear and two proportional measurements were made (Fig 2):

1) Intercanine width: the distance between canine clinical bracket points.

2) Intermolar width: the distance between first molar clinical bracket points.

Table 1 - Sex and age comparisons between North American and Turkish samples.

		North American (n = 160)	Turkish (n = 132)	p value
Total % (n)	Male	47.5 (76)	43.9 (58)	0.54 NS
	Female	52.5 (84)	56.1 (74)	
Class I % (n)	Male	38.3 (23)	35.3 (12)	0.77 NS
	Female	61.7 (37)	64.7 (22)	
Class II % (n)	Male	52.0 (26)	51.7 (30)	0.97 NS
	Female	48.0 (24)	48.3 (28)	
Class III % (n)	Male	54.0 (27)	40.0 (16)	0.18 NS
	Female	46.0 (23)	60.0 (24)	
Age (years) Mean (SD)	Total	15.4 (5.2)	13.9 (2.5)	
	Class I	16.6 (5.9)	13.8 (2.5)	
	Class II	14.7 (4.7)	14.4 (1.9)	
	Class III	14.5 (4.3)	13.4 (3.2)	

$p > 0.05$, NS = non-significant, Chi-square test.

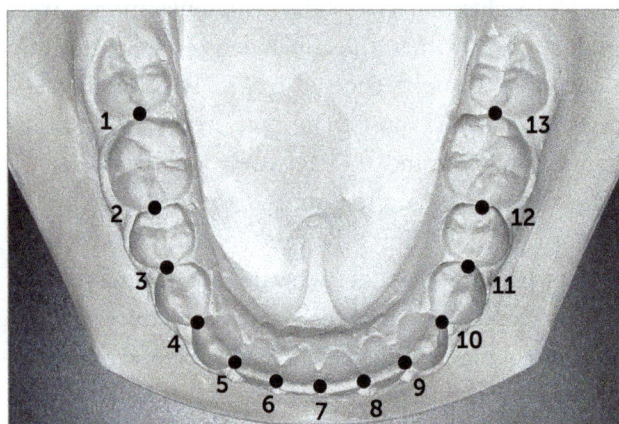

Figure 1 - Points digitized on the occlusal photocopy. These points represent the most facial portions of 13 proximal contact areas.
Modified from: Nojima et al.[14], 2001.

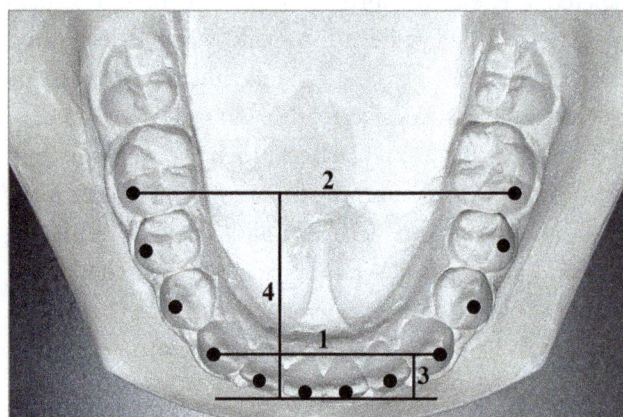

Figure 2 - Twelve clinical bracket points, four linear and two proportional measurements of arch dimensions: **1)** intercanine width; **2)** intermolar width; **3)** canine depth; **4)** molar depth; **5)** canine W/D ratio; and **6)** molar WD ratio.
Modified from: Nojima et al.[14], 2001.

3) Canine depth: the shortest distance from a line connecting the canine clinical bracket points to the origin between central incisors.

4) Molar depth: the shortest distance from a line connecting the first molar clinical bracket points to the origin between central incisors.

5) Canine width-depth (W/D) ratio: the ratio of intercanine width and canine depth.

6) Molar W/D ratio: the ratio of intermolar width and molar depth.

In addition, 12 clinical bracket points were printed per patient at full size to select, from square, ovoid and tapered arch forms (OrthoForm; 3M Unitek, Monrovia, California, USA), the arch form that best fits the eight clinical bracket points from first premolar to first premolar (Fig 2).

STATISTICAL ANALYSIS

Power analysis showed that, for this study, $\alpha = 0.01$; $\beta = 0.20$ ($1-\beta = 0.80$; power = 0.8225); and power of 82 % were needed, so as to detect a difference of 1 mm. Power analysis showed that 32 patients were required in each group. Statistical evaluation was performed with SPSS 16.0 software (SPSS Inc., Chicago, IL, USA).

Chi-square test was used to assess the association between sex and the two ethnic groups: North American and Turkish groups. The association between arch form and ethnic group was also assessed by means of chi-square test. Analysis of variance (ANOVA) was performed to compare the adjusted means of arch dimensions between the two ethnic groups by Angle classification and arch form separately. The results of the continuous variables were compared by ANOVA (for three subgroups) or by two-sample t-test for differences in means (for two subgroups). All analyses were tested at a significance level of 0.05.

RESULTS

Measurement errors were assessed by statistically analyzing the difference between duplicate measurements taken at least two weeks apart on 24 casts selected at random. Measurement errors were generally small (less than 5% of the measured mean value) and within acceptable limits.

Tables 2 and 3 depict the arch dimension measurements and results of the t-test for the North American and Turkish Class I, II, and III samples. The Turkish group showed significantly smaller molar depth and bigger molar W/D ratio in all three Angle classifications. In addition, the Turkish group also showed a significantly larger intercanine width in Class III malocclusion and intermolar width in Class II malocclusion. When Class I, II, and III malocclusions were combined, statistically significant differences were observed in canine depth, molar depth, canine W/D ratio and molar W/D ratio between the two ethnic groups.

Table 4 shows the frequency distributions of the three forms and the results of the chi-square test for the North American and Turkish groups. In the former group, ovoid and tapered arch forms together made up more than 80% of the sample; but in the Turkish group, only 69% of the sample had ovoid and tapered arch forms. Square arch forms made up 30.3% of the Turkish group, but only 18.1% of the North American group. The most frequent arch forms seen were the ovoid arch form in the Turkish group and the tapered form in the North American group. The square arch form had the lowest frequency distribution in the Class I and Class II groups in both Turkish and North American groups; however, in the North American Class III samples, square arch forms were found at the highest frequency of 44% while ovoid arch forms were found at the highest frequency of 45% of the Class III samples in the Turkish.

Table 5 depicts arch dimension measurements and results of t-test obtained by regrouping the subjects into square, ovoid and tapered arch form samples. The Turkish had significantly narrower intercanine widths than the North American in the square arch form groups, and significantly larger intercanine widths than the North American in the ovoid and tapered arch form groups. The North American groups had significantly higher values for intermolar width in the square arch form and lower values for intermolar width in the tapered and ovoid arch form compared with the Turkish sample. Both ethnic groups showed significant increases in molar depth as the mandibular arches changed in form from square to ovoid to tapered.

Table 2 - Complete sample comparison between North American white and Turkish groups.

Variable	White (n = 160) Mean (SD)	Turkish (n = 132) Mean (SD)	p value
Intercanine width (mm)	29.07 (1.39)	29.19 (1.67)	> 0.05
Intermolar width (mm)	49.42 (2.61)	49.77 (2.71)	> 0.05
Canine depth (mm)	6.26 (1.13)	5.84 (1.00)	< 0.05*
Molar depth (mm)	27.08 (2.07)	25.37 (1.87)	< 0.01**
Canine W/D ratio	4.79 (0.85)	4.92 (0.77)	< 0.05*
Molar W/D ratio	1.84 (0.17)	1.97 (0.17)	< 0.05*

*p < 0.05; **p < 0.01, Two-sample t-test for difference in means.

Table 3 - Comparison between North American and Turkish groups by Angle classification. Values presented as: Mean (SD).

Variable	Class I (n = 94)			Class II (n = 108)			Class III (n = 90)		
	White (n = 60)	Turkish (n = 34)	p value	White (n = 50)	Turkish (n = 58)	p value	White (n = 50)	Turkish (n = 40)	p value
Intercanine width (mm)	29.01 (1.26)	28.96 (1.36)	> 0.05	28.92 (1.22)	28.87 (1.88)	> 0.05	29.29 (1.68)	29.74 (1.56)	< 0.05*
Intermolar width (mm)	49.17 (2.29)	48.97 (2.29)	> 0.05	48.5 (2.53)	49.25 (2.24)	< 0.05*	50.62 (2.65)	49.75 (3.46)	> 0.05
Canine depth (mm)	6.3 (0.88)	6.33 (0.92)	> 0.05	6.79 (1.12)	6.85 (0.81)	> 0.05	5.69 (1.15)	3.95 (0.94)	< 0.01**
Molar depth (mm)	26.84 (1.62)	25.63 (1.64)	< 0.05*	27.3 (2.12)	26.03 (1.80)	< 0.05*	27.02 (2.59)	24.20 (1.63)	< 0.05*
Canine W/D ratio	4.68 (0.56)	4.59 (0.62)	> 0.05	4.37 (0.7)	4.35 (0.50)	> 0.05	5.34 (1.0)	6,02 (0.91)	< 0.01**
Molar W/D ratio	1.84 (0.11)	1.91 (0.14)	< 0.05*	1.78 (0.16)	1.89 (0.51)	< 0.05*	1.89 (0.21)	2.06 (0.20)	< 0.05*

*$p < 0.05$; **$p < 0.01$, Two-sample t-test for difference in means.

Table 4 - Distribution of arch forms by race and Angle classifications. Values presented as: percentage (n).

		White	Turkish	p value
Total	Square	18.1 (29)	30.3 (40)	
	Ovoid	38.1 (61)	42.4 (56)	0.006*
	Tapered	43.8 (70)	27.3 (36)	
Class I	Square	8.3 (5)	23.5 (8)	
	Ovoid	45.0 (27)	47.1 (16)	0.073 NS
	Tapered	46.7 (28)	29.4 (10)	
Class II	Square	4.0 (2)	27.6 (16)	
	Ovoid	36.0 (18)	37.9 (22)	0.002*
	Tapered	60.0 (30)	34.5 (20)	
Class III	Square	44.0 (22)	40.0 (16)	
	Ovoid	32.0 (16)	45.0 (18)	0.372 NS
	Tapered	24.0 (12)	15.0 (6)	

$p > 0.05$, NS = non-significant, *$p < 0.01$, Chi-square test.

Table 5 - Comparison between North American and Turkish groups, by arch forms. Values presented as: Mean (SD).

	Square (n = 69)			Ovoid (n = 117)			Tapered (n = 106)		
	White (n = 29)	Turkish (n = 40)	p value	White (n = 61)	Turkish (n = 56)	p value	White (n = 70)	Turkish (n = 36)	p value
Intercanine width (mm)	29.96 (1.69)	29.23 (1.47)	< 0.05*	29.37 (1.34)	29.54 (1.68)	< 0.05*	28.44 (0.97)	28.60 (1.86)	> 0.05 NS
Intermolar width (mm)	52.24 (2.01)	50.18 (3.07)	< 0.05*	49.81 (2.27)	50.03 (2.69)	> 0.05	47.90 (1.95)	48.89 (2.12)	< 0.05*
Canine depth (mm)	5.26 (1.11)	5.49 (0.71)	< 0.05*	6.05 (0.76)	6.17 (0.99)	> 0.05	6.85 (1.06)	5.71 (1.08)	< 0.01**
Molar depth (mm)	26.16 (2.71)	24.69 (1.39)	< 0.05*	27.02 (1.78)	25.41 (1.98)	< 0.05*	27.52 (1.90)	26.07 (1.93)	< 0.05*
Canine W/D ratio	5.86 (0.92)	5.36 (0.70)	< 0.05*	4.91 (0.48)	4.73 (0.78)	> 0.05	4.24 (0.57)	4.73 (0.67)	< 0.05*
Molar W/D ratio	2.02 (0.19)	2.04 (0.20)	> 0.05	1.85 (0.12)	1.97 (0.16)	< 0.05*	1.75 (0.12)	1.88 (0.13)	< 0.05*

$p > 0.05$, NS = non-significant, *$p < 0.05$; **$p < 0.01$. ANOVA, 2-sample t-test.

DISCUSSION

Some studies have reported on dental arch form, and a number of researchers have tried to establish the form unique to certain malocclusions, ethnic groups, and sex.[17,18]

Several classification schemes have been suggested, but the three basic arch forms that are commonly described by clinicians are tapered, ovoid and square arch forms.[19] Clinically, it is important that arch form does not change during orthodontic treatment because occlusal stability depends on preservation of patient's original arch form.[3,20]

Preformed arch wires have been used frequently, although many reports have brought up the fact that application of the same arch wire in all cases can negatively affect post-treatment occlusal stability.[21,22] Most manufacturers produce their arch wires based on North American or European arch forms; however, focusing on ethnic groups outside of these groups is more than a scholarly exercise.

Several studies have described the shape of the dental arch by using different mathematical methods[23,24,25] or by characterizing arch form through various measurements using the incisal edges and cusp tips as landmarks.[7,26] These landmarks were used in studies carried out by Burris and Harris[27] and Ling and Wong.[28] Some researchers;[13,14,29,30] however, used clinical bracket points as landmarks in their studies. Clinical bracket points corresponding to a bracket slot were used in this study, according to a method described in recent reports.[15,16,31,32]

These bracket points corresponded to bracket slot points that were mathematically estimated from the most facial portion of the proximal contact area of each tooth. Kook et al[13] argued that using clinical bracket points as landmarks for measurement of dental arch shapes was of greater value for modern orthodontic treatment than the conventional incisal edge and cusp tip landmarks, since preformed superelastic arch wires are frequently used for clinical treatment.

The results of the current study clearly indicate that North American people have deeper arch forms in both canine and molar regions in comparison to the Turkish. Similar results were reported by both Gafni et al[29] and Nojima et al.[14] In the study by Nojima et al,[14] the transverse widths of canines and molars were statistically significant larger for the Japanese than for the North American whites, and the ratio of anteroposterior lengths to canine and molar widths was also greater for the Japanese than for the North American whites. However, no statistically significant difference existed for the transverse widths of canines and molars between Turkish and white subjects.

One can rank the total sample of Turkish mandibular arch dimension in relation to both North American whites and Japanese in the following order: North American whites < Turkish < Japanese.

Braun et al[31] stated, in their report on differences in arch dimensions between Angle classifications, that Class II mandibular arches exhibited generalized reduced arch width and depth compared with Class I arches, and that Class III mandibular arches had smaller arch depth and greater arch width than Class I arches. Our study showed that Class II canine and molar depth of the Turkish population was greater than in Class I and Class III subjects. This could be explained by the more tapered anterior curvature of Class II arches, which directly influences both canine and molar depth parameters. Class III arches showed significantly larger intercanine and molar widths than did the Class I and Class II arches in whites; this was consistent with previous reports.[13,14] For both Turkish and North American whites, these findings also correlate with those of Nojima et al[14] regarding Japanese subjects.

Felton et al[3] reported little difference between the arch forms of Class I and Class II malocclusion groups. Our results showed that Class II arches for North American and Turkish groups were associated with a decreased frequency of the ovoid arch form and an increased frequency of the tapered arch form compared with Class I arches. For the Turkish group, similar results have been obtained in studies performed by Olmez et al.[11]

For Class III arches, the frequency of square arch form was the highest in all three groups, followed by ovoid and tapered arch forms. For both Turkish and North American whites, these findings also correlate with those of Nojima et al,[14] regarding the Japanese sample. This can be similarity explained by the common developmental pattern of Class III malocclusion and the resultant dental compensation by lingual tipping of mandibular anterior teeth, which causes the anterior part of the mandibular arch to flatten.

Table 5 shows significant difference between white and Turkish groups when comparing them only within each arch form type. Square arch forms had significant differences in size, except for molar W/D ratio. Ovoid arch forms showed significant differences in intercanine width, molar depth, and molar W/D ratio. Tapered arch

forms were totally different in all areas, except for intercanine width.

Multiple studies have already reported differences in arch forms of subjects from various ethnic backgrounds.[13,14,29]

This study was the first comparison of arch forms between Turkish and North American white subjects. A study comparing the mandibular arches of Hispanic and Caucasian samples found that the square arch form was most prevalent in the Hispanic population (44%), followed by ovoid and tapering (28% each).[32] Tapering arch form (44%) was more common in Caucasians, followed by ovoid (38%) and square (18%);[32] thus, supporting that this anatomical guideline changes with race. Similar findings were reported by Nojima et al.[14] The most frequent arch form was square in the Japanese group (45.6%), followed by ovoid (42.5%) and tapering (11.9%). A study on a Korean sample found ovoid (49.02%) to be the most frequent, followed by square (42.06%) and tapering (8.82%).[33]

The results of this study on a Turkish population, using a subjective method for arch form evaluation, reports that the most frequent arch form was ovoid (42%), followed by square (30%), with only 27% of tapered arch forms.

Since there are differences in both arch dimension and frequency of arch form between Turkish and white subjects, as well as among malocclusion types, it is essential to select the best fit arch form for non-adaptable wires and to individualize the arch form in wires that can be altered in order to minimize round tripping of the dentition and to enhance stability of orthodontic results.

CONCLUSION

This study demonstrates that when treating Turkish patients, one should expect to use preformed ovoid arch form orthodontic wires in a significant percentage of patients. It is hoped that the arch form classification method will provide a practical guide in designing and fabricating preformed archwire forms for the Turkish population.

Acknowledgments

The authors thank Dr Richard P. McLaughlin, Clinical professor, Department of Orthodontics, University of Southern California, Los Angeles; private practice, San Diego, California, for his valuable contributions.

REFERENCES

1. Ricketts RM. A detailed consideration of the line of occlusion. Angle Orthod. 1978 Oct;48(4):274-82.

2. McLaughlin RP, Bennett JC. Arch form considerations for stability and esthetics. Rev Esp Orthod. 1999;29(3):46-63.

3. Felton JM, Sinclair PM, Jones DL, Alexander RG. A computerized analysis of the shape and stability of mandibular arch form. Am J Orthod Dentofacial Orthop. 1987 Dec;92(6):478-83.

4. Vaden JL, Dale JG, Klontz HA. The Tweed-Merrifield edgewise appliance: philosophy, diagnosis and treatment. In: Graber MT, Vanarsdall RL Jr. Orthodontics:current principles and techniques. 2nd ed. St. Louis: Mosby; 1994. p. 579-635.

5. Raberin M, Laumon B, Martin JL, Brunner F. Dimensions and form of dental arches in subjects with normal occlusions. Am J Orthod Dentofacial Orthop. 1993 July;104(1):67-72.

6. Braun S, Hnat WP, Leschinsky R, Legan HL. An evaluation of the shape of some popular nickel titanium alloy preformed arch wires. Am J Orthod Dentofacial Orthop. 1999 July;116(1):1-12.

7. Nummikoski P, Prihoda T, Langlais RP, McDavid WD, Welander U, Tronje G. Dental and mandibular arch widths in three ethnic groups in Texas: a radiographic study. Oral Surg Oral Med Oral Pathol. 1988 May;65(5):609-17.

8. Kim SC. A study on the configurations of Korean normal dental arches for preformed arch wire. Korean J Orthod. 1984;14(1):93-100.

9. Lee YC, Park YC. A study on the dental arch by occlusogram in normal occlusion. Korean J Orthod 1987;17(2):279-86.

10. Hickey J, Zarb G, Bolender C. Boucher's prosthodontic treatment for edentulous patients. St Louis: C.V. Mosby; 1985.

11. Olmez S, Dogan S. Comparison of the arch forms and dimensions in various malocclusions of the Turkish population. Open J Stomatol. 2011;1(4):158-64.

12. Chuck GC. Ideal arch form. Angle Orthod. 1932;4(4):312-27.

13. Kook YA, Nojima K, Moon HB, McLaughlin RP, Sinclair PM. Comparison of arch forms between Korean and North American white populations. Am J Orthod Dentofacial Orthop. 2004 Dec;126(6):680-6.

14. Nojima K, McLaughlin RP, Isshiki Y, Sinclair PM. A comparative study of Caucasian and Japanese mandibular clinical arch forms. Angle Orthod. 2001 Jun;71(3):195-200.

15. Celebi AA, Tan E, Gelgor IE, Colak T, Ayyildiz E. Comparison of soft tissue cephalometric norms between Turkish and European-American adults. Sci World J. 2013;2013:806203.

16. Andrews LF. Straight Wire - The concept and appliance. San Diego: LA Wells; 1989.

17. Ferrario VF, Sforza C, Miani A Jr, Tartaglia G. Human dental arch shape evaluated by euclidean-distance matrix analysis. Am J Phys Anthropol. 1993 Apr;90(4):445-53.

18. Cassidy KM, Harris EF, Tolley EA, Keim RG. Genetic influence on dental arch form in orthodontic patients. Angle Orthod. 1998 Oct;68(5):445-54.

19. McLaughlin RP, Bennett JCD, Trevisi HJ. Systemized orthodontic treatment mechanics. Edinburgh : Mosby; 2001.

20. de la Cruz A, Sampson P, Little RM, Artun J, Shapiro PA. Long-term changes in arch form after orthodontic treatment and retention. Am J Orthod Dentofacial Orthop. 1995 May;107(5):518-30.

21. Strang RHW. The fallacy of denture expansion as a treatment procedure. Angle Orthod. 1949;19(1):12-7.

22. Gardner SD, Chaconas SJ. Posttreatment and postretention changes following orthodontic therapy. Angle Orthod. 1976 Apr;46(2):151-61.

23. Bonwill WGA. Geometrical and mechanical laws of articulation. Tr Odont Soc Penn. 1884-1885:119–33.

24. Camporesi M, Franchi L, Baccetti T, Antonini A. Thin-plate spline analysis of arch form in a Southern European population with an ideal natural occlusion. Eur J Orthod. 2006 Apr;28(2):135-40.

25. Noroozi H, Nik TH, Saeeda R. The dental arch form revisited. Angle Orthod. 2001 Oct;71(5):386-9.

26. Aoki H, Tsuta A, Ukiya M, Reitz P. A morphological study and comparison of the dental arch form of Japanese and American adults: detailed measurements of the transverse width. Bull Tokyo Dent Coll. 1971 Feb;12(1):9-14.

27. Burris BG, Harris EF. Maxillary arch size and shape in American blacks and whites. Angle Orthod. 2000 Aug;70(4):297-302.

28. Ling JY, Wong RW. Dental arch widths of Southern Chinese. Angle Orthod. 2009 Jan;79(1):54-63.

29. Gafni Y, Tzur-Gadassi L, Nojima K, McLaughlin RP, Abed Y, Redlich M. Comparison of arch forms between Israeli and North American white populations. Am J Orthod Dentofacial Orthop. 2011 Mar;139(3):339-44.

30. Bayome M, Sameshima GT, Kim Y, Nojima K, Baek SH, Kook YA. Comparison of arch forms between Egyptian and North American white populations. Am J Orthod Dentofacial Orthop. 2011 Mar;139(3):e245-52.

31. Braun S, Hnat WP, Fender DE, Legan HL. The form of the human dental arch. Angle Orthod. 1998 Feb;68(1):29-36.

32. Gimlen AA. Comparative study of Caucasian and Hispanic mandibular clinical arch forms Cranio-Facial Biology. Los Angeles: University of Southern California; 2007.

33. Yun YK, Mo SS, Kim JG. Mandibular clinical arch forms in Korean with normal occlusion. Korean J Orthod. 2004;36:481-7.

25

Predisposing factors to severe external root resorption associated to orthodontic treatment

Gracemia Vasconcelos Picanço[1], Karina Maria Salvatore de Freitas[2], Rodrigo Hermont Cançado[3], Fabricio Pinelli Valarelli[4], Paulo Roberto Barroso Picanço[5], Camila Pontes Feijão[6]

Objective: The aim of this study was to evaluate predisposing factors among patients who developed moderate or severe external root resorption (Malmgren's grades 3 and 4), on the maxillary incisors, during fixed orthodontic treatment in the permanent dentition. **Methods:** Ninety-nine patients who underwent orthodontic treatment with fixed edgewise appliances were selected. Patients were divided into two groups: G1 – 50 patients with no root resorption or presenting only apical irregularities (Malmgren's grades 0 and 1) at the end of the treatment, with mean initial age of 16.79 years and mean treatment time of 3.21 years; G2 – 49 patients presenting moderate or severe root resorption (Malmgren's grades 3 and 4) at the end of treatment on the maxillary incisors, with mean initial age of 19.92 years and mean treatment time of 3.98 years. Periapical radiographs and lateral cephalograms were evaluated. Factors that could influence the occurrence of severe root resorption were also recorded. Statistical analysis included chi-square tests, Fisher's exact test and independent *t* tests. **Results:** The results demonstrated significant difference between the groups for the variables: Extractions, initial degree of root resorption, root length and crown/root ratio at the beginning, and cortical thickness of the alveolar bone. **Conclusion:** It can be concluded that: Presence of root resorption before the beginning of treatment, extractions, reduced root length, decreased crown/root ratio and thin alveolar bone represent risk factors for severe root resorption in maxillary incisors during orthodontic treatment.

Keywords: Root resorption. Tooth movement. Orthodontics.

[1] MSc in Orthodontics, UNINGA.
[2] Post-Doc in Orthodontics, UNINGÁ.
[3] PhD in Orthodontics, FOB-USP.
[4] PhD in Orthodontics, UNINGÁ.
[5] MSc in Orthodontics, UNINGÁ.
[6] Specialist in Orthodontics, UVA-CE.

» The authors report no commercial, proprietary or financial interest in the products or companies described in this article.

Karina Maria Salvatore de Freitas
Rua Jamil Gebara, 1-25 – Apto 111 – Brazil
CEP: 17017-150 – Bauru/SP – E-mail: kmsf@uol.com.br

INTRODUCTION

The external root resorption (ERR) is frequently observed by orthodontists and are usually diagnosed in clinical practice when radiographs (panoramic or periapical) are performed. ERR are usually asymptomatic, and when the loss of root structure by resorption become severe the physiology and retention of the affected teeth may be compromised.[14]

The anterior teeth are more affected by root resorption, probably because they are single-rooted with tapered roots, conducting the orthodontic force directly to the apex. They are also constantly moved during orthodontic treatment. Moreover, they are more exposed to external factors, such as trauma, making these teeth a good reference for the magnitude of root resorption during orthodontic treatments.[22]

The literature about root resorption is extensive but very controversial in relation to the factors that actually influence the occurrence and severity of resorption during orthodontic treatment. In this context, this study was conducted in order to evaluate which factors are commonly observed in patients who develop moderate or severe degrees of resorption in maxillary incisors during orthodontic treatment.

MATERIAL AND METHODS
Material

The sample consisted of 99 patients from the Paulo Picanço Advanced Orthodontics Center, Fortaleza-CE, who underwent orthodontic treatment with fixed appliance (Edgewise technique) in the permanent dentition, and met the following requirements: Good oral and systemic health, no tooth loss in the region from canine to canine in the maxillary arch, absence of vertical bone loss and periodontal disease, and no prosthesis. Patients who developed grade 2 resorption[26] at the end of treatment was excluded from the study. Only patients who had complete treatment records, medical records, initial cephalogram and initial and final periapical radiographs of maxillary incisors in good conditions were included in the sample.

Teeth with endodontic treatment, incomplete development of the root apex, tooth agenesis, supernumerary teeth and patients with incomplete initial records were excluded from the sample. Radiographs with distortion or blur were also eliminated.

Sample division:
» Group 1 (Patients who had degree 0 or 1 of root resorption of the maxillary incisors at the end of treatment): 50 patients, 26 without and 24 with extractions (13 first premolars; 8 second premolars and 3 first molars). The mean age at the beginning of the treatment was 16.79 years, the mean age at the end of treatment was 20.00 years. The mean treatment time was 3.21 years.
» Group 2 (patients who had degree 3 or 4 of root resorption in maxillary incisors at the end of treatment): 49 patients, 26 without and 24 with extractions (31 first premolars, 9 second premolars, 2 first molars) The mean age at the beginning of the treatment was 19.92 years and the mean age at the end of treatment was 23.90 years. The mean treatment time was 3.98 years.

Methods

In order to evaluate the variables, initial and final periapical radiographs and initial cephalograms were used of each patient. The radiographs were scanned with a scanner (Microtek ScanMaker i800, Microtek International, Inc., Carson, USA) and coupled to a Pentium computer. The images were transferred to the software Dolphin Imaging Premium 10.5 (Dolphin Imaging & Management Solutions, Chatsworth, USA) through which the images were digitized, the points were marked and cephalometric measurements were performed automatically by the software Dolphin.

The periapical radiographs were analyzed as follows: The degree of initial and final, based on the classification proposed by Malmgren: Grade 0 (no resorption), grade 1 (presence of apical irregularities), grade 2 (presence of resorption by 2 mm), grade 3 (presence of resorption between 2 mm and a third of the original length), grade 4 (the presence of root resorption greater than one third of the original length of the root) (Fig 1).[7,8]

The bone crest was classified based on the observation of periapical radiographs as follows: Flat (width greater than 1 mm, representing the crest of a rectangular shape) and sharp (width less than or equal to 1 mm, representing the crest of triangular shape) (Fig 2).

The evaluation of the root shape was performed based on the classification proposed by Consolaro[9] as follows: Triangular (T), rhomboid (R), pipette (P) and dilacerated (D) (Fig 3).

The root length was obtained by measuring the distance from the apex to the cementoenamel junction, following the long axis of the incisor (Fig 4). This measurement was performed in both initial and final periapical radiographs.

Cephalometric variables used are shown in Figures 5, 6 and 7, and described in Table 1.

Method error

For the evaluation of the intraexaminer error, the measurements were performed on 20 patients randomly selected, after a month interval. It was applied the dependent t test to obtain the systematic

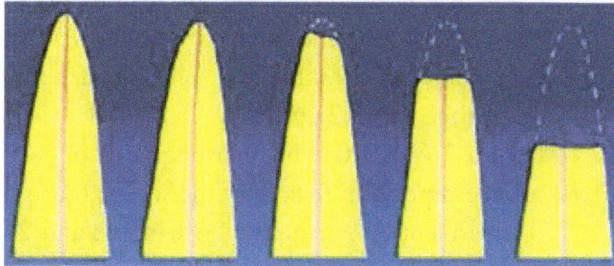

Figure 1 - Malmgren[7,8] classification.

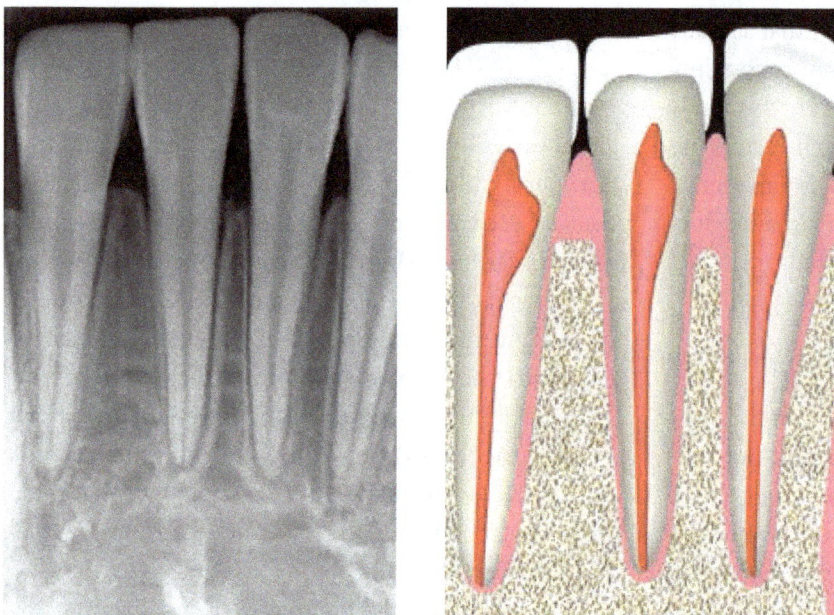

Figure 2 - Alveolar crest bone morphology.

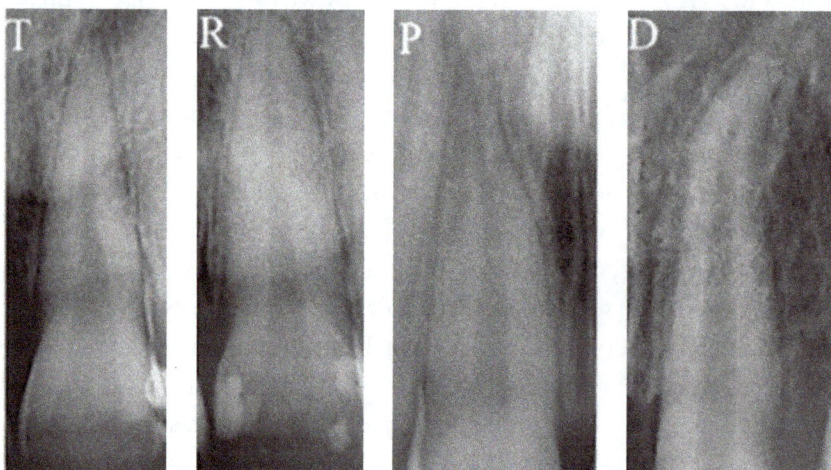

Figure 3 - Root morphologies: triangular (T), rhomboid (R), pipette (P) and dilacerated (D).

Root/crown proportion

Example of Grade 4
Crown: 11 mm
Root: 10 mm
11 ----- 100%
10 ----- X
X = 0.9

Proportion = 1:0.9

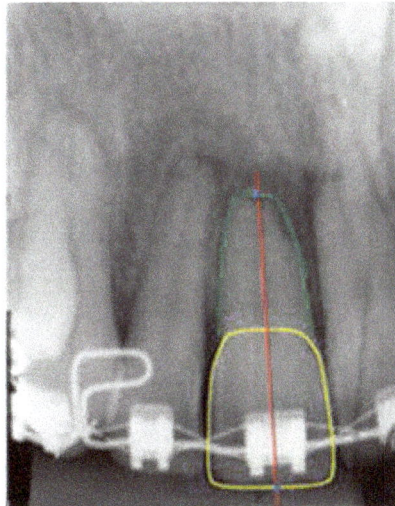

Figure 4 - Evaluation of the crown/root proportion.

error and Dahlberg[11] formula to estimate the random error. To evaluate the error of the score of root resorption, the Kappa test was used.

Statistical analysis

It was used the following statistical tests: Chi-square test for intergroup comparison of gender, type of malocclusion, treatment with or without extraction, shape of the root and bone crest; independent *t* test for comparison of the ages, treatment time and cephalometric variables between the two groups. All tests were performed with Statistica software (Statistica for Windows, versão 7.0, Statsoft). Results were considered significant when $p < 0.05$.

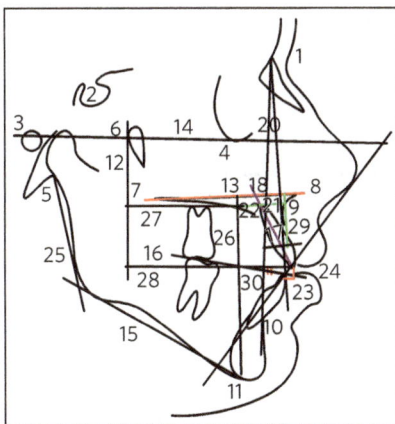

Figure 5 - Cephalometric variables used.

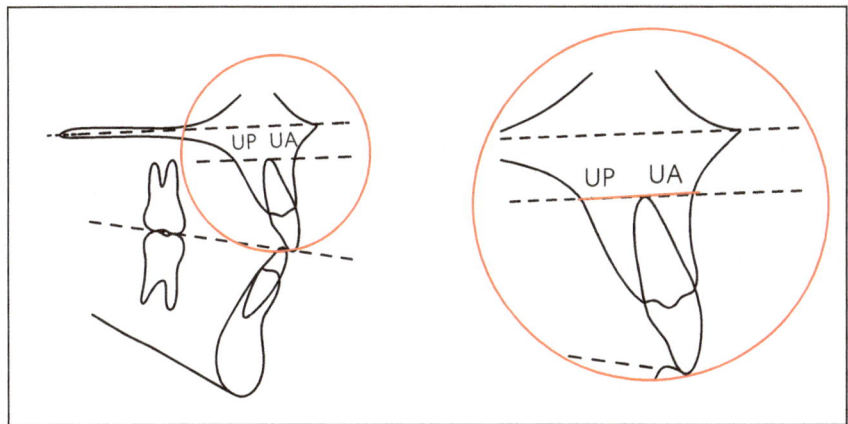

Figure 6 - UA+UP distance, parallel to the palatal plane (ANS-PNS).

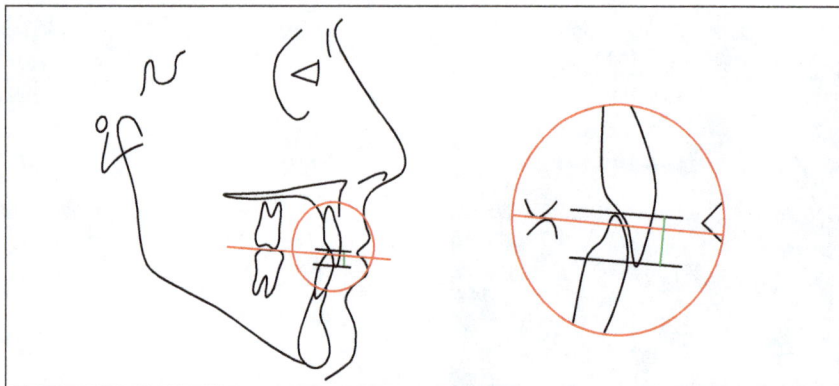

Figure 7 - Overbite.

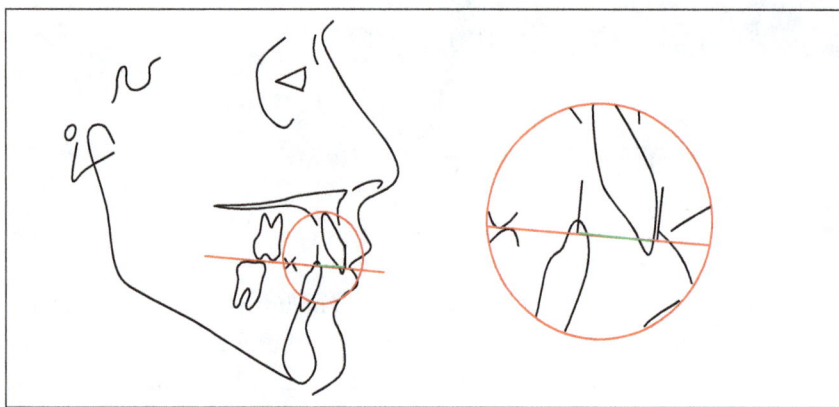

Figure 8 - Overjet.

Table 1 - Cephalometric variables used.

1-PTV INC (mm)	Distance of the incisal of the maxillary central incisor to the PTV line (line vertical to the pterygoid fossa, perpendicular to Frankfurt).
1-PTV APIC (mm)	Distance of the apical root of the maxillary central incisor to the PTV line (line vertical to the pterygoid fossa, perpendicular to Frankfurt).
1.NA (degrees)	Angle between the long axis of the maxillary central incisor and the line NA.
FMA (degrees)	Angle formed by the horizontal planes of Frankfurt and mandibular (GoMe)
PFH/AFH (mm)	Proportion between the posterior face height (S-Go) and the anterior face height (N-Me).
ANB (degrees)	Angle formed by the lines NA and NB.
Wits (mm)	Distance between the points A and B projected perpendicularly to the functional occlusal plane.
Overjet (mm)	Distance between the incisal edges of the maxillary and mandibular central incisors projected perpendicularly to the occlusal plane.
Overbite (mm)	Distance between the incisal edges of the maxillary and mandibular central incisors measured perpendicularly to the occlusal plane.
H-11 (mm)	Total length of the maxillary central incisor, including crown and root.
UA+UP (mm)	Sum of the thickness of the anterior (buccal) and posterior (palatal) alveolar crest bone.

RESULTS

The largest linear random error found, was for the variable 1-PTV apical (1.36 mm), and angular for the measure 1.NA (1.41°) and the largest systematic error was 0.12 mm of the variable Overjet. The percentage of agreement was substantial (87%) and Kappa coefficient was 0.794.

Increased age and longer treatment was significantly related to the occurrence of severe root resorption (Table 2).

Gender, type of malocclusion, morphology of the root and the bone crest are not risk factors for developing severe root resorption (Table 3). The treatment protocol with extractions increases the risk of severe apical root resorption (Table 3).

The short root length and the decreased proportion of the crown/root ratio at the beginning of treatment increases the chance of developing severe resorption (Table 4).

Patients with thin maxillary alveolar cortical bone are more likely to develop severe resorption than patients with good bone thickness (Table 5).

Table 2 - Intergroup comparison of the ages and treatment time (independent t test).

Variables	Group 1 absent or light resorption (n = 50)		Group 2 moderate or severe resorption (n = 49)		p
	Mean	SD	Mean	SD	
Initial age (years)	16.79	5.47	19.92	6.94	0.014*
Final age (years)	20.00	5.46	23.90	7.05	0.002*
Treatment time (years)	3.21	0.84	3.98	1.01	0.000*

* Statistically significant p < 0.05.

Table 3 - Intergroup comparison of the gender, type of malocclusion, root morphology, alveolar crest and presence of initial resorption (chi-square).

Variables		Group 1 absent or light resorption (n = 50)	Group 2 moderate or severe resorption (n = 49)	λ	DF	p
Gender	Male	18.18%	13.13%	1.03	1	0.309
	Female	32.32%	36.36%			
Malocclusion	Class I	8.08%	12.12%	3.45	2	0.179
	Class II	29.29%	31.31%			
	Class III	13.13%	6.06%			
Type of treatment	Without extraction	26.26%	9.09%	2.24	1	0.000*
	With extraction	24.24%	40.40%			
Root morphology	Triangular	4.04%	4.04%	0.97	3	0.806
	Rhomboid	34.34%	29.29%			
	Pipette	10.10%	13.13%			
	Dilacerated	2.02%	3.03%			
Alveolar crest	Flat	29.29%	35.35%	1.95	1	0.162
	Sharp	21.21%	14.14%			
Initial degree of resorption	0	48.48%	30.30%	17.91	1	0.000*
	1	2,02%	19,19%			

* Statistically significant p < 0.05.

Table 4 - Intergroup comparison of the root length and the crown/root proportion in T_1, T_2 and T_2-T_1 (independent t test).

Variables	Group 1 absent or light resorption (n = 50)		Group 2 moderate or severe resorption (n = 49)		p
	Mean	SD	Mean	SD	
Root length T_1 (mm)	16.69	2.06	15.90	1.58	0.033*
Root length T_2 (mm)	16.05	2.04	12.44	1.74	0.000*
Root length T_2-T_1	-0.64	0.49	-3.45	1.40	0.000*
Crown/root Initial proportion	1:1.82	0.24	1:1.69	0.21	0.005*
Crown/root Final proportion	1:1.78	0.24	1:1.37	0.20	0.000*
Crown/root T_2-T_1	-0.03	0.04	-0.31	0.15	0.000*

* Statistically significant p < 0.05.

Table 5 - Intergroup comparison of the cephalometric variables (independent *t* test).

VARIABLES	Group 1 absent or light resorption (n = 50)		Group 2 moderate or severe resorption (n = 49)		p
	Mean	SD	Mean	SD	
1-PTV INC (mm)	59.83	5.96	61.84	5.01	0.073
1-PTV APIC (mm)	49.65	7.76	51.15	3.66	0.224
1.NA (degrees)	26.68	8.98	29.73	6.84	0.060
FMA (degrees)	27.36	7.45	26.29	6.07	0.438
PFH/AFH (mm)	0.72	0.11	0.74	0.11	0.378
ANB (degree)	2.20	2.27	2.54	2.11	0.441
Wits (mm)	-1.03	10.67	-0.81	5.43	0.900
Overjet (mm)	1.14	1.48	2.53	5.68	0.097
Overbite (mm)	3.43	2.52	4.17	4.48	0.315
H-11 (mm)	20.04	3.15	20.23	4.61	0.810
UA+UP (mm)	14.26	4.65	12.31	3.02	0.015*

* Statistically significant p < 0.05.

DISCUSSION

Sample

The sample of this study was obtained from Paulo Picanço Orthodontics Center. Initially, periapical radiographs were examined to obtain the degree of resorption and then the patients were divided into two groups. At this time, it was excluded patients with absences in the region from canine to canine in the maxilla, presence of vertical bone loss, patients with resorption grade 2, patients with incomplete, damaged or without final orthodontic records. After the selection, 165 patients from all subjects had completed files available. After checking the periapical radiographs, the evaluation of the orthodontic records was made, noting that many patients had incomplete records, absence of final orthodontic records, lack of signed informed consent, incomplete permanent dentition. At the end, a final sample of 99 patients attended the inclusion criteria.

Although the control group (group 1, with resorption grade 0 or 1 at the end of treatment) have more patients, this was the most difficult to collect, especially patients with grade 0 who fulfilled all the requirements of research, since the literature affirms that the resorption in orthodontically treated patients is 100%.[3,4,19,22,36]

To collect the ideal sample was the greatest challenge of this study, however, the number of subjects was considered good, because of the strict selection criteria.

Method

In this study only the maxillary incisors were evaluated, because previous studies showed that these teeth have more susceptibility to develop resorption during orthodontic treatment. Incisors are the more constantly moved, for example, during retraction and intrusion.[8,12,22] Moreover, incisors are single-rooted elements and easier for obtaining images without distortion or image overlays.[15,18,23,33]

The most common radiographic examination used for the detection of resorption is periapical x-ray. For Sameshima and Asgarifar[33] this type of radiograph shows finer detail, allowing visualization of anatomical details such as the cementoenamel junction and have less distortion and overlap when compared to panoramic and cephalometric radiographs.[26] In this study the standardized technique for periapical radiographs used was the parallelism, and the fact that all patients in the study underwent radiographic follow-up at the Paulo Picanço Orthodontics Center, ensuring greater standardization of radiographs. The choice for this technique is the fact that it allows greater standardization of the image for pre- and post-treatment, what is not possible by the bisection technique, since the average angle of incidence of x-rays is more difficult to reproduce even hindering over the accuracy of quantitative measurements.[32]

Age

The results were significant in relation to age, because the group 1 presented younger patients when compared to group 2. It can be affirmed that older patients have a higher risk of developing moderate or severe root resorption during orthodontic treatment (Table 2).

Some authors mentioned that age does not influence root resorption.[1,9,19] However, corroborating the results of this study, Sameshima and Sinclair[34,35] observed that the resorption is most prevalent in adults than in children.

Adults seem more susceptible to resorption because, with aging, the periodontal membrane becomes less vascularized, inelastic, more narrow and the cementum becomes thicker, and also the fact that the apical third of the root is more firmly anchored in adult patients, creating a difficulty in tooth movement and predisposing to resorption.[3,4,6]

However, the results of this study must be interpreted with caution, since the age difference between the groups 1 and 2 was only about three years, and both patients in group 1 and group 2 were considered "young adults" (Table 2).

Treatment time

The results showed that a longer treatment is a risk factor to the occurrence of severe root resorption, as the group 1 showed a significantly shorter treatment time compared to group 2 (Table 2).

These results are opposite to those authors who suggest no relation between the duration of treatment and the degree of resorption.[2,13,37]

According to Sameshima and Sinclair,[34,35] the duration of treatment and the amount of horizontal displacement of the apical root of the maxillary incisors had strong correlation with root resorption.

Brin et al[5] evaluated the root resorption in patients with Class II malocclusion treated in only one phase or with treatment divided into two phases, observed that patients undergoing a single phase of treatment had a proportion of moderate to severe resorption slightly larger than the group with two phases of treatment.

Gender

In this study no significant relationships were found between severe resorption and the gender (Table 3), agreeing with the results of most authors.[9,19,20,31,34,35,36]

Type of malocclusion

Regarding the type of malocclusion and orthodontic techniques, many studies have shown that there is no relationship between root resorption and type of malocclusion.[6,19,30] The results of this study also found no significant relationship (Table 3).

Type of treatment (with or without extraction)

The results of this study showed that patients treated with extraction were more likely to develop severe root resorption than patients whose treatment did not include extraction (Table 3).

Many studies showed that patients treated with extractions showed more resorption and with more severe degree, because mechanical retraction of anterior teeth cause greater movement of the root apex and the need for longer treatment.[12,16,29,34,35]

Root and bone crest morphology

The results of this study showed no relationship between the morphology of the root and the bone crest to the occurrence of severe resorption during orthodontic treatment (Table 3).

Most authors consider, regarding the root morphology, that teeth with atypical root have a higher risk of root resorption.[25,29,30,34,35]

It is likely that this result is due to the fact that most of the sample presented rhomboid root and tapered bone crest, which according to most authors, reduce the risk of resorption.

Degree of initial resorption

The results have shown that patients with some degree of root resorption at the beginning of treatment have a greater predisposition and an increased risk of developing severe root resorption during orthodontic treatment (Table 3).

Some authors believe that patients with minimal or no resorption present little risk to severe resorption, patients with moderate resorption have regular risk to severe and extreme resorption, while patients starting orthodontic treatment with severe resorption has a high risk of extreme resorption at the end of treatment.[6,36]

Root length and crown/root proportion

In this study, the root length decreased significantly more during treatment in patients with severe resorption compared to the group with mild resorption (Table 4), as expected, because of the criterion for group division. However, the root length of group 2 was already smaller than the group 1 before the beginning of treatment (Table 4). This can be considered an indication that a smaller root length at the beginning of treatment is a risk factor for increased occurrence of root resorption during orthodontic treatment. Likewise, the crown/root proportion at the beginning of treatment was lower in group 2 than in group 1, and continued lower at the end of treatment (Table 4). Furthermore, the crown/root proportion suffered a greater decrease in group 2 (Table 4), as expected.

The root length and crown/root proportion seem to influence the tendency to resorption. A large crown will tend to concentrate force on certain focal points, thus short roots tend to suffer more resorption during orthodontic movements.

In cases of patients with severe resorption the professional should be very careful with the root length, teeth with roots length less than or equal to 9 mm have a higher risk of teeth mobility.[27] According to Kalkwarf et al,[24] the reduction of 3 mm in apical tooth structure corresponds to the loss of alveolar bone crest of 1 mm.

Incisor position

Variables related to the position of the maxillary incisor showed no statistically significant difference between the groups, indicating no relationship among the protrusion and buccal tipping of the incisors and the occurrence of severe root resorption (Table 5).

The results showed no statistically significant difference between the groups for the protrusion and initial inclination of the incisors, indicating that they are not risk factors to the occurrence of severe root resorption, although group 2 showed a greater buccal inclination of the incisors at the beginning of treatment, but not statistically significant (Table 5).

FMA and PFH/AFH

The FMA angle showed no statistically significant difference between the groups, indicating no relationship between the vertical pattern of the patients and the occurrence of severe root resorption (Table 5). The proportion PFH/AFH showed

no statistically significant difference between the groups, indicating no relationship between the facial pattern of the patients and the occurrence of severe root resorption (Table 5).

Handelman[17] analyzed the variable SN-MP that, represents the relationship between the cranial base and the mandibular plane and found positive association between this variable and root resorption.

Harris, Kineret and Tolley[19] also conducted a study to evaluate the relationship between FMA and root resorption and found a relatively high correlation between them.

ANB and WITS

The results of this study demonstrate that the maxillomandibular relationship was not significantly different between the groups, indicating that this variable is not a risk factor for the occurrence of severe root resorption (Table 5). It is likely that this result is due to the fact that the present sample does not show large maxillomandibular discrepancies.

In a study by Harris, Kineret and Tolley[19], these two variables (ANB and Wits) were evaluated and it was observed that both have strong relationship with the occurrence of resorption, as higher maxillomandibular discrepancies tend to require greater retraction of anterior teeth and therefore enhance the risk of resorption.

Overjet and Overbite

The results of this study showed no statistically significant difference between the groups for overjet and overbite, indicating that, at the beginning of treatment, these variables are not a risk factor to the occurrence of severe root resorption (Table 5). These findings, however, contradict most of the authors and the justification for this is the absence of great skeletal discrepancies and also the absence of a significant number of cases with open bite and/or deep bite.

There is a consensus in considering the overjet as a risk factor for resorption, because the correction requires the retraction of anterior teeth, and the greater the magnitude of this malocclusion, the greater the amount of movement, increasing the risk and severity of resorption.[2,5,28,31] Freitas et al[12] observed a great degree of resorption for correction of great amount of overjet.

H-11

The results showed no significant difference between the groups for this variable, indicating that the position of the incisors in relation to the palatal plane at the beginning of treatment is not a risk factor for the occurrence of severe root resorption.

Some studies show that the intrusion with lingual torque movement, horizontal movement of the apex increase the chance of root resorption.[1,10,30,31] For Parker and Harris,[31] extrusion movements are also risk factors, but less aggressive than the intrusion. For Freitas et al,[12] anteroposterior movement, is a risk factor found in 29% of the resorptions observed in patients during orthodontic treatment.

Bone thickness

The bone thickness (UA + UP) showed a statistically significant result (Table 5) confirming the authors hypothesis about the increased risk of resorption in patients with thin cortical.[10,17]

According to Handelman,[17] the dimension of the alveolus (UA + UP) seems to set limits to orthodontic treatment and challenge these limits can accelerate iatrogenic fenestrations and root resorption. Horiuchi, Hotokezaka and Kobayashi[21] observed that the proximity of the apex to the palatal cortex also influences the resorption. To these authors, the maxillary width insufficient to tooth movement can be considered a risk associated to root resorption.

CONCLUSIONS

According to the methodology applied and the conditions established in this study, it can be conclude that cases treated with extraction have a higher chance of presenting severe root resorption than patients treated without extractions. Short root length and crown/root proportion at the beginning of treatment increases the chance of developing severe resorption. Patients with thin cortical alveolar bone are more likely to develop severe resorption than patients with good bone thickness.

REFERENCES

1. Baumrind S, Korn EL, Boyd RL. Apical root resorption in orthodontically treated adults. Am J Orthod Dentofacial Orthop. 1996;110(3):311-20.

2. Beck BW, Harris EF. Apical root resorption in orthodontically treated subjects: analysis of edgewise and light wire mechanics. Am J Orthod Dentofacial Orthop. 1994;105(4):350-61.

3. Brezniak N, Wasserstein A. Root resorption after orthodontic treatment: Part 1. Literature review. Am J Orthod Dentofacial Orthop. 1993;103(1):62-6.

4. Brezniak N, Wasserstein A. Root resorption after orthodontic treatment: Part 2. Literature review. Am J Orthod Dentofacial Orthop. 1993;103(2):138-46.

5. Brin I, Tulloch JF, Koroluk L, Philips C. External apical root resorption in Class II malocclusion: a retrospective review of 1- versus 2-phase treatment. Am J Orthod Dentofacial Orthop. 2003;124(2):151-6.

6. Capelozza Filho L, Silva Filho OG. Reabsorção radicular na clínica ortodôntica: atitudes para uma conduta preventiva. Rev Dental Press Ortod Ortop Facial. 1998;3(1):104-26.

7. Chiqueto K, Martins DR, Janson G. Effects of accentuated and reversed curve of Spee on apical root resorption. Am J Orthod Dentofacial Orthop. 2008;133(2):261-8.

8. Chiqueto K. Influência da mecânica intrusiva de acentuação e reversão da curva de spee no grau de reabsorção radicular [dissertação]. Bauru (SP): Universidade de São Paulo; 2005.

9. Consolaro A. Reabsorções dentárias nas especialidades clínicas. 2ª ed. Maringá: Dental Press; 2005.

10. Costopoulos G, Nanda R. An evaluation of root resorption incident to orthodontic intrusion. Am J Orthod Dentofacial Orthop. 1996;109(5):543-8.

11. Dahlberg G. Statistical methods for medical and biological students. London: George Allen and Unwin; 1940.

12. de Freitas MR, Beltrão RT, Janson G, Henriques JF, Chiqueto K. Evaluation of root resorption after open bite treatment with and without extractions. Am J Orthod Dentofacial Orthop. 2007;132(2):143.e15-22.

13. Dermaut LR, De Munck A. Apical root resorption of upper incisors caused by intrusive tooth movement: a radiographic study. Am J Orthod Dentofacial Orthop. 1986;90(4):321-6.

14. Dudic A, Giannopoulou C, Leuzinger M, Kiliaridis S. Detection of apical root resorption after orthodontic treatment by using panoramic radiography and cone-beam computed tomography of super-high resolution. Am J Orthod Dentofacial Orthop. 2009;135(4):434-7.

15. Furquim LZ. Perfil endocrinológico de pacientes ortodônticos com e sem reabsorções dentárias: correlação com a morfologia radicular e da crista óssea. [tese]. Bauru (SP): Faculdade de Odontologia de Bauru; 2002.

16. Gadben JMA, Ribeiro A, Generoso R, Armond MC, Marques LS. Avaliação radiográfica periapical dos níveis de reabsorção radicular de incisivos superiores após tratamento ortodôntico. Arq Odontol. 2006;42(4):257-336.

17. Handelman CS. The anterior alveolus: its importance in limiting orthodontic treatment and its influence on the occurrence of iatrogenic sequelae. Angle Orthod. 1996;66(2):95-109.

18. Harris EF, Baker WC. Loss of root length and crestal bone height before and during treatment in adolescent and adult orthodontic patients. Am J Orthod Dentofacial Orthop. 1990;98(5):463-9.

19. Harris EF, Kineret SE, Tolley EA. A heritable component for external apical root resorption in patients treated orthodontically. Am J Orthod Dentofacial Orthop. 1997;111(3):301-9.

20. Hendrix I, Carels C, Kuijpers-Jagtman AM, Van 'T Hof M. A radiographic study of posterior apical root resorption in orthodontic patients. Am J Orthod Dentofacial Orthop. 1994;105(4):345-9.

21. Horiuchi A, Hotokezaka H, Kobayashi K. Correlation between cortical plate proximity and apical root resorption. Am J Orthod Dentofacial Orthop. 1998;114(3):311-8.

22. Janson GR, De Luca Canto G, Martins DR, Henriques JF, De Freitas MR. A radiographic comparison of apical root resorption after orthodontic treatment with 3 different fixed appliance techniques. Am J Orthod Dentofacial Orthop. 2000;118(3):262-73.

23. Kaley J, Phillips C. Factors related to root resorption in edgewise practice. Angle Orthod. 1991;61(2):125-32.

24. Kalkwarf KL, Krejci RF, Pao YC. Effect of apical root resorption on periodontal support. J Prosthet Dent. 1986;56(3):317-9.

25. Kjaer I. Morphological characteristics of dentitions developing excessive root resorption during orthodontic treatment. Eur J Orthod. 1995;17(1):25-34.

26. Levander E, Malmgren O. Evaluation of the risk of root resorption during orthodontic treatment: a study of upper incisors. Eur J Orthod. 1988;10(1):30-8.

27. Levander E, Malmgren O. Long-term follow-up of maxillary incisors with severe apical root resorption. Eur J Orthod. 2000;22(1):85-92.

28. Linge L, Linge BO. Patient characteristics and treatment variables associated with apical root resorption during orthodontic treatment. Am J Orthod Dentofacial Orthop. 1991;99(1):35-43.

29. Marques LS, Ramos-Jorge ML, Rey AC, Armond MC, Ruellas AC. Severe root resorption in orthodontic patients treated with the edgewise method: Prevalence and predictive factors. Am J Orthod Dentofacial Orthop. 2010;137(3):384-8.

30. Mirabella AD, Artun J. Risk factors for apical root resorption of maxillary anterior teeth in adult orthodontic patients. Am J Orthod Dentofacial Orthop. 1995;108(1):48-55.

31. Parker RJ, Harris EF. Directions of orthodontic tooth movements associated with external apical root resorption of the maxillary central incisor. Am J Orthod Dentofacial Orthop. 1998;114(6):677-83.

32. Remington DN, Joondeph DR, Artun J, Riedel RA, Chapko MK. Long-term evaluation of root resorption occurring during orthodontic treatment. Am J Orthod Dentofacial Orthop. 1989;96(1):43-6.

33. Sameshima GT, Asgarifar K. O. Assessment of root resorption and root shape: periapical vs panoramic films. Angle Orthod. 2011;71(3):185-9.

34. Sameshima GT, Sinclair PM. Predicting and preventing root resorption: Part I. Diagnostic factors. Am J Orthod Dentofacial Orthop. 2001;119(5):505-10.

35. Sameshima GT, Sinclair PM. Predicting and preventing root resorption: Part II. Treatment factors. Am J Orthod Dentofacial Orthop. 2001;119(5): 511-5.

36. Silva Filho OG, Berreta EC, Cavassan AO, Capelozza Filho L. Estimativa da reabsorção radicular em 50 anos casos ortodônticos bem finalizados. Ortodontia. 1993;26(1):24-35.

37. Taner T, Ciğer S, Sençift Y. Evaluation of apical root resorption following extraction therapy in subjects with Class I and Class II malocclusions. Eur J Orthod. 1999;21(5):491-6.

26

Changes on facial profile in the mixed dentition, from natural growth and induced by Balters' bionator appliance

Denise Rocha Goes Landázuri[1], Dirceu Barnabé Raveli[2], Ary dos Santos-Pinto[2], Luana Paz Sampaio Dib[3], Savana Maia[4]

Objective: The purpose of this study was to evaluate the facial profile changes induced by Balters' bionator appliance in Class II division 1 patients, at mixed dentition stage. **Methods:** The sample consisted of 28 pre-pubertal individuals at stages 1 and 2 of skeletal maturation (CVM), which were divided in two groups. The experimental group consisted of 14 individuals (7 boys and 7 girls, initial mean age of 8y12m) which were treated with Balters' bionator appliance for 14.7 months. The effects of treatment were compared to a control group of 14 subjects (7 boys and 7 girls, initial mean age of 8y5m) with Class II malocclusion, division 1, not orthodontically treated, which were followed up for 15.4 months. The statistical analysis was performed using Student's t test, at a significance level of 5%. **Results:** The results showed that the Balters' bionator appliance promoted a significant increase on the mentolabial angle, in addition to demonstrating a tendency to reduce the facial skeletal convexity, to restrict the maxillary growth and to increase the nasolabial angle and the lower anterior facial height. **Conclusion:** It can be concluded that the Balters' bionator appliance improved the facial profile of children treated at mixed dentition stage.

Keywords: Activator appliances. Angle Class II malocclusion. Cephalometry.

[1] Master and Doctor in Orthodontics, Dental School of Araraquara - State University of São Paulo (FOA-UNESP).
[2] Associate Professor of Orthodontics, FOA-UNESP.
[3] Doctor in Orthodontics, FOA-UNESP. Associate professor at the specialization program in Orthodontics, FAMOSP – GESTOS.
[4] Doctor in Orthodontics, FOA-UNESP. Professor at the State University of Amazonas.

» The authors report no commercial, proprietary or financial interest in the products or companies described in this article.

Denise Rocha Goes Landázuri
Av. Portugal, 887 – Centro – Araraquara/SP, Brazil
CEP: 14.801-075 – E-mail: denisergoes@gmail.com

INTRODUCTION

Achieving an esthetically pleasing face is one of the main goals of orthodontic treatment, and since the beginning of orthodontics, great researchers such as Kingsley,[16] Case[10] and Angle[3] emphasized the importance of the interrelation between esthetics and this specialty. However, to achieve this goal, it is necessary that the orthodontist deeply understand not only the biomechanical aspects related to tooth movement, but also the continuous changes that occur during facial growth and development of natural individuals.[27]

The introduction of cephalostat in dentistry[9] allowed the standardization of lateral teleradiography and allowed the accomplishment of more accurate dentoskeletal and facial profile assessments. Thus, combining the results of cephalometric analysis associated to clinical and subjective examination by each professional will enable the achievement of an ideal occlusion with functional stability and facial esthetic.[1,20,26]

Despite the various cephalometric analysis proposed in literature, initially, little emphasis was given to the analysis of the soft tissue profile, due to the inadequate concept that changes on soft tissue would accurately follow the repositioning of subjacent skeletal and dental tissues.[19] Currently, it is known that due to the large variability inherent to soft tissues — such as thickness and tonicity, especially of the lips —, they can mitigate or protrude the contours of the subjacent anatomical structures.

The concept of the ideal profile has been discussed in literature[8,14,23,25] and despite of accepting variations due to differences among races, countries, culture and time, the straight or slightly convex profile is still synonymous of beauty. As the aspect of the facial profile in patients with Class II malocclusion, division 1, with mandibular retrusion is quite convex, one of the main goals of this treatment is to improve facial aesthetics, by reducing the profile convexity.[22]

Class II malocclusions are characterized by an imbalance between bone bases in the anteroposterior direction, which can result in maxillary basal protrusion, maxillary dentoalveolar protrusion, mandibular deficiency, mandibular dentoalveolar retrusion or a combination of these factors.[12,15] This maxillomandibular discrepancy is present in a significant percentage of the population,[18,30] and is considered the most frequent in orthodontics practice. In Brazil, according to an epidemiological study conducted by Silva Filho et al,[29] with 2,016 children of 07-11

years-old, both genders, Class II malocclusion showed a prevalence of 42 %, being 27 % of dental origin and 15 % considered as skeletal Class II. Thus, it explains the large number of patients with this clinical feature who seek orthodontic clinics to address the esthetic and functional problems triggered by this malocclusion.

The treatment of Class II malocclusion, division 1, with mandibular deficiency in growing patients aims the mandibular advancement, to achieve better relations between bone bases and improve the convex facial profile. Among the functional orthodontic devices intended for this purpose, Balters' bionator is highlighted. It was developed by Wilhelm Balters in the 50's.[13] He believed that improper posture of the tongue, which was placed in a retruded manner, would be responsible for a disturbance in cervical region, change in respiratory function, atypical deglutition and consequent impairment of mandibular growth.[5] Therefore, Balters designed a device to promote an anterior mandibular positioning, enabling the tongue to occupy a normal intraoral position and, also, lip competence.[19]

The few data reported in the literature about possible changes on facial profile of children with Class II malocclusion, division 1, due to mandibular retrusion treated with Balters' bionator, led us to evaluate the effect of treatment with this device.

PURPOSE

The aim of this study was to provide data to assess changes in the facial profile resulting from natural growth and induced by the use of Balters' bionator device in children, before the growth peak of the pre-pubertal period, more specifically in stages 1 and 2 of skeletal maturation, observed through the analysis of cervical vertebrae.

MATERIAL AND METHODS
Material

The sample used in this study was obtained from two distinct populations: Brazilian and Canadian. Individuals were divided into two groups: the experimental group treated with Balters' bionator and a control group that received no orthodontic treatment.

Experimental group

The experimental group consisted of 14 patients treated with Balters' bionator, 7 males and 7 females. The inclusion criteria used were: Class II division 1 facial pattern, associated with mandibular retrusion; Class II, division 1, dental relation; permanent upper and lower central and lateral incisors erupted or erupting, no mandibular crowding, 5-7 mm overjet, mixed dentition and absence of cross-sectional problems.

All patients were treated with Balters' bionator, which was based on the original design proposed by Balters[5] and adapted by Ascher,[2] having the acrylic extension of the lower arch deeper than the original, and covering the incisal and cusps of the incisors and canines, respectively (Fig 1), so that the effect of inclination of the lower incisors was decreased.

The mandibular advancement was carried out in a unique way to obtain a cusp to cusp relation with incisors and, for patients whose overjet was more accentuated, the reference was the canine relation in Class I. For these cases, the treatment was carried out in two phases: The first phase with canine relation in Class I, and the second phase with the incisors in a cusp to cusp relation.

Control group

The control group was selected from the documentation files of the Burlington Growth Centre, located in the Department of Orthodontics, Faculty of Dentistry, University of Toronto, Canada. This sample consisted of 14 individuals, 7 males and 7 females, randomly selected from a group of 20 individuals. Selection criteria for this group were: Class II division 1 facial pattern, associated with mandibular retrusion; Class II division 1 dental relation; upper and lower central incisors erupted, mixed dentition and no previous orthodontic treatment.

These individuals were randomly paired with patients of the same gender from the experimental group, and selected the observation times that corresponded to the age, in complete years, of the respective pair.

The descriptive data about age and time of treatment for the experimental and control groups are shown in Tables 1 and 2, respectively.

Determination of skeletal maturation

The determination of skeletal age was verified through lateral teleradiographies, using the indicators of skeletal maturation of cervical vertebrae. The bone age determination was performed by the same operator and in a blind study, i.e., without identification of the patient evaluated, which reduces the subjectivity of this evaluation. Thus, the selected individuals were located in the maturation stages 1 and 2, i.e., before the growth peak of pre-pubertal period, according to Baccetti, Franchi, McNamara;[4] O'Reilly and Yanniello.[21]

METHODS

For each individual, it were obtained two lateral cephalograms, called T_1 (beginning of treatment) and T_2 (end of treatment), for the experimental group; and T_1 (beginning of the observation period) and T_2 (end of the observation period) for the control group.

Although the radiographs had been obtained by different X-ray equipments, it was not performed a correction for image magnification. The difference of

Table 1 - Descriptive data of patients' ages in experimental and control groups, according to gender and treatment stage.

		Experimental		Control	
		Mean	SD	Mean	SD
Female					
	Baseline	8y 9m	6m	8y 3m	6m
	End	10y 2m	4m	9y 9m	6m
Male					
	Baseline	9y 2m	5m	8y 7m	6m
	End	10y 3m	5m	9y 9m	6m
Both					
	Baseline	8y 12m	6m	8y 5m	6m
	End	10y 3m	5m	9y 9m	6m

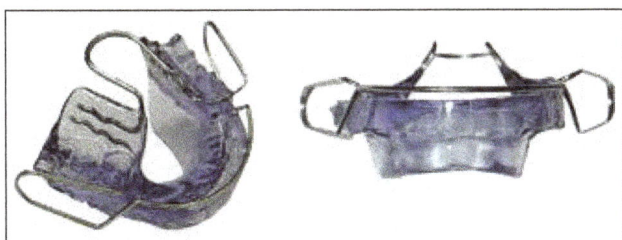

Figure 1 - Side and front view of Balters' bionator.

Table 2 - Descriptive data of treatment period, in months, of the patients in experimental and control groups, according to gender.

	Experimental		Control	
	Mean	SD	Mean	SD
Female	16.7	4.6	17.1	6.4
Male	12.4	1.7	13.7	4.5
Both	14.6	4.0	15.4	5.6

magnification percentage between samples would be 0.16 %, which would not affect the comparison of the variables displayed in radiographs obtained by different X-ray devices. This difference in image magnification corresponds to a difference in magnification between X-rays of 0.0016 cm (0.016 mm).

All radiographs were traced by hand by the same operator, the cephalometric points were digitized on a Numonics AccuGrid tablet, and evaluated through Dentofacial Planner Plus 2.01 computer software for obtaining cephalometric measurements.

Obtaining cephalometric measurements

The cephalometric measures used in this study are shown in Table 3 and Figure 2.

Statistical analysis

To evaluate the data, the following statistical tests were performed:

» Student's t-test for the equality of means of two independent populations: To examine the hypothesis that the mean of each measure in the control group did not differ from the mean of the experimental group at baseline (Table 4).

» Student's t-test for the equality of means of two populations with independent samples: To examine the hypothesis that the changes observed in a cephalometric measure between times 1 and 2 do not differ, in terms of means, in the control group and the experimental group (Table 5).

Table 3 - Cephalometric measures evaluated.

Cephalometric measures	Definition
1) Convex	Supplement of the angle that measures the convexity of the bone profile
2) LAFH	Linear measure that represents the height of the lower anterior facial third
3) SNA	Represents the anteroposterior position of the maxilla in relation to the anterior cranial base
4) SNB	Represents the anteroposterior position of the mandible in relation to the anterior cranial base
5) U1PP	Angle formed by the long axis of the upper incisor and the palatal plane
6) L1MP	Angle formed by the long axis of the lower incisor and the mandibular plane
7) U1L1	Angle formed by the long axis of the upper incisor and the long axis of the lower incisor
8) NL	Angle formed by the columella line and the upper lip
9) ML	Supplement of the angle formed by the line of the lower lip and the chin
10) UL_E	Linear measure between the most prominent point of the upper lip and the line E
11) LL_E	Linear measure between the most prominent point of the lower lip and the line E

RESULTS

To compare the changes that have occurred in the measurements, with and without treatment, it was necessary to eliminate the effect of the difference in time between the measurements performed in the experimental and control groups. For this reason, the changes in the measures were annualized (Table 5). The representation of the skeletal, dental and soft tissue changes is presented in Figure 3.

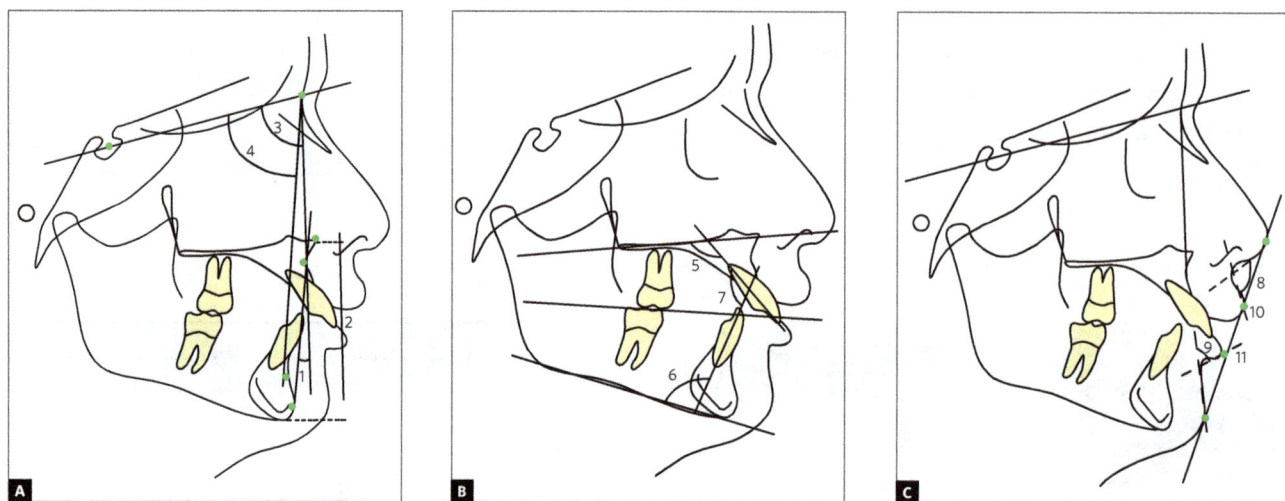

Figure 2 - Skeletal (**A**), dental (**B**) and soft tissue (**C**) cephalometric measures.

Table 4 - Means and standard deviations of measures at baseline for each group, Levene's test for comparison of variances and Student's t-test to compare the means of the two groups.

Measures	Experimental group		Control group		Levene's test		Student's t-test		
	Mean	SD	Mean	SD	F	p	t	df	p
Convex	8.8	4.91	8.0	4.45	0.02	0.884	0.47	26	0.645
LAFH	61.4	3.34	59.8	3.53	0.07	0.793	1.24	26	0.224
U1PP	113.9	9.02	112.5	5.49	2.68	0.114	0.49	26	0.630
L1MP	97.5	5.51	98.0	6.25	0.46	0.505	-0.21	26	0.834
NL	108.9	10.68	105.4	9.90	0.06	0.804	0.90	26	0.376
ML	**5.5**	**1.27**	**4.2**	**1.10**	1.00	0.327	**3.00**	**26**	**0.006**
UL_E	**0.5**	**2.38**	**-1.9**	**1.64**	1.11	0.304	**2.98**	**24**	**0.006**
LL_E	0.2	2.37	-1.5	2.15	0.78	0.386	1.90	26	0.069
U1L1	120.9	11.70	122.3	8.31	0.57	0.456	-0.36	26	0.719
SNA	82.0	5.07	79.6	3.69	1.30	0.265	1.47	26	0.155
SNB	77.3	3.95	75.0	2.38	2.65	0.115	1.81	26	0.082

Table 5 - Means and standard deviations of annualized changes of measures for each group, Levene's test results for equality of variances and Student's t-test for equality of mean changes.

Measurement	Experimental group		Control group		Levene's test		Student's t-test		
	Mean	SD	Mean	SD	F	p	t	df	P
Convex	-0.9	2.91	0.0	2.36	1.81	0.190	-0.86	26	0.396
LAFH	1.4	1.20	0.7	1.20	0.05	0.828	1.48	26	0.151
U1PP	-4.5	7.59	-0.6	2.95	2.88	0.102	-1.80	26	0.084
L1MP	1.5	4.13	0.9	4.55	0.00	0.994	0.34	26	0.735
NL	4.3	8.23	1.6	6.44	2.10	0.159	0.97	26	0.340
ML	**-0.8**	**0.94**	**0.1**	**0.58**	3.49	0.073	**-3.10**	**26**	**0.005**
UL_E	-0.7	1.21	0.0	1.24	0.03	0.866	-1.50	26	0.145
LL_E	0.3	1.26	0.5	1.03	0.04	0.845	-0.44	26	0.662
U1L1	3.0	6.97	0.2	4.96	2.48	0.127	1.21	26	0.236
SNA	-0.6	1.55	0.4	1.91	0.04	0.843	-1.45	26	0.160
SNB	0.2	1.16	0.4	1.32	0.20	0.658	-0.41	26	0.684

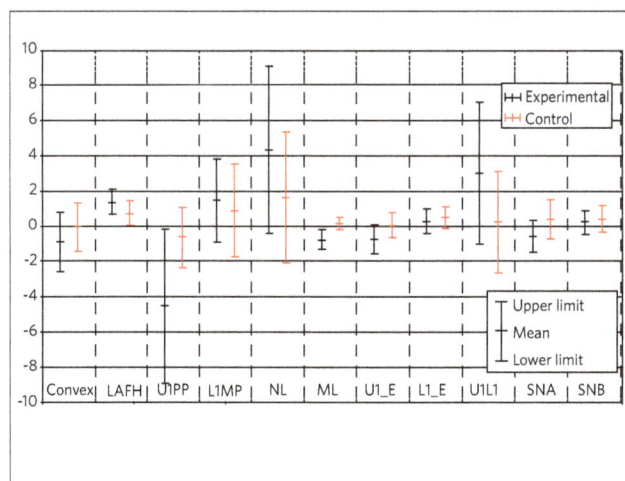

Figure 3 - Annualized changes: sample means and 95% confidence intervals for the populational means.

DISCUSSION

The present study aimed to evaluate the changes in the facial profile of pre-pubertal individuals with Class II, division 1, mandibular retrusion, treated with Balters' bionator. In order to discriminate alterations induced by treatment from those deriving from natural growth, a control group was used from the Burlington Growth Centre, Toronto, Canada, which did not receive orthodontic treatment.

The knowledge about the growth process and natural craniofacial development is essential for distinguishing changes that truly occur by means of the established treatment, from those that occur regardless of the use of orthodontic appliances. However, one of the major methodological difficulties in clinical research, in the field of orthodontics, is the composition of a control group orthodontically untreated with similar characteristics to the experimental group.[11] In the present study, it was used a control group from Canada, so it was possible to preserve the ethics, providing orthodontic treatment to all screened patients and eliminating a common bias for clinical work which is the absence of a control group.

In order to identify the actual stage of skeletal age, indicators of cervical vertebrae skeletal maturation were used based on the lateral teleradiographs, which are already part of the routine orthodontic records and therefore do not expose patients to additional X-rays,[24] as it happens when hand and wrist radiographs are requested. In this study, all individuals were located in stages 1 or 2 of maturation, i.e. before pubertal growth peak period.[4,21]

The assessment of equivalency between the experimental and control groups on measures targeted at baseline (Table 4) showed great cephalometric similarities before treatment between groups, since only 2 of the 11 variables were statistically different.

Finally, it will be discussed the changes on the facial profile that occurred due to the functional orthopedic treatment (experimental group) and without interference from any device (control group).

Effects of treatment

After the trial period of one year, it was observed that the supplementary angle to skeletal convexity (Convex) showed a nonsignificant reduction of 0.9° per year in the experimental group (Fig 3), while the control group did not change (0.0° per year), i.e. Balters' bionator provided a tendency towards improvement of facial convexity. These findings are in agreement with Melo[19] whose studies about the changes on skeletal angle of convexity (NAPg) showed an increase of 2.52° per year in children treated with bionator.

Considering that this angle is strongly influenced by the dislocation of the jaw bones during craniofacial growth and development, the behavior of anteroposterior jaw relative to the cranial base (SNA) was evaluated. It was identified that there was a tendency towards restriction of maxillary growth, known as extraoral effect, in the treated group (-0.6° per year), while the control group showed an increase of 0.4° per year (Fig 3). These data confirm the findings of Brandão[7] who verified the decrease of SNA in patients treated with bionator. As for the jaw, the SNB angle showed no statistically significant change.

The balance in the relation between the upper lip and the nose is quite evident by the nasolabial angle, which is often associated with the characterization of facial esthetics. In this experiment, there was an increase of 4.3° per year in the experimental group and 1.6° per year in the control group (Fig 3). The data shows that there was a tendency for this angle to become more opened in the group receiving treatment and are in agreement with the findings of Silva and Dominguez-Rodriguez,[28] who observed an increase of 9.83° per year on a sample treated with bionator.

A determinant factor in the nasolabial angle is the postural position of the upper lip, which was assessed by checking the inclination of the upper incisor (U1PP). In the treated group, it was found a decrease of 4.5° per year, highlighting the tendency towards vertical of maxillary incisors, whereas in the control group this decrease occurred on a much smaller scale (-0.6° per year). As for the lower incisors, they tended to proclination, with a not statistically significant slight increase of 1.5 mm per year in group 1 and 0.9 mm per year in group 2 (Fig 1). We also assessed the interincisal angle (U1L1), which confirmed these aforementioned findings, with an increase of 3.0° per year in the group receiving treatment and a slight increase of 0.2° per year in the untreated group. Despite of lower incisors proclination being an undesired side effect of this treatment, this may contribute to postural correction of the lower lip.[19]

Assessing the behavior of the supplementary angle to mentolabial (ML), it was observed a statistically significant decrease (p< 0.05) of 0.8 mm per year for the treated group, whereas there was a tendency to an increase of 0.1 mm per year in the control group (Fig 3). This means that there was a significant improvement in the mentolabial angle for the treated group. These results are in agreement with the study of Silva and Dominguez-Rodriguez,[28] who observed an increase of 6.85° in patients treated with bionator for 18 months. According to Blanchette et al,[6] the mentum/labial sulcus of Class II children, with horizontal growth pattern and not submitted to orthodontic or orthopedic treatment, deepens naturally, which can be explained by the lower lip retracted and positioned between upper and lower incisors.

Evaluating the performance of the variable LAFH, there was a non-significant increase in the treated group of 1.4 mm per year, while in the control group this increase occurred in a lower manner (0.7 mm per year), which means that there was a trend to increased lower anterior facial height, a fact also confirmed by Melo,[19] who observed an increase in skeletal lower facial third of 1.37 mm per year in children treated with bionator.

Adding up the nose to the facial profile analysis, it was observed that the position of the upper lip to the line E (UL_E) showed a negative change of 0.8 mm per year (treatment group), while the control group did not show any alteration (0.0 mm per year). Then, there was a tendency to retrusion of the upper lip, a fact confirmed by Lange et al[17] who demonstrated the existence of an upper lip retrusion of 1.0 mm per year in patients treated with Balters' bionator. Regarding the lower lip (LL_E), there was a slight tendency to protrusion of the lower lip in both groups, being higher in the group that received no treatment (0.5 mm/year).

The statistical analysis at a significance level of 5% could not detect differences among most of the studied measures, except for the ML measure. It is noteworthy that, after a certain type of treatment, it is possible to find clinically detectable changes, but statistically insignificant, due to some factors such as the high variability of middle and/or high standard deviation, that may interfere on the effectiveness of the test used to identify these differences.

CONCLUSION

Considering the present study, it can be concluded that the effects produced by Balters' bionator on facial profile of children treated in the mixed dentition stage were:

» Increase of mentolabial angle.
» Tendency to decreased skeletal facial convexity.
» Tendency to maxillary growth restriction.
» Tendency to increased nasolabial angle.
» Tendency to verticalization of the upper incisors.
» Tendency to proclination of the lower incisors.
» Tendency to retrusion of the upper lip.
» Tendency to increased anterior facial height.

REFERENCES

1. Ackerman JL. Orthodontics: art, science or transcience? Angle Orthod. 1974;44(3):243-50.
2. Ascher F. The bionator in functional orthodontics. Inf Orthod Kieferorthop. 1984;16(3):215-46.
3. Angle EH. Classification of malocclusion. Dent Cosmos. 1899;41(3):248-64.
4. Baccetti T, Franchi L, McNamara JA. The cervical vertebral maturation (CVM) method for the assessment of optimal treatment timing in dentofacial orthopedics. Semin Orthod. 2005;11:119-29.
5. Balters W. Betrachtugen uber Sinn und Zweck bei der funktionelli entwicklung des mundhohlenbereicher. Zahanartliche Welt, Heidelberg. 1950;5:460-3.
6. Blanchette ME, Nanda RS, Currier GF, Ghosh J, Nanda SK. A longitudinal cephalometric study of the soft-tissue profile of short and long face syndromes from 7 to 17 years. Am J Orthod Dentofacial Orthop. 1996;109(2):116-31.
7. Brandão RC. Avaliação cefalométrica do comportamento da mandíbula na interceptação da má oclusão classe II divisão 1 de Angle, com o Bionator [tese]. Araraquara (SP): Universidade Estadual Paulista; 2000.
8. Burstone CJ. The integumental profile. Am J Orthod. 1958;44(1):1-25.
9. Broadent H. A new x-ray technique and its application to Orthodontia. Angle Orthod. 1931;1(2):45-66.
10. Case CS. Facial and oral deformities. Chicago: CS Case; 1986.
11. Cozza P, Baccetti T, Franchi L, De Toffol L, McNamara JA Jr. Mandibular changes produced by functional appliances in class II malocclusion: A systematic review. Am J Orthod Dentofacial Orthop. 2006;129(5):599. e1-12; discussion e1-6.
12. Dale J. Interceptive guidance of occlusion with emphasis on diagnosis. In: Graber TM, Vanarsdall RL. Orthodontics, current principles and techniques. 2nd ed. St. Louis: Mosby; 1994. p. 375-469.
13. Eirew HL. The Bionator. Br J Orthod. 1981;8(1):33-6.
14. Hambleton RS. The soft tissue covering of the skeletal face as related to orthodontic problems. Am J Orthod Dentofacial Orthop. 1964;50(6):405-20.
15. Henry RG. A classification of Class II division 1 malocclusion. Angle Orthod. 1957;27(3):83-92.
16. Nanda RS, Ghosh J. Facial soft-tissue harmony and growth in orthodontic treatment. Semin Orthod. 1981;1(2):67-81.
17. Lange DW, Kalra V, Broadbent BH Jr, Powers M, Nelson S. Changes in soft tissue profile following treatment with the bionator appliance. Angle Orthod. 1995;65(6):423-30.

18. Martins JCR, Sinimbú CMB, Dinelli TCS, Martins LPM, Raveli DB. Prevalência da má oclusão em pré-escolares de Araraquara: relação da dentição decídua com hábitos bucais e nível socioeconômico. Rev Dental Press Ortod Ortop Facial. 1998;3(6):35-43.

19. Melo ACM. Mudanças no perfil facial de crianças com má oclusão classe II, divisão 1 decorrentes do crescimento normal e induzidas pelo Bionator de Balters [tese]. Araraquara (SP): Universidade Estadual Paulista; 2003.

20. Nguyen DD, Turley PK. Changes in the Caucasian male profile as depicted in fashion magazines during the twentieth century. Am J Orthod Dentofacial Orthop. 1998;114(2):208-17.

21. O'Reilly MT, Yanniello GJ. Mandibular growth changes and maturation of cervical vertebrae – a longitudinal cephalometric study. Angle Orthod. 1988;58(2):179-84.

22. Pancherz H, Anehus-Pancherz M. Facial profile changes during and after Herbst appliance treatment. Eur J Orthod. 1994;16(4):275-86.

23. Peck H, Peck S. A concept of facial esthetics. Angle Orthod. 1970;40(4):284-317.

24. Raveli DB, Goes DR, Dib LPS. Avaliação da maturidade esquelética através das vértebras cervicais. Ortodontia SPO. 2006;34(4):362-64.

25. Riedel RA. An analysis of dentofacial relationships. Am J Orthod Dentofacial Orthop. 1957;43(2):103-19.

26. Romani KL, Agahi F, Nanda R, Zernik JH. Evaluation of horizontal and vertical differences in facial profiles by orthodontists and lay people. Angle Orthod. 1993;63(3):175-82.

27. Scavone Jr H. O perfil facial tegumentar dos 13 aos 18 anos de idade [tese]. Bauru (SP): Universidade de São Paulo; 1996.

28. Silva SV, Dominguez-Rodriguez GC. Estudo comparativo cefalométrico radiográfico das mudanças do perfil tegumentar de adolescentes com má oclusão de classe II, divisão 1ª e retrognatismo mandibular, tratados com bionator de Balters. Ortodontia. 2002;38(3):43-56.

29. Silva Filho OG, Freitas SF, Cavassan AO. Prevalência de oclusão normal e má oclusão na dentadura mista em escalares da cidade de Bauru (São Paulo). Rev Assoc Paul Cir Dent. 1989;43:287-90.

30. Silva Filho OG, Silva PRB, Rego MVNN, Silva FPL, Cavassan AO. Epidemiologia da má oclusão na dentadura decídua. Ortodontia. 2002;33(2):22-33.

27

Periodontal and dental effects of surgically assisted rapid maxillary expansion, assessed by using digital study models

Danilo Furquim Siqueira[1], Mauricio de Almeida Cardoso[2], Leopoldino Capelozza Filho[2], Dov Charles Goldenberg[3], Mariana dos Santos Fernandes[4]

Objective: The present study assessed the maxillary dental arch changes produced by surgically assisted rapid maxillary expansion (SARME). **Methods:** Dental casts from 18 patients (mean age of 23.3 years) were obtained at treatment onset (T_1), three months after SARME (T_2) and 6 months after expansion (T_3). The casts were scanned in a 3D scanner (D-250, 3Shape, Copenhagen, Denmark). Maxillary dental arch width, dental crown tipping and height were measured and assessed by ANOVA and Tukey's test. **Results:** Increased transversal widths from T_1 and T_2 and the maintenance of these values from T_2 and T_3 were observed. Buccal teeth tipping also showed statistically significant differences, with an increase in all teeth from T_1 to T_2 and a decrease from T_2 to T_3. No statistically significant difference was found for dental crown height, except for left first and second molars, although clinically irrelevant. **Conclusion:** SARME proved to be an effective and stable procedure, with minimum periodontal hazards.

Keywords: Orthodontics. Periodontics. Palatal expansion technique. Dental casts.

[1] Coordinator of the Postgraduate course in Orthodontics, Sociedade Paulista de Ortodontia, Botucatu, São Paulo, Brazil.
[2] Professor of Orthodontics, Universidade Sagrado Coração (USC), Bauru, São Paulo, Brazil.
[3] Full professor, Universidade de São Paulo (USP), School of Medicine, Department of Surgery, São Paulo, São Paulo, Brazil.
[4] MSc in Orthodontics, Universidade Metodista de São Paulo (UMESP), São Bernardo do Campo, São Paulo, Brazil.

» The authors report no commercial, proprietary or financial interest in the products or companies described in this article.

Danilo Furquim Siqueira
Rua Moyses Leme da Silva, 8-38, Jd América, Bauru, SP, Brazil
E-mail: danilofurquim@uol.com.br

INTRODUCTION

Proper maxillary transverse dimension is a key component of optimal, stable occlusion. Rapid maxillary expansion (RME) is a procedure commonly employed by orthodontists treating transverse issues.[1-5] Despite being successful in children and adolescents, this procedure fails when performed in patients in the final growth phase and in adults.[1,2,6,7,8]

After growth ends, the amount of force required to split the midpalatal suture is relatively high due to increases both in the complexity of this suture and in the rigidity of adjacent facial structures. Thus, enlarging the maxillary complex by nonsurgical expansion in adults can cause side effects, such as higher relapse rates, tipping of support teeth, severe pain and gingival recession,[1,2,6,9] since the forces delivered during expansion may produce buccal tipping of teeth, thereby generating areas of compression in the periodontal ligament of support teeth.[10,11] In these cases, midpalatal suture splitting must be combined with a surgical procedure known as surgically assisted rapid maxillary expansion (SARME) which breaks down sutural resistance and enables maxillary expansion without the aforementioned side effects.[1,3,4,6,9,12,13]

The benefits of treating transverse maxillary deficiency include improvements in dental and skeletal stability, decreased need for extractions to perform alignment and leveling, increased teeth visibility at smiling, and, occasionally, improvements in nasal breathing.[5,12,14,15]

There are numerous ways to assess changes resulting from SARME, but in the last two decades, thanks to remarkable technological advances in Dentistry, cutting edge analysis tools have emerged. In Orthodontics, these advances have primarily occurred in diagnostic elements, such as the use of photography and digital radiography. The use of digital dental casts was introduced by the orthodontic industry as a component of the new, now fully digitized and highly accurate orthodontic records.[7,16-23] Thus, this study aims at analyzing, with the aid of digital models, the major changes produced in the transverse dimension and tipping of maxillary teeth, as well as the potential impact of this procedure on adult patients undergoing SARME.

MATERIAL AND METHODS

This project was submitted to Universidade Metodista de São Paulo Institutional Review Board, and approved under protocol number 142.170/07.

This is a retrospective study of which sample comprised 54 maxillary dental casts obtained from 18 adult patients with maxillary atresia, 6 men and 12 women, with a mean age of 23.3 years (minimum of 18 and maximum of 35 years old) from the Postgraduate Clinic of Universidade Metodista de São Paulo. All subjects underwent SARME.

To perform the expansion procedure, a 13-mm Hyrax expansion screw was used.[24] Moreover, a conservative surgical technique consisting of LeFort I osteotomy was employed to approach the midpalatal suture without involving the pterygopalatine suture.[25] All surgeries were conducted by the same surgeon.

The expansion screw was first activated on the third day after surgery, and patients were instructed to make two daily activations, one in the morning (1/4 turn) and one at night (1/4 turn), until the screw was fully opened, or until it reached the desired overcorrection (palatal cusp of the maxillary first molar edge-to-edge with the buccal cusp of the mandibular first molar).

The appliance (Hyrax) remained in the oral cavity for three months, functioning as a retainer. After this period, the expander was removed and an acrylic plate (with retention clips between premolars) was inserted and remained in place for three months until a fixed orthodontic appliance was placed.

For variables assessment, dental casts were scanned with a 3D scanner (D-250, 3Shape, Copenhagen, Denmark). Only the maxillary models during phases T_1 (initial), T_2 (three months post-expansion) and T_3 (six months post-expansion) were used.

Linear measurements were taken by means of Geomagic Studio 5™ (Research Triangle Park, USA), a software that allows viewing and manipulating digital representations on a computer screen. Transverse changes resulting from SARME were assessed by means of intercanine, interpremolar and intermolar widths (Fig 1), using the points described by Currier[26] and Berger et al[27] as reference.

The height of the clinical crown of canines, premolars and molars was measured based on the distance between the buccal cusp and the most apical point of the gingival margin,[5,9] as shown in Figure 2.

Angular measurements were taken with the aid of OrthoDesigner™ software (3Shape, Copenhagen, Denmark) which also features tools to assist in obtaining angular measurements and slicing dental casts.

Intercanine, interpremolar and intermolar tipping was calculated using the following references[5]: Line a= distance between the left and right midpoints of the deepest region of buccal and palatal surfaces in the gingival margin; Line b= distance between the geometric midpoint on the right side of the center of buccal and palatal cusps, and the midpoint of the deepest region in the gingival margin; Line c= distance from the left side of the geometric midpoint at the center of buccal and palatal cusps, and the midpoints of the deepest buccal and palatal portions of the gingival margin. With these reference lines, the internal angles formed by lines a-b and a-c were calculated with the aid of the software. After this definition, the bilateral angulation of posterior teeth was calculated (Fig 3).

To this end, it was necessary to create a clipping plane in the models (Fig 4) to allow teeth to be viewed mesially. The reference plane met the aforementioned criteria.

In selecting the clipping plane, the tool "enable clipping plane" was used. This allowed the mesial viewing of the models, as it excluded their anterior portion (Fig 5). The changes in each parameter occurring during treatment were calculated in the models at the times described before.

Statistical analysis

To determine the error of the method, 30% of the sample was randomly selected and measured after at least one week, using the same material and applying the same aforementioned criteria. Paired t-test was used to determine intraexaminer systematic error. Random error was calculated by Dahlberg's formula.[28]

In order to compare the three assessment periods, analysis of variance (ANOVA) was used with a criterion

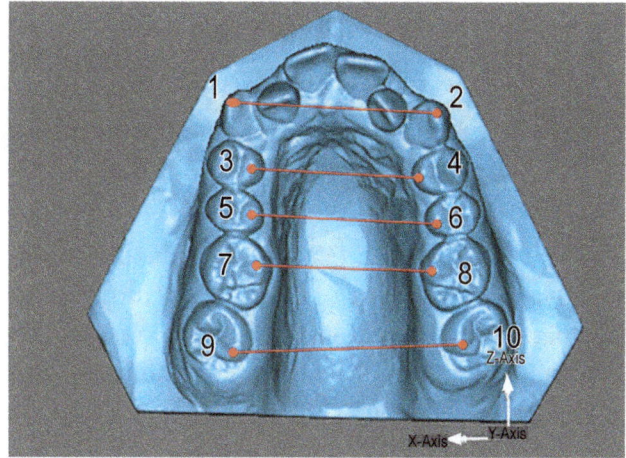

Figure 1 - Points and transverse widths in the digital models: **1**) Cusp tip of right canine; **2**) Cusp tip of left canine; **3**) Palatal cusp tip of right maxillary first premolar; **4**) Palatal cusp tip of left maxillary first premolar; **5**) Palatal cusp tip of right maxillary second premolar; **6**) Palatal cusp tip of left maxillary second premolar; **7**) Mesio-palatal cusp tip of right maxillary first molar; **8**) Mesio-palatal cusp tip of left maxillary first molar; **9**) Mesio-palatal cusp tip of right maxillary second molar; **10**) Mesio-palatal cusp tip of left maxillary second molar.

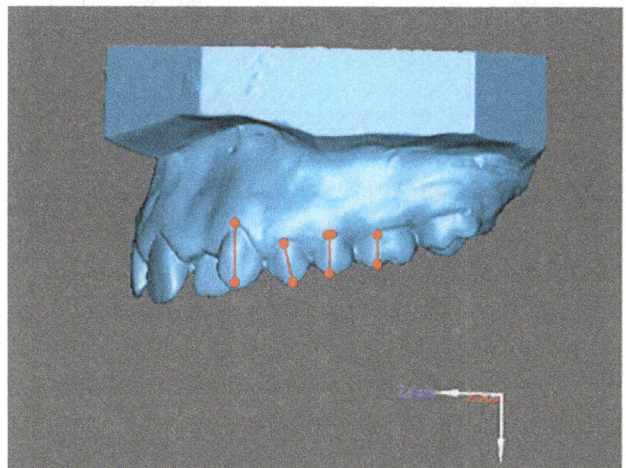

Figure 2 - Height of clinical crowns.

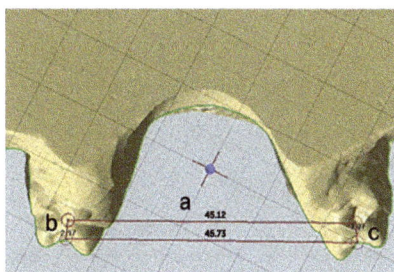

Figure 3 - Defining lines a, b and c

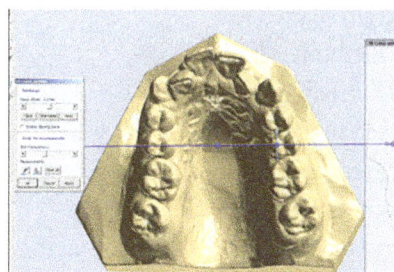

Figure 4 - Defining clipping plane.

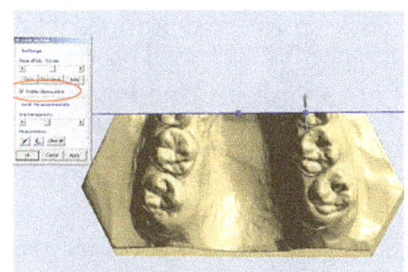

Figure 5 - Enabling clipping plane tool, shown in red.

for repeated measurements. When ANOVA revealed statistically significant difference, Tukey's test for multiple comparisons was applied. A level of significance of 5% (p < 0.05) was adopted for all tests.

RESULTS

From the foregoing, one can argue that the results found in this study are reliable, since, after further measurements were carried out in the dental casts of five randomly selected patients, no intraexaminer errors that might compromise this research were identified. Measurements of tooth tipping are more error-prone due to inconsistencies in (a) the location of points, (b) trimming of casts, and (c) construction of lines.

Table 1 depicts means and standard deviation values of transverse widths in the upper dental arch, expressed in millimeters, at the three evaluation periods, and results from ANOVA and Tukey's test. It shows an increase in transverse width with means of 9.26 mm for first molars, 5.4 mm for second molars, 9.8 mm for first premolars, 9.49 mm for second premolars, and 5.87 mm for canines from T_1 to T_2. These values remained unchanged from T_2 to T_3.

Table 2 presents the mean size of crowns in the maxillary arch, expressed in millimeters, at T_1, T_2 and T_3, and the results of ANOVA and Tukey's test showing differences only in left first and second molars.

Table 3 shows means and standard deviation values of maxillary teeth tipping, expressed in degrees, at T_1, T_2 and T_3, and the results of ANOVA and Tukey's test. All values increased, thereby pointing to buccal tipping, although significant only in some teeth.

DISCUSSION

The literature presents different methods to assess changes induced by SARME in dental casts, namely: assessment with a bow compass,[27] digital calipter[4] and laser-scanned models. Laser scanning is common in industrial engineering and medicine as a noninvasive alternative to generate 3D images. The measurement method using a 3D scanner has been studied and proved reliable and convenient.[7,18,21] It has also been proven that analyses in digital models can be performed in both clinical practice and research, with extremely accurate outcomes.[16,17,19,20]

Digital models have the added advantage of allowing images to be sliced, providing superior viewing of points not visible in dental casts. Furthermore, they can

Table 1 - Means and standard deviation values of transverse widths in the upper dental arch, in mm, at the three assessment periods, and results of ANOVA and Tukey's test.

Tooth	T_1	T_2	T_3	p
1stM	35.94 ± 4.43[a]	45.20 ± 3.96[b]	45.26 ± 4.41[b]	< 0.001*
2ndM	43.45 ± 4.58[a]	48.85 ± 4.53[b]	48.82 ± 4.72[b]	< 0.001*
1stPM	26.02 ± 2.56[a]	35.82 ± 2.97[b]	35.47 ± 2.69[b]	< 0.001*
2ndPM	31.28 ± 3.24[a]	40.77 ± 3.05[b]	40.73 ± 3.20[b]	< 0.001*
C	30.56 ± 2.39[a]	36.43 ± 2.41[b]	36.14 ± 2.57[b]	< 0.001*

*Statistically significant difference found by ANOVA (p < 0.05).
Periods of time with the same letter are not statistically different (Tukey's test).

Table 2 - Means and standard deviation values of crown heights in the upper dental arch, in mm, at the three assessment periods, and results of ANOVA and Tukey's test.

Tooth	T_1	T_2	T_3	p
1stM right	7.25 ± 1.08	7.25 ± 0.84	7.23 ± 0.81	0.996 ns
2ndM right	6.88 ± 1.00	7.19 ± 0.78	7.05 ± 0.79	0.182 ns
1stPM right	7.66 ± 0.89	7.92 ± 0.94	8.04 ± 0.88	0.062 ns
2ndPM right	6.88 ± 1.11	6.88 ± 1.15	6.98 ± 0.94	0.754 ns
C right	9.29 ± 1.15	9.47 ± 1.14	9.40 ± 0.98	0.492 ns
1stM left	6.96 ± 0.74[a]	7.17 ± 1.03[ab]	7.39 ± 1.11[b]	0.035*
2ndM left	6.45 ± 0.78[a]	6.89 ± 0.89[b]	6.87 ± 0.91[b]	0.006*
1stPM left	7.92 ± 1.03	8.00 ± 0.79	8.03 ± 0.70	0.748 ns
2ndPM left	6.81 ± 0.99	6.84 ± 0.93	6.84 ± 0.97	0.930 ns
C left	9.21 ± 1.00	9.35 ± 1.15	9.38 ± 0.99	0.597 ns

ns = No statistically significant difference.
*Statistically significant difference found by ANOVA (p < 0.05).
Periods of time with the same letter are not statistically different (Tukey's test).

Table 3 - Means and standard deviation values of tipping of teeth in the upper dental arch, in mm, at the three assessment periods, and results of ANOVA and Tukey's test.

Tooth	T_1	T_2	T_3	p
1stM right	98.96 ± 9.47	102.76 ± 5.63	102.61 ± 4.90	0.120 ns
2ndM right	106.98 ± 7.50[a]	110.82 ± 8.73[b]	109.41 ± 7.69[ab]	0.041*
1stPM right	88.18 ± 8.00[a]	96.37 ± 8.19[b]	95.48 ± 7.15[b]	< 0.001*
2ndPM right	92.20 ± 8.85[a]	101.54 ± 8.77[b]	100.34 ± 5.48[b]	< 0.001*
C right	100.17 ± 8.77	99.33 ± 8.11	98.76 ± 8.95	0.644 ns
1stM left	102.07 ± 7.10[a]	106.40 ± 7.46[b]	104.62 ± 5.72[ab]	0.019*
2ndM left	112.18 ± 6.28	113.70 ± 6.05	110.47 ± 6.34	0.154 ns
1stPM left	94.24 ± 6.53	96.17 ± 7.13	96.68 ± 6.30	0.312 ns
2PM left	93.33 ± 6.37[a]	103.84 ± 5.78[b]	101.45 ± 6.70[b]	< 0.001*
C left	103.29 ± 7.17	104.06 ± 7.84	100.17 ± 5.13	0.084 ns

ns – No statistically significant difference.
*Statistically significant difference found by ANOVA (p < 0.05)
Periods of time with the same letter are not statistically different (Tukey's test).

be superimposed, which facilitates viewing of the mechanics used in a given treatment.[21]

The time spent while taking measurements in the digital models was relatively shorter, given the user-friendliness of the programs and the measuring resources available, which yield very accurate measurements.[23]

Treatment including SARME proved successful for adult patients requiring maxillary expansion, a finding reported by several authors.[2,4,6,12,13,25]

The present study disclosed an increase in transverse width in all teeth from T_1 to T_2, with measurements remaining unchanged from T_2 to T_3 (Table 1). Thus, it is reasonable to assert that SARME demonstrated effectiveness and stability during the assessment period (6 months).

The slight increase found in intercanine width can be attributed to the fact that patients with indication for SARME often have canines in infralabioversion. As anterior space is gained, these teeth tend to align, consequently taking on a more lingual position and not showing so much increase in width.[1,4,13,27]

In comparison to first molars, there was less increase in transverse width in second molars (5.4 mm and 9.4 mm, respectively). This difference can be probably linked to release of the pterygopalatine process due to the surgical technique employed, and also to the fact that this tooth was not included in the appliance.[25]

In adults, both surgical and nonsurgical procedures can correct maxillary transverse deficiency and achieve stability,[4,5,8,9] but comparison showed greater transverse increase in surgical cases.

SARME did not interfere in gingival attachment at the three assessment periods, except for first and second molars on the left side. Bassareli, Dalstra and Melsen[5] as well as Handelman et al[8] reported that nonsurgical maxillary expansion is effective in adults. However, these studies demonstrated greater dentoalveolar compensation due to increased tipping. Furthermore, they found no connection between the development of gingival recession and the amount of transverse expansion in adults, since there was no change in clinical crown height. In comparing the two types of treatment, i.e., SARME *versus* nonsurgical expansion, Carmen et al[9] found that these treatment modalities result in increased transverse dimension and show no statistically significant differences in the development of gingival recession. Nevertheless, SARME proved more effective and

less harmful to the periodontium, thereby corroborating Northway and Meade,[4] who argued that crown length displayed greater increase in nonsurgical patients.

The literature has shown that bone dehiscence can be produced in the alveolar bone when teeth are tipped bucally, but orthodontic movement would not necessarily be accompanied by loss of connective tissue.[10,11]

It has been acknowledged that teeth positioned or moved bucally, bone dehiscence and the presence of thin and brittle keratinized mucosa are the main predisposing factors of gingival recession.[15,29] Gingival recession, however, is only triggered by mechanical trauma caused by brushing, or inflammation induced by the presence of plaque.[15] Therefore, the quality of the keratinized mucosa and tooth brushing in particular should be closely monitored in patients undergoing SARME.

The surgical procedure resulted in dentoalveolar tipping, with statistical significance (Table 3), in the second molar, first and second premolars on the right side, and first molar and second premolars on the left side from T_1 to T_2. From T_2 to T_3, tipping remained unchanged. In this study, crown tipping was calculated by means of the angle formed by the long axis of the tooth with a line that connects the buccal and lingual surfaces of the gingival most points. Thus, calculating tipping was less dependent on crown morphology,[5] since other methods are influenced by changes in cusp height.[1,4]

This difference in the amount of tipping may be related to the way in which expansive force is delivered. Second premolars experienced expansion forces through contact between the lingual connection wire and its homonymous surface. With simple force applied to the crown, away from the center of resistance, a moment of force was created in the buccal direction, ultimately yielding some tipping component. Furthermore, anchorage teeth received expansion forces by means of bands rigidly fixed to the appliance. As the screw was activated, the bands, which were wide in the cervico-occlusal direction, resisted the tendency to tip by moving the anchorage teeth predominantly through a bodily movement in buccal direction.[15] This clearly shows that overcorrection was necessary due to relapse induced by the effects of tipping.[3,4,8]

CONCLUSION

SARME proved to be an effective and stable procedure, with minimum periodontal hazards.

REFERENCES

1. Adkins MD, Nanda RS, Currier GF. Arch perimeter changes on rapid palatal expansion. Am J Orthod Dentofacial Orthop. 1990;97(3):194-9.

2. Atac ATA, Karasu HA, Aytac D. Surgically assisted rapid maxillary expansion compared with orthopedic rapid maxillary expansion. Angle Orthod. 2006;76(3):353-9.

3. Chung C, Goldman AM. Dental tipping and rotation immediately after surgically assisted rapid palatal expansion. Eur J Orthod. 2003;25(4):353-8.

4. Northway WM, Meade JB Jr. Surgically assisted rapid expansion: a comparison of technique, response, and stability. Angle Orthod. 1997;67(4):309-20.

5. Bassarelli T, Dalstra M, Melsen B. Changes in clinical crown height as a result of transverse expansion of the maxilla in adults. Eur J Orthod. 2005;27(2):121-8.

6. Bays R, Greco JM. Surgically assisted rapid palatal expansion: an outpatient technique with long-term stability. J Oral Maxillofac Surg. 1992;50(2):110-5.

7. Bell A, Ayoub F, Siebert P. Assessment of the accuracy of a three-dimensional imaging system for archiving dental study models. J Orthod. 2003;30(3):219-23.

8. Handelman CS, Wang L, BeGole EA, Haas AJ. Nonsurgical rapid maxillary expansion in adults: report on 47 cases using the Haas expander. Angle Orthod. 2000;70(2):129-44.

9. Carmem M, Marcella P, Giuseppe C, Roberto A. Periodontal evaluation in patients undergoing maxillary expansion. J Craniofac Surg. 2000;11(5):491-4.

10. Garib DG, Henriques JFC, Janson G, Freitas MR, Fernandes AY. Periodontal effects of rapid maxillary expansion with tooth-tissue-borne and tooth-borne expanders: a computed tomography evaluation. Am J Orthod Dentofacial Orthop. 2006;129(6):749-58.

11. Steiner GG, Pearson JK, Ainamo J. Changes of the marginal periodontium as a result of labial tooth movement in monkeys. J Periodontol. 1981;52(6):314-20.

12. Betts NJ, Vanarsdall RL, Barber HD, Higgns-Barber K, Fonseca RJ. Diagnosis and treatment of transverse maxillary deficiency. Int J Adult Orthodon Orthognath Surg. 1995;10(2):75-96.

13. Byloff FK, Mossaz CF. Skeletal and dental changes following surgically assisted rapid palatal expansion. Eur J Orthod. 2004;26(4):403-9.

14. Haas A. Long-term post treatment evaluation of rapid palatal expansion. Angle Orthod. 1980;50(3):189-217.

15. Garib DG, Henriques JFC, Janson G, Freitas MR, Coelho RA. Rapid maxillary expansion — tooth-tissue-borne versus tooth-borne expanders: a computed tomography evaluation of dentoskeletal effects. Angle Orthod. 2005;75(4):548-57.

16. DeLong R, Heinzen M, Hodges JS, Ko CC, Douglas WH. Accuracy of a system for creating 3D computer models of dental arches. J Dent Res. 2003;82(6):438-42.

17. Hayasaki H, Martins RP, Gandini LG Jr, Saitoh I, Nonaka K. A new way of analyzing occlusion 3 dimensionally. Am J Orthod Dentofacial Orthop. 2005;128(1):128-32.

18. Kusnoto B, Evans CA. Reliability of a 3D surface laser scanner for orthodontic applications. Am J Orthod Dentofacial Orthop. 2002;122(4):342-8.

19. Motohashi N, Kuroda T. A 3D computer-aided design system applied to diagnosis and treatment planning in orthodontics and orthognathic surgery. Eur J Orthod. 1999;21(3):263-74.

20. Okumura H, Chen L, Tsutsumi S, Oka M. Three-dimensional virtual imaging of facial skeleton and dental morphologic condition for treatment planning in orthognathic surgery. Am J Orthod Dentofacial Orthop. 1999;116(2):126-31.

21. Oliveira NL, Silveira ACd, Kusnoto B, Viana G. Three-dimensional assessment of morphologic changes of the maxilla: A comparison of 2 kinds of palatal expanders. Am J Orthod Dentofacial Orthop. 2004;126(3):354-62.

22. Stevens DR, Flores-Mir C, Nebbe B, Raboud DW, Heo G, Major PW. Validity, reliability, and reproducibility of plaster vs digital study models: comparison of peer assessment rating and Bolton analysis and their constituent measurements. Am J Orthod Dentofacial Orthop. 2006;129(6):794-803.

23. Sousa MVS, Vasconcelos EC, Janson G, Garib D, Pinzan A. Accuracy and reproducibility of 3-dimensional digital model measurements. Am J Orthod Dentofacial Orthop 2012;142(2):269-73.

24. Biederman W. A hygienic appliance for rapid expansion. JPO, J Pract Orthod. 1968;2(2):67-70.

25. Goldenberg DC, Alonso N, Goldenberg FC, Gebrin E, Amaral TS, Scanavini MA, et al. Using computed tomography to evaluate maxillary changes after surgically assisted rapid palatal expansion. J Craniofacial Surg 2007;18(2):302-11.

26. Currier JHA. A computerized geometric analysis of human dental arch form. Am J Orthod. 1969;56(2):164-79.

27. Berger JL, Pangrazio-Kulbersh V, Borgula T, Kaczynski R. Stability of orthopedic and surgically assisted rapid palatal expansion over time. Am J Orthod Dentofacial Orthop. 1998;114(6):638-45.

28. Houston WJB. The analysis of errors in orthodontic measurements. Am J Orthod. 1983;83(5):382-90.

29. Joss-Vassalli, Grebenstein C, Topouzelis N, Sculean A, Katsaros C. Orthodontic therapy and gingival recession: a systematic review. Orthod Craniofac Res. 2010;13(3):127-41.

The effects of binge-pattern alcohol consumption on orthodontic tooth movement

Cristiano Miranda de Araujo[1], Aline Cristina Batista Rodrigues Johann[2], Elisa Souza Camargo[3], Orlando Motohiro Tanaka[3]

Objective: This study aimed to assess tissue changes during orthodontic movement after binge-pattern ethanol 20% exposure. **Methods:** Male Wistar rats (n = 54) were divided into two groups. The control group (CG) received 0.9% saline solution, while the experimental group (EG) received 20% ethanol in 0.9% saline solution (3 g/kg/day). On the 30th day, a force of 25 cN was applied with a nickel-titanium closed coil spring to move the maxillary right first molar mesially. The groups were further divided into three subgroups (2, 14 and 28 days). Tartrate-resistant acid phosphatase and picrosirius were used to assess bone resorption and neoformation, respectively. Data were compared by two-way ANOVA, Tukey's HSD, Games-Howell and chi-square test. Significance level was set at 5%. **Results:** There was a decrease in the number of osteoclasts in EG at day 28. The percentage of collagen showed no interaction between group and time. **Conclusion:** Binge-pattern 20% ethanol promoted less bone resorption at the end of tooth movement, thereby suggesting delay in tooth movement.

Keywords: Tooth movement. Orthodontics. Bone remodeling.

» The authors report no commercial, proprietary or financial interest in the products or companies described in this article.

Orlando Motohiro Tanaka
Rua Imaculada Conceição, 1155 – Bairro Prado Velho
CEP: 80215-901 – Curitiba/PR — Brazil
Email: tanakaom@gmail.com

[1] PhD resident in Dentistry, Catholic University of Paraná (PUC-PR).
[2] Associate professor, School of Dentistry, PUC-PR.
[3] Full professor, School of Dentistry, PUC-PR.

INTRODUCTION

Alcohol abuse affects approximately 14 million North Americans.[1] Ethanol is the main component of alcoholic beverages, and it is considered to be toxic not only to vital organs, but also to hard tissues, such as bones. Chronic alcohol consumption is associated with pathological effects on bone and tissue integrity, which complicates post-injury or surgery repair processes in addition to acceleration of osteoblast apoptosis.[2,3]

Binge-pattern alcohol consumption in humans is characterized by excessive consumption within a short period of time, with approximately five or more drinks on a single occasion for men and four for women.[4,5] According to Callaci et al,[6] experimental binge-pattern ethanol consumption can be mimicked by administering ethanol injections four days a week, followed by three days during which no alcohol is administered. Intraperitoneal (IP) injections are well tolerated by rats and cause minimal stress. Another advantage of this route is that it achieves a high concentration of alcohol in blood and in a controlled environment. Additionally, it has minimal effects on rat's body weight.

Callaci et al[7] administered 20% binge-pattern ethanol in rats and found decreased mineral density in the vertebrae, both in cortical and cancellous regions, as well as decreased compressive strength. Similarly, they reported that treatment with 20% ethanol had varying effects on different bone regions, i.e., lumbar vertebrae proved more resistant than the tibia. Callaci et al[6] also observed that, from the third week of binge-pattern 20% ethanol exposure on, bone mineral density of the femur and lumbar spine decreased significantly.

Orthodontic tooth movement (OTM) is characterized by sequential reactions to biomechanical forces that induce changes in periodontal tissue and are related to bone remodeling by activation of alveolar bone resorption on the pressure side and consequent bone apposition on the traction side.[9,10,11] Ethanol-induced imbalance between the processes of bone formation and resorption directly affect bone repair.[15] To date, there have been no reports in the literature regarding the influence of ethanol on OTM.

Therefore, the objective of our study was to assess the tissue changes occurring during OTM in the periodontal ligament and alveolar bone adjacent to the mesial and distal areas of maxillary right first molar after administration of 20% ethanol. We particularly assessed bone resorption and neoformation.

MATERIAL AND METHODS

This project was approved by PUC-PR Ethics Committee on Animal Use. A total of 54 male, 9-week-old Wistar rats (*Rattus norvegicus albinus*), weighting approximately 300-350 g, was used. Temperature remained between 19 °C and 22 °C with a 12/12-hour light/dark photoperiod. The rats were provided with crushed food and water *ad libitum*. To observe changes in weight, the animals were weighed weekly with the aid of an electronic precision scale (Gehaka - BG 4001, São Paulo, Brazil).

The animals were randomly divided into two groups (27 rats per group): The control group (CG) received 0.9% saline solution in a volume similar to that given to the experimental group, whereas the experimental group (EG) received 20% ethanol (w/v) in 0.9% saline solution (3 g/kg/day).[6] These groups were further subdivided into three subgroups (2, 14 and 28 days; n = 9/group),which corresponded to the day of animal death after applying orthodontic force, so as to characterize the evolution of OTM over time.

Administration of solutions began 30 days before the orthodontic appliance was installed and continued until animal's sacrifice. It was performed intraperitoneally and designed so as to mimic binge drinking. Ethanol was administered four days a week, followed by three days of abstinence.[6]

The device used to induce OTM consisted of a nickel-titanium closed coil spring (G&H® Wire - Franklin, Indiana, USA) attached to maxillary right first molar and central incisors of all animals, which produced a 25-cN reciprocal force.[14] Measurement of the force produced by the coil spring was standardized by means of a calibrated dynamometer (Haag-Streit AG, Switzerland Koeniz, Switzerland). After initial activation, the coil spring was not reactivated during the experimental period; however, its position was checked on a daily basis.

The animals were sacrificed with an intraperitoneal overdose of anesthetic (5.4 ml/kg ketamine). Then, the mandible of each animal was removed, dissected and sectioned at the midline. Right hemimaxilla remained in 10% formaldehyde solution for 24 hours for proper fixation. After two months of demineralization, animals' maxilla was further fixed in 4.13% ethylenediamine tetraacetic acid solution (Biotec Analytical Reagents, Pinhais, Brazil), processed and embedded in paraffin. A total of 15 cross-sections were cut on the cervical third of the mesiobuccal root of maxillary first molars with a microtome at 4 μm, the occlusal surface of the molar parallel to the microtome and 60-μm intervals between sections.

The slides were stained with picrosirius and tartrate-resistant acid phosphatase (TRAP). Five sections were used for each technique.

Picrosirius staining was performed as follows: After deparaffinization in xylene, the sections were hydrated in ethanol and incubated for 1 hour in a solution of Sirius Red (Direct Red 80, diluted to 0.19% in saturated picric acid, Aldrich Chemical Company, Milwaukee, USA) at room temperature, followed by washing with distilled water, counterstaining with Harris hematoxylin, dehydrating in increasing alcohol solutions, deparaffinizing in xylene and mounting in Entellan.

For the TRAP technique, we used the TRAP Sigma 387A kit (Sigma-Aldrich Chemicals, St. Louis, Missouri, USA), following the manufacturer's recommendations.

Picrosirius-treated histological slides were assessed under light microscopy. Images were obtained using an Olympus BX-50 microscope (Olympus, Tokyo, Japan) equipped with Olympus U-Pot® polarized lens (Olympus, Tokyo, Japan) coupled to a Dino-Lite® microcamera (AmMo Electronics Corporation, New Taipei City, Taiwan) at a magnification of 100x. Images were analyzed with the Image Pro Plus morphometry program version 4.5 (Media Cybernetics, Rockville, Maryland, USA) to determine the percentage of areas of immature and mature collagen.[13] Type I collagen (mature) appeared red-orange, while type III collagen (immature) was yellowish-green.[15] The bone adjacent to the distal surface of the root was chosen for evaluation, as, during OTM, bone is deposited in the alveolar wall on the traction side.[13]

The TRAP-stained sections were used to identify osteoclasts and to determine bone resorption quantitatively. Thus, TRAP-positive multinucleated cells in the periodontal ligament adjacent to the alveolar bone were considered as functional osteoclasts. These cells were quantified[16] by means of obtaining five images of the mesial region of the root, totaling an area of 942,813.00 μm² of the periodontal ligament. An Olympus BX-50 microscope (Olympus, Tokyo, Japan) coupled to a Dino-Lite® microcamera at 400 x magnification.[17] Images were analyzed with Image Pro Plus software, version 4.5 (Media Cybernetics, Silver Spring, Maryland, USA), using a counting grid. We calculated the mean of the five sections to obtain the average number of osteoclasts.

Reproducibility power was analyzed. Dahlberg error was less than 1.8%, thereby indicating that the estimate of random error was reliable.

Statistical analysis was performed using SPSS software (version 16.0, SPSS IBM, Armonk, New York, USA). Significance level for all tests was set at 0.05.

To compare the mean values of dependent variables, in other words, the percentage of type I collagen in bone tissue and the number of osteoclasts according to the interaction between group and time, we initially tested the data for normal distribution and homogeneity of variances among the different treatments. To this end, Shapiro-Wilk test and Levene's test were used.

Since groups showed normal distribution ($P > 0.05$), mean values were compared by means of two-way ANOVA (group and time) with full factorial design. When ANOVA revealed differences and when treatment presented homogeneity of variance, we performed Tukey's HSD test for multiple comparison. For heterogeneous variance, we employed Games-Howell multiple comparison tests.

RESULTS

Bone resorption

The interaction between group and time revealed statistically significant difference ($P < 0.05$). EG showed a smaller number of osteoclasts than CG when they were compared on day 28 (Table 1, Fig 1).

Bone neoformation

When the percentage of type I collagen was assessed, no statistically significant difference ($P > 0.05$) was observed based on group-time interaction (Table 1, Fig 2).

Weight

We found statistically significant weight difference between EG and CG on day 2 (P < 0.05) (Table 1).

DISCUSSION

Alcohol consumption during adolescence and young adulthood is considered an important public health issue in the United States.[18,19] However, despite evidence showing that a significant number of adolescents and young people tend to binge drink ethanol, most studies about the effects of ethanol action on bone metabolism have used chronic consumption models.[8] Based on these data, we decided to investigate binge pattern which is a more common pattern of alcohol consumption among teenagers and college students,[19] an age group which often undergo orthodontic treatment.

The methods described in the literature have employed varying concentrations of ethanol and

Table 1 - Variables mean and standard deviation: Number of osteoclasts, percentage of type I collagen and weight variation in control (CG) and experimental (EG) groups.

Groups/Variables	Mean ± SD		Comparison
	CG	EG	CG x EG
Number of osteoclasts			
2 days	1.7375 ± 2.05492	2.6286 ± 1.17716	0.971
14 days	4.7250 ± 3.24643	3.8571 ± 2.36492	0.999
28 days	7.0000 ± 3.92641	2.1571 ± 1.72516	0.012*
Percentage of type I collagen			
2 days	86.1425 ± 8.48060	66.1814 ± 15.9878	0.179
14 days	78.5175 ± 17.6788	70.1642 ± 18.7859	0.968
28 days	85.7328 ± 9.10578	75.8685 ± 15.2132	0.932
Weight variation			
2 days	15.7863 ± 4.25056	6.0014 ± 5.31286	0.005*
14 days	10.5050 ± 22.8312	14.1914 ± 4.39931	0.852
28 days	14.2486 ± 2.22475	6.1529 ± 5.77777	0.055

* P < 0.05.

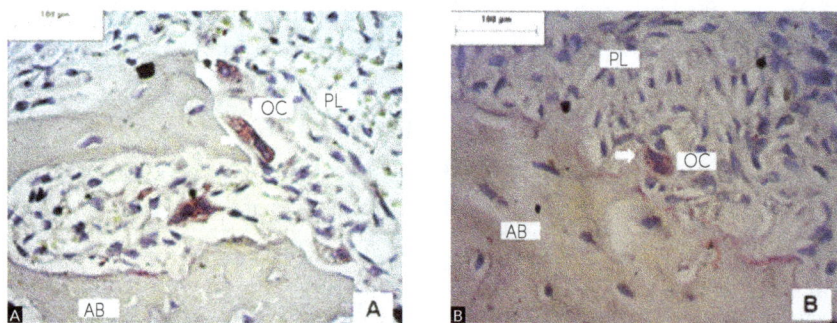

Figure 1 - Photomicrographs of histological slides in CG (**A**) and EG (**B**) on the 28th day after orthodontic appliance installation. Fewer osteoclasts were observed in the EG on the side where pressure was applied to the periodontal ligament of the mesiobuccal root of the right maxillary first molar. AB: alveolar bone; PL: periodontal ligament; OC: osteoclasts. White arrows indicate TRAP-positive cells (TRAP, magnification 400x).

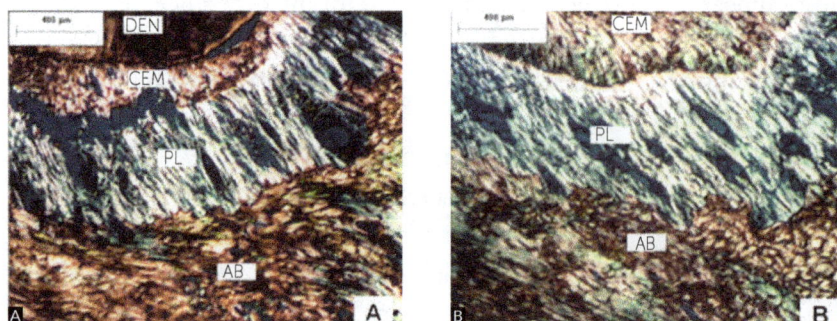

Figure 2 - Photomicrographs of histological slides on the distal surface of mesiobuccal root of right maxillary first molar in control (**A**) and experimental (**B**) groups on the 28th day after orthodontic appliance installation. There were no statistically significant differences in the group-time interaction. DEN: dentin; CEM: cementum; PL: periodontal ligament; AB: alveolar bone (picrosirius, magnification 100x).

different application times to assess the effects of ethanol on bone tissue and neoformation. Studies on the effects of ethanol on bone tissue have used concentrations ranging from 5% to 20% for periods of 4 to 12 weeks.[2,7,8,20,21] No reports associating the effects of ethanol and OTM were found; thus, we used 20% ethanol of which effects on bone neoformation are widely known.[2,6,7,8,22]

OTM is predominantly mediated by the periodontal ligament. For this reason, periodontal health is essential for OTM to occur without causing deleterious effects to the patient. Dantas et al[23] stated that ethanol consumption is a risk factor for periodontal health as it promotes local inflammation in gingival tissues. Nevertheless, Liberman et al[24] reported a dose-dependent relationship between bone loss and ethanol consumption. They also found that low concentrations of ethanol do not significantly lead to alveolar bone loss. Conversely, high concentrations may aggravate bones loss, even in the absence of stainless steel ligature ties which may induce periodontal disease. Accordingly, Souza et al[25] and Porto et al[26] also detected the harmful potential of ethanol in periodontal bone tissues.

In the present study, we observed that on the 28th day after the orthodontic appliance was installed, there was a decrease in the number of osteoclasts in the EG group (P < 0.05) compared to the CG group. There have been reports that ethanol promotes increased resorptive activity; however, the maximal time of application in these studies was four weeks.[6,7,8] Preedy et al[27] assessed the influence of ethanol applied for more than four weeks, and found a decrease in urinary DPD excretion after six weeks of consumption. Accordingly, we observed a statistically significant decrease in the number of osteoclasts at day 28, after six weeks of ethanol exposure. These changes suggest that OTM could be delayed by decreased bone resorption and that ethanol could influence osteoclast activity over time.

Approximately 90% of organic bone matrix consists of type I collagen degraded during bone resorption and replaced by immature fibers composed of type III collagen.[16,24] Callaci et al[6] assessed the effects of ethanol on bone metabolism and found an increase in type I collagen degradation and a corresponding decrease in bone mineral density.

Conversely, Maran et al[25] found that there was no reduction in type I collagen. Similarly, we did not find differences in the percentage of type I collagen in alveolar bone (P ≥ 0.05). These results suggest that ethanol does not influence the processes of collagen deposition and bone neoformation.

We observed statistically significant differences in weight (P < 0.05) at day 2. EG II group showed greater weight variation than CG. Lauing et al[8] reported that factors such as animal health after intraperitoneal injection, reduced food intake of animals exposed to ethanol and the direct effect of ethanol on the ability of rats to transform dietary nutrients into body weight might have directly influenced the difference in weight gain between control and experimental groups.

The effects of ethanol on bone remodeling remain controversial, but the common hypothesis is that ethanol affects bone metabolism. Differences in variables such as age and time of ethanol consumption could explain discrepant results. In addition, no consensus has yet been reached on which factor, whether increased resorption or decreased neoformation, acts as the major mediator inducing bone loss as a result of ethanol consumption.[12] Nevertheless, we found that ethanol promoted an imbalance in bone resorption. Additionally, its effects must be thoroughly considered from an orthodontic viewpoint, since tooth movement is a bone-dependent process.

Further studies should be performed in order to find out how ethanol affects bone remodeling. In the present study, we showed that 20% ethanol influences bone metabolism due to decreasing the number of osteoclasts when an orthodontic force is applied. Caution should be taken when applying orthodontic force in individuals who binge drink ethanol, as this substance can delay bone remodeling processes and possibly increase orthodontic treatment total time.

CONCLUSION

Ethanol does not influence the processes of collagen deposition or bone neoformation.

Binge-pattern 20% ethanol consumption promotes a decrease in resorption at the end of OTM.

Ethanol affects bone metabolism, thereby suggesting delay in OTM.

REFERENCES

1. Grant BF, Dawson DA, Stinson FS, Chou SP, Dufour MC, Pickering RP. The 12-month prevalence and trends in DSM-IV alcohol abuse and dependence: United States, 1991-1992 and 2001-2002. Drug Alcohol Depend. 2004;74:223-34.

2. Soares EV, Favaro WJ, Cagnon VH, Bertran CA, Camilli JA. Effects of alcohol and nicotine on the mechanical resistance of bone and bone neoformation around hydroxyapatite implants. J Bone Miner Metab. 2010;28:101-7.

3. Klein RF. Alcohol-induced bone disease: impact of ethanol on osteoblast proliferation. Alcohol Clin Exp Res. 1997;21(3):392-9.

4. Wezeman FH, Juknelis D, Himes R, Callaci JJ. Vitamin D and ibandronate prevent cancellous bone loss associated with binge alcohol treatment in male rats. Bone. 2007;41(4):639-45.

5. Wechsler H, Nelson TF. Binge drinking and the American college student: what's five drinks? Psychol Addict Behav. 2001;15(4):287-91.

6. Callaci JJ, Juknelis D, Patwardhan A, Sartori M, Frost N, Wezeman FH. The effects of binge alcohol exposure on bone resorption and biomechanical and structural properties are offset by concurrent bisphosphonate treatment. Alcohol Clin Exp Res. 2004;28(1):182-91.

7. Callaci JJ, Juknelis D, Patwardhan A, Wezeman FH. Binge alcohol treatment increases vertebral bone loss following ovariectomy: compensation by intermittent parathyroid hormone. Alcohol Clin Exp Res. 2006;30(4):665-72.

8. Lauing K, Himes R, Rachwalski M, Strotman P, Callaci JJ. Binge alcohol treatment of adolescent rats followed by alcohol abstinence is associated with site-specific differences in bone loss and incomplete recovery of bone mass and strength. Alcohol. 2008;42(8):649-56.

9. Macapanpan LC, Weinmann JP. The influence of injury to the periodontal membrane on the spread of gingival inflammation. J Dent Res. 1954;33(2):263-72.

10. Heller IJ, Nanda R. Effect of metabolic alteration of periodontal fibers on orthodontic tooth movement. An experimental study. Am J Orthod. 1979;75(3):239-58.

11. Hamaya M, Mizoguchi I, Sakakura Y, Yajima T, Abiko Y. Cell death of osteocytes occurs in rat alveolar bone during experimental tooth movement. Calcif Tissue Int. 2002;70(2):117-26.

12. Dai J, Lin D, Zhang J, Habib P, Smith P, Murtha J, et al. Chronic alcohol ingestion induces osteoclastogenesis and bone loss through IL-6 in mice. J Clin Invest. 2000 Oct;106(7):887-95.

13. Retamoso L, Knop L, Shintcovsk R, Maciel JV, Machado MA, Tanaka O. Influence of anti-inflammatory administration in collagen maturation process during orthodontic tooth movement. Microsc Res Tech. 2011;74(8):709-13.

14. Hashimoto M, Hotokezaka H, Sirisoontorn I, Nakano T, Arita K, Tanaka M, et al. The effect of bone morphometric changes on orthodontic tooth movement in an osteoporotic animal model. Angle Orthod. 2013;83(5):766-73.

15. Borges LF, Gutierrez PS, Marana HR, Taboga SR. Picrosirius-polarization staining method as an efficient histopathological tool for collagenolysis detection in vesical prolapse lesions. Micron. 2007;38(6):580-3. Epub 2006 Nov 13.

16. Marquezan M, Bolognese AM, Araujo MT. Effects of two low-intensity laser therapy protocols on experimental tooth movement. Photomed Laser Surg. 2010;28(6):757-62.

17. Braga SM, Taddei SR, Andrade Jr I, Queiroz-Junior CM, Garlet GP, Repeke CE, et al. Effect of diabetes on orthodontic tooth movement in a mouse model. Eur J Oral Sci. 2011;119(1):7-14.

18. Naimi TS, Brewer RD, Mokdad A, Denny C, Serdula MK, Marks JS. Binge drinking among US adults. JAMA. 2003;289(1):70-5.

19. Windle M. Alcohol use among adolescents and young adults. Alcohol Res Health. 2003;27:79-85.

20. Lima CC, Silva TD, Santos L, Nakagaki WR, Loyola YC, Resck MC, et al. Effects of ethanol on the osteogenesis around porous hydroxyapatite implants. Braz J Biol. 2011;71(1):115-9.

21. Sampson HW, Gallager S, Lange J, Chondra W, Hogan HA. Binge drinking and bone metabolism in a young actively growing rat model. Alcohol Clin Exp Res. 1999;23(7):1228-31.

22. Volkmer DL, Sears B, Lauing KL, Nauer RK, Roper PM, Yong S, et al. Antioxidant therapy attenuates deficient bone fracture repair associated with binge alcohol exposure. J Orthop Trauma. 2011;25(8):516-21.

23. Dantas AM, Mohn CE, Burdet B, Zorrilla Zubilete M, Mandalunis PM, Elverdin JC, et al. Ethanol consumption enhances periodontal inflammatory markers in rats. Arch Oral Biol. 2012;57(9):1211-7

24. Liberman DN, Pilau RM, Gaio EJ, Orlandini LF, Rosing CK. Low concentration alcohol intake may inhibit spontaneous alveolar bone loss in Wistar rats. Arch Oral Biol. 2011;56(2):109-13.

25. Souza DM, Ricardo LH, Kantoski KZ, Rocha RF. Influence of alcohol consumption on alveolar bone level associated with ligature-induced periodontitis in rats. Braz Oral Res. 2009;23(3):326-32.

26. Porto AN, Semenoff Segundo A, Vedove Semenoff TA, Pedro FM, Borges AH, Cortelli JR, et al. Effects of forced alcohol intake associated with chronic stress on the severity of periodontitis: an animal model study. Int J Dent. 2012;2012:465698.

27. Preedy VR, Sherwood RA, Akpoguma CI, Black D. The urinary excretion of the collagen degradation markers pyridinoline and deoxypyridinoline in an experimental rat model of alcoholic bone disease. Alcohol Alcohol. 1991;26(2):191-8.

28. Eriksen EF, Charles P, Melsen F, Mosekilde L, Risteli L, Risteli J. Serum markers of type I collagen formation and degradation in metabolic bone disease: correlation with bone histomorphometry. J Bone Miner Res. 1993;8(2):127-32.

29. Maran A, Zhang M, Spelsberg TC, Turner RT. The dose-response effects of ethanol on the human fetal osteoblastic cell line. J Bone Miner Res. 2001;16(2):270-6.

Permissions

The contributors of this book come from diverse backgrounds, making this book a truly international effort. This book will bring forth new frontiers with its revolutionizing research information and detailed analysis of the nascent developments around the world.

We would like to thank all the contributing authors for lending their expertise to make the book truly unique. They have played a crucial role in the development of this book. Without their invaluable contributions this book wouldn't have been possible. They have made vital efforts to compile up to date information on the varied aspects of this subject to make this book a valuable addition to the collection of many professionals and students.

This book was conceptualized with the vision of imparting up-to-date information and advanced data in this field. To ensure the same, a matchless editorial board was set up. Every individual on the board went through rigorous rounds of assessment to prove their worth. After which they invested a large part of their time researching and compiling the most relevant data for our readers.

The editorial board has been involved in producing this book since its inception. They have spent rigorous hours researching and exploring the diverse topics which have resulted in the successful publishing of this book. They have passed on their knowledge of decades through this book. To expedite this challenging task, the publisher supported the team at every step. A small team of assistant editors was also appointed to further simplify the editing procedure and attain best results for the readers.

Apart from the editorial board, the designing team has also invested a significant amount of their time in understanding the subject and creating the most relevant covers. They scrutinized every image to scout for the most suitable representation of the subject and create an appropriate cover for the book.

The publishing team has been an ardent support to the editorial, designing and production team. Their endless efforts to recruit the best for this project, has resulted in the accomplishment of this book. They are a veteran in the field of academics and their pool of knowledge is as vast as their experience in printing. Their expertise and guidance has proved useful at every step. Their uncompromising quality standards have made this book an exceptional effort. Their encouragement from time to time has been an inspiration for everyone.

The publisher and the editorial board hope that this book will prove to be a valuable piece of knowledge for researchers, students, practitioners and scholars across the globe.

List of Contributors

Érika Machado Caldeira and Felipe Giacomet
MSc in Orthodontics, Department of Pediatric Dentistry and Orthodontics, Federal University of Rio de Janeiro (UFRJ)

Antonio de Moraes Izquierdo
Doctorate Student in Orthodontics, Department of Pediatric Dentistry and Orthodontics, Federal University of Rio de Janeiro (UFRJ)

Eduardo Franzotti Sant'Anna and Antônio Carlos de Oliveira Ruellas
Adjunct professor, Department of Pediatric Dentistry and Orthodontics, Federal University of Rio de Janeiro (UFRJ)

Tomas Salomão Muniz and Saulo Henrique de Andrade
Private practice, Bragança Paulista, São Paulo, Brazil

Maurilo de Mello Lemos
Full professor, Universidade Guarulhos, Department of Orthodontics, Guarulhos, São Paulo, Brazil

Shirley Shizue Nagata Pignatari
Adjunct professor of Otolaryngology, Universidade Federal de São Paulo, Department of Otolaryngology, Head and Neck Surgery, São Paulo, São Paulo, Brazil

Márcio Alexandre Homem
MSc in Dentistry, Federal University of the Jequitinhonha and Mucuri Valleys (UFVJM)

Raquel Gonçalves Vieira-Andrade and Leandro Silva Marques
PhD Resident in Dentistry, Federal University of Minas Gerais (UFMG)

Saulo Gabriel Moreira Falci
Visiting professor, Federal University of the Jequitinhonha and Mucuri Valleys (UFVJM)

Maria Letícia Ramos-Jorge
Adjunct professor, Department of Dentistry, Federal University of the Jequitinhonha and Mucuri Valleys (UFVJM)

Murilo Fernando Neuppmann Feres
Associate professor, Universidade São Francisco, Department of Orthodontics, Bragança Paulista, São Paulo, Brazil

Marcelo de Castellucci
Professor, Specialization Course in Orthodontics and Facial Orthopedics, School of Dentistry, UFBA

Shreya Gupta
Senior lecturer, Index Institute of Dental Science, Department of Orthodontics and Dentofacial Orthopedics, Rau, Indore (M.P.), India

Anuradha Deoskar
Senior Lecturer, Hitkarini Dental College and Hospital, Department of Orthodontics and Dentofacial Orthopedics, Jabalpur, (M.P.), India

Puneet Gupta
MDS Public Health Dentistry, Government College of Dentistry, Department of Public Health Dentistry, Indore (M.P.), India

Sandhya Jain
Professor and Head, Government College of Dentistry, Department of Orthodontics and Dentofacial Orthopedics, Indore (M.P.), India

Gracemia Vasconcelos Picanço
MSc in Orthodontics, UNINGA

Karina Maria Salvatore de Freitas
Post-Doc in Orthodontics, UNINGÁ

Rodrigo Hermont Cançado
PhD in Orthodontics, FOB-USP

Fabricio Pinelli Valarelli
PhD in Orthodontics, UNINGÁ

Paulo Roberto Barroso Picanço
MSc in Orthodontics, UNINGÁ

Camila Pontes Feijão
Specialist in Orthodontics, UVA-CE

Marianna Mendonca Brandão
Postgraduate student in Orthodontics and Facial Orthopedics, Universidade Federal da Bahia (UFBA), Salvador, Bahia, Brazil

Marcio Costal Sobral
Professor, Universidade Federal da Bahia (UFBA), Postgraduate Program, Salvador, Bahia, Brazil

Carlos Jorge Vogel
PhD in Orthodontics, Universidade de São Paulo (USP), São Paulo, São Paulo, Brazil

Enio Ribeiro Cotrim
Specialist in Orthodontics, Sérgio Feitosa Institute for Health Studies and Management (IES)

Átila Valadares Vasconcelos Júnior and Ana Cristina Soares Santos Haddad
Assistant professor, IES

Sílvia Augusta Braga Reis
Assistant professor, UMESP

Ahmet A. Celebi
Assistant professor, Zirve University, Department of Orthodontics, School of Dentistry, Gaziantep, Turkey

Hakan Keklik
Postgraduate student, Kirikkale University, Department of Orthodontics, School of Dentistry, Kirikkale, Turkey

Enes Tan
Assistant professor, Kirikkale University, Department of Orthodontics, School of Dentistry, Kirikkale, Turkey

Faruk I. Ucar
Assistant professor, Selcuk University, Department of Orthodontics, School of Dentistry, Konya, Turkey

Matheus Melo Pithon
Professor, Department of Orthodontics, State University of Southwestern Bahia (UESB)

Rogério Lacerda dos Santos
Professor, Department of Orthodontics, Federal University of Campina Grande (UFCG)

Pedro Henrique Bomfim Magalhães
DDS, State University of Southwestern Bahia (UESB)

Raildo da Silva Coqueiro
Professor, Department of Epidemiology, State University of Southwestern Bahia (UESB)

Sissy Maria Mendes Machado
Professor, Specialization Course of Orthodontics, Brazilian Dental Association - Pará (ABO-PA)

Diego Bruno Pinho do Nascimento and Robson Costa Silva
Student of the Specialization Course of Orthodontics, ABO-PA

Sandro Cordeiro Loretto
Associate Professor of Dentistry. Professor of the MSc Program of the School of Dentistry, Federal University of Pará (UFPa)

David Normando
Associate Professor, Division of Orthodontics, School of Dentistry, Federal University of Pará (UFPa), Professor of the Specialization Program of Orthodontics, ABO-PA

Bruna de Rezende Marins
Graduate student in Oral and Maxillofacial Surgery, Universidade Estadual do Oeste do Paraná (UNIOESTE), School of Dentistry, Cascavel, Paraná, Brazil

Suy Ellen Pramiu
Undergraduate student, Universidade Estadual do Oeste do Paraná (UNIOESTE), School of Dentistry, Cascavel, Paraná, Brazil

Mauro Carlos Agner Busato and Luiz Carlos Marchi
Professor, Universidade Estadual do Oeste do Paraná (UNIOESTE), Department of Orthodontics, School of Dentistry, Cascavel, Paraná, Brazil

Adriane Yaeko Togashi
Professor of Periodontology and Oral Implantology, Universidade Estadual do Oeste do Paraná (UNIOESTE), Department of Implantology, School of Dentistry, Cascavel, Paraná, Brazil

Giovanni Modesto Vieira
PhD resident in Medical Sciences, University of Brasília (UnB)

Matheus Miotello Valieri
MSc in Orthodontics, Ingá College (UNINGÁ)

Karina Maria Salvatore de Freitas
Coordinator of the Master's program in Orthodontics, Ingá University (UNINGÁ)

Fabricio Pinelli Valarelli and Rodrigo Hermont Cançado
Adjunct professor, Department of Orthodontics, Master's program, Ingá College (UNINGÁ)

Danilo Furquim Siqueira
Coordinator of the Postgraduate course in Orthodontics, Sociedade Paulista de Ortodontia, Botucatu, São Paulo, Brazil

Mauricio de Almeida Cardoso and Leopoldino Capelozza Filho
Professor of Orthodontics, Universidade Sagrado Coração (USC), Bauru, São Paulo, Brazil

Dov Charles Goldenberg
Full professor, Universidade de São Paulo (USP), School of Medicine, Department of Surgery, São Paulo, São Paulo, Brazil

Mariana dos Santos Fernandes
MSc in Orthodontics, Universidade Metodista de São Paulo (UMESP), São Bernardo do Campo, São Paulo, Brazil

Fabricio Batistin Zanatta and Thiago Machado Ardenghi
Associate professor, Department of Stomatology, Federal University of Santa Maria (UFSM)

Raquel Pippi Antoniazzi and Tatiana Militz Perrone Pinto
Assistant professor, Franciscano University Center (UNIFRA)

Cassiano Kuchenbecker Rösing
Postdoc in Periodontics, Adjunct professor, Federal University of Rio Grande do Sul, (UFRGS)

Rafael Ribeiro Maya
MSc in Orthodontics, Universidade Ceuma (UNICEUMA), São Luís, Maranhão, Brazil

Célia Regina Maio Pinzan-Vercelino and Julio de Araujo Gurgel
Professor, Universidade Ceuma (UNICEUMA), Masters Program in Dentistry, São Luis, Maranhão, Brazil

Arthur Costa Rodrigues Farias
Orthodontist of the Unit of Face Deformities of UFRN

Maria Cristina Teixeira Cangussu
Associate professor, Department of Social and Pediatric Dentistry, UFBA

Rogério Frederico Alves Ferreira
Associate professor of Orthodontics, UFBA

Caio Biasi
PhD Resident, Veterinary Medicine, University of São Paulo (USP)

Jesualdo Luiz Rossi
Postdoc in Materials Science and Engineering, University of Surrey

Jose Luis Munoz Pedraza
Private practice (Rio de Janeiro/RJ, Brazil)

Mariana Marquezan
Universidade Federal de Santa Maria, Departamento de Estomatologia, Disciplina de Ortodontia (Santa Maria/RS, Brazil)

Lincoln Issamu Nojima and Matilde da Cunha Gonçalves Nojima
Universidade Federal do Rio de Janeiro, Faculdade de Odontologia, Departamento de Ortodontia e Odontopediatria (Rio de Janeiro/RJ, Brazil)
Case Western Reserve University, Department of Orthodontics (Cleveland, USA)

Denise Rocha Goes Landázuri
Master and Doctor in Orthodontics, Dental School of Araraquara – State University of São Paulo (FOA-UNESP)

Dirceu Barnabé Raveli and Ary dos Santos-Pinto
Associate Professor of Orthodontics, FOA-UNESP

Luana Paz Sampaio Dib
Doctor in Orthodontics, FOA-UNESP. Associate professor at the specialization program in Orthodontics, FAMOSP – GESTOS

Savana Maia
Doctor in Orthodontics, FOA-UNESP. Professor at the State University of Amazonas

Leanne Matias Portela Leal
Masters student in Orthodontics, Sacred Heart University (USC)

Marcus Vinicius Neiva Nunes do Rego
Professor of Orthodontics at the Graduate and Postgraduate programs, UNINOVAFAPI. Professor of Orthodontics at the Postgraduate program, Federal University of Piauí (UFPI)

Cosme José Albergaria da Silva Filho
Graduated in Dentistry, UNINOVAFAPI

Leopoldino Capelozza Filho
PhD in Orthodontics, College of Dentistry — Bauru/USP. Professor of Orthodontics at the Graduate and Postgraduate (specialization and Masters courses) programs, USC

Mauricio de Almeida Cardoso
PhD in Orthodontics, State University of São Paulo (UNESP). Professor of Orthodontics at the Graduate and Postgraduate (specialization and Masters courses) programs, USC

Bilal Al-Falahi, Ahmad Mohammad Hafez and Maher Fouda
Mansoura University, Faculty of Dentistry, Department of Orthodontics (Mansoura, Egypt)

Tulio Silva Lara
PhD in Orthodontics, UNESP

Melissa Lancia
Masters student in Rehabilitation Sciences, Hospital for Rehabilitation of Craniofacial Anomalies/University of São Paulo (USP)

Omar Gabriel da Silva Filho
MSc in Orthodontics, UNESP

Daniela Gamba Garib
Full professor in Orthodontics, FOB-USP

Terumi Okada Ozawa
PhD in Orthodontics, UNESP

Thais Maria Freire Fernandes
PhD and Postdoc in Orthodontics, Bauru Dental School - University of São Paulo (FOB-USP)

Arnaldo Pinzan
Associate Professor, Department of Pediatric Dentistry, Orthodontics and Public Health, Bauru Dental School, FOB-USP

Renata Sathler
MSc in Orthodontics, USP

Marcos Roberto de Freitas and Guilherme Janson
Head Professor, Department of Pediatric Dentistry, Orthodontics and Public Health, FOB-USP

Fabiano Paiva Vieira
Head Professor, Department of Pediatric Dentistry, Orthodontics and Public Health, FOB-USP

Marcos Porto Trein
Specialist in Orthodontics, Federal University of Rio Grande do Sul (UFRGS)

Karina Santos Mundstock
PhD in Orthodontics, State University of São Paulo (UNESP). Associate professor of Orthodontics,UFRGS

Leonardo Maciel and Jaqueline Rachor
Undergraduate student of Dentistry, UFRGS

Gustavo Hauber Gameiro
PhD in Orthodontics, University of Campinas (UNICAMP). Associate professor of Physiology, UFRGS

Patrícia Gomide de Souza Andrade Oliveira
Specialist in Orthodontics

Rubens Rodrigues Tavares
Professor of the Orthodontics Specialization Program at the Brazilian Dental Association - Goiás Section (ABO-GO)

Jairo Curado de Freitas
Head of the Orthodontics Specialization Program, ABO-GO

Samaneh Nakhaei
Assistant Professor, Department of Orthodontics, Birjand Dental School, Birjand University of Medical Science, Birjand, Iran

Raha Habib Agahi
Oral and Dental Disease Research Center, Kerman Dental School, Kerman University of Medical Science, Kerman, Iran

Amin Aminian
Assistant Professor, Oral and Dental Diseases Research center, Department of Orthodontics, Kerman Dental School, Kerman University of Medical Science, Kerman, Iran

Masoud Rezaeizadeh
Assistant Professor, Graduate University of Advanced Technology, Mechanical Engineering Department, Kerman, Iran

Klaus Barretto Lopes
Postdoc in Orthodontics, State University of Rio de Janeiro (UERJ)

Gladys Cristina Dominguez
Full professor, Department of Orthodontics, College of Dentistry, University of São Paulo (USP)

Cristiano Miranda de Araujo
PhD resident in Dentistry, Catholic University of Paraná (PUC-PR)

Aline Cristina Batista Rodrigues Johann
Associate professor, School of Dentistry, PUC-PR

Elisa Souza Camargo and Orlando Motohiro Tanaka
Full professor, School of Dentistry, PUC-PR

Index